Worst Case Bioethics

ALSO BY THE AUTHOR

The Rights of Patients
Judging Medicine
Standard of Care: The Law of American Bioethics
Some Choice: Law, Medicine, and the Market
American Bioethics: Crossing Human Rights and Health Law Boundaries

Coauthored

Informed Consent to Human Experimentation:
The Subject's Dilemma
(with Leonard Glantz and Barbara Katz)
The Rights of Doctors, Nurses and Allied Health Professionals
(with Leonard Glantz and Barbara Katz)
Reproductive Genetics and the Law
(with Sherman Elias)
American Health Law
(with Sylvia Law, Rand Rosenblatt, and Ken Wing)
Public Health Law
(with Wendy Mariner, Ken Wing, and Dan Strouse)

Coedited

Genetics and the Law
Genetics and the Law II
Genetics and the Law III
(with Aubrey Milunsky)
The Nazi Doctors and the Nuremberg Code:
Human Rights in Human Experimentation
(with Michael Grodin)
Gene Mapping: Using Law and Ethics as Guides
(with Sherman Elias)
Health and Human Rights: A Reader
(with Jonathan Mann, Sofia Gruskin, and Michael Grodin)
Perspectives in Health and Human Rights
(with Sofia Gruskin, Michael Grodin, and Stephen Marks)

George J. Annas

. . . .

WORST CASE
BIOETHICS

. . . .

Death, Disaster, and

Public Health

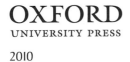

OXFORD
UNIVERSITY PRESS

2010

OXFORD
UNIVERSITY PRESS

Oxford University Press, Inc., publishes works that further
Oxford University's objective of excellence
in research, scholarship, and education.

Oxford   New York
Auckland   Cape Town   Dar es Salaam   Hong Kong   Karachi
Kuala Lumpur   Madrid   Melbourne   Mexico City   Nairobi
New Delhi   Shanghai   Taipei   Toronto

With offices in
Argentina   Austria   Brazil   Chile   Czech Republic   France   Greece
Guatemala   Hungary   Italy   Japan   Poland   Portugal   Singapore
South Korea   Switzerland   Thailand   Turkey   Ukraine   Vietnam

Published by Oxford University Press, Inc.
198 Madison Avenue, New York, New York 10016

www.oup.com

Oxford is a registered trademark of Oxford University Press, Inc.

Library of congress Cataloging-in-Publication Data
Annas, George J.
Worst case bioethics : death, disaster, and public health / George J. Annas.
p. ; cm.
Includes bibliographical references and index.
ISBN 978-0-19-539173-2
1. Medical ethics—United States.   2. Medical care—United States.
3. Public health—United States.   4. Medical policy—United States.   I. Title.
Published by Oxford University Press, Inc.
[DNLM: 1. Bioethics—United States. 2.   Attitude to Death—United States.
3. Disasters—United States. 4.   Health Policy—United States.
5. Human Rights—United States.   6. Jurisprudence—United States.
WB 60 A613w 2010]
R724.A67 2010
174.2—dc22
                                                      2009029993

9   8   7   6   5   4   3   2   1

Printed in the United States of America
on acid-free paper

To

Gust Annas (WWI & WWII)
Joseph Pallansch (WWI)

George J. Annas, Sr. (WWII)
Michael Pallansch (WWII)
George (Junior) Schroeder (WWII)
Jack Walter (WWII)

William Eddy (Cuban Missile Crisis)

Contents

. . . this is what we fear — no sight, no sound,
No touch or taste or smell, nothing to think with,
Nothing to love or link with,
The anesthetic from which none come round.

Philip Larkin (1922–1985)
"Aubade"

Introduction

Scared to Death

Death is almost everyone's personal worst case scenario. Society's worst case scenario, at least in America, is the disaster of large numbers of Americans killed by terrorists, a second 9/11. Denial in the face of death, including the belief that modern medicine and scientific progress may somehow provide us with an indefinite postponement, allows us to go on with our lives believing that our government can prevent a future terrorist attack permits us to engage in day-to-day activities and care for our families. Fixating on death and disaster, especially in the form of worst case scenarios, on the other hand, produces mostly fear and anxiety, which leads to rash acts or mental illness, or simply wasting time and money, and distorting our priorities.

In *Worst Case Bioethics,* I use bioethics cases involving death and disaster to illustrate and explore radical changes in human rights, public health doctrine, and the application of constitutional law to the practice of medicine. These real life cases lead to the conclusion that worst case scenarios are almost always counterproductive as planning exercises, and that their use as a government tool must be reconceptualized.

There is also a worst case scenario narrative—worst case scenarios lead to more worst case imaginings which, in turn, produce either over-reactions, unintended consequences, or even unanticipated disaster. Worst case scenario's traveling companion, "all-hazards preparedness," is equally destructive, and predictably guarantees that real disasters will be made even worse and that manageable incidents will more likely become unmanageable disasters.

On a recent visit to the Hiroshima Memorial Museum I couldn't help but think that this is what it must feel like to be a German touring the Dachau Concentration Camp today. Not that I felt personally responsible for dropping the atomic bomb on Hiroshima—I was less than a month old on August 6, 1945—but I do feel responsible for what is done in the name of my country. Of course there are major differences between the 20th century's two worst case scenarios, the Holocaust and Hiroshima. One is that many, if not most, Americans continue to insist that Hiroshima was justified. No sane German justifies the Holocaust. Another difference is that the Holocaust was exclusively about killing. Hiroshima, on the other hand, is justified as a military necessity that "saved lives." As Paul Tibbits, the pilot of the *Enola Gay* that dropped the bomb on Hiroshima, put it, "The fact that we killed so many people so quickly was just unheard of, it was terrible. But on the other hand, that had to be done, and it was done, to save millions of lives."

It is no accident that in the Department of Homeland Security's list of 15 National Planning Scenarios, the detonation of a 10-kiloton improvised nuclear device (approximately the size of the Hiroshima bomb) is listed first. Nor is it surprising that this worst case scenario has been on the mind of top US officials since 9/11. As former Vice President Dick Cheney put it to Tim Russert in 2006: "If on 9/11 they'd had a nuke instead of airplanes, you'd have been looking at a casualty toll that would rival all the deaths in all the wars fought by America in 230 years. That's the threat we have to deal with, and that drove our thinking in the aftermath of 9/11 and does today."

Cheney had been playing worst case scenario games for a long time. For the past three decades, federal officials have role-played surviving a nuclear exchange by holing up for weeks in secret caves outside of Washington, D. C. The idea behind the exercise is to retain "continuity of government" after a doomsday event. Since 9/11, similar play-acting drills, like Dark Winter (a simulated smallpox attack), have been used to suggest how the government and its people might react to other horrors. Dark Winter led Cheney and President Bush to attempt to have the entire country vaccinated against smallpox. Overreactions to 9/11, including

Department of Homeland Security Planning Scenarios

1. Nuclear Detonation – 10-Kiloton Improvised Nuclear
2. Biological Attack – Aerosol Anthrax
3. Biological Disease Outbreak – Pandemic Influenza
4. Biological Attack – Plague
5. Chemical Attack – Blister Agent
6. Chemical Attack – Toxic Industrial Chemicals
7. Chemical Attack – Nerve Agent
8. Chemical Attack – Chlorine Tank Explosion
9. Natural Disaster – Major Earthquake
10. Natural Disaster – Major Hurricane
11. Radiological Attack – Radiological Dispersal Devices
12. Explosive Attack – Bombing Using Improvised Explosive Device
13. Biological Attack – Food Contamination
14. Biological Attack – Foreign Animal Disease (Foot-and-Mouth Disease)
15. Cyber Attack

launching a war with Iraq—again, based on worst case scenario thinking—have been legion. Likewise, saving lives remains the all-purpose justification. Asked, after he left office, how he could justify the torture technique known as waterboarding, for example, Cheney's reprised Tibbets: "I'm convinced, absolutely convinced, that we saved thousands, perhaps hundreds of thousands, of lives."

Saving lives is a powerful mantra in its own right, but draws much of its appeal from its unstated opposite: death. We humans are the only species on the planet who know we are going to die, and we construct strong defenses to avoid thinking about death and attempt to transcend it. Psychologists Tom Pyszczynski, Sheldon Solomon, and Jeff Greenberg have termed our ways of dealing with our pending deaths "terror management," and the strategies we adopt to manage the terror "anxiety-buffering worldviews." These worldviews can be either religious or secular, are usually very fragile, and "require constant validation." Those who disagree with us threaten to undermine our defenses against death anxiety, and the "promise of literal or symbolic immortality afforded by them." This anxiety in turn, "drives the hostility and hatred we often feel toward those who view the world differently than we do." In his book, *The Political Brain*, Drew Westen argues that the terror management theory has direct application to contemporary politics. He concludes that when people are reminded of death they tend to "cling more tenaciously to the worldviews they hold dear," and "become less tolerant toward people who differ with them in religion, more nationalistic, and harsher in the way they punish those who transgress traditional moral values." Use of the mythical "death panels" to oppose healthcare reform in 2009 elicited just such a reaction.

We really do want to avoid thinking about death, but there are limits. As Eliezer Yudkowsky has suggested, we care deeply about our own death and that of our families and friends, and even of our fellow Americans. As horrible as the annihilation of an entire city, like Paris, might be to us, we feel "still greater horror on hearing the doctor say that our child has cancer." Even though our death is too horrible to contemplate, Yudkowsky suggests that we can nonetheless "discuss the extinction of humanity with perfect calm." He continues, "the phrase 'extinction of humanity'...appears in fictional novels [and] philosophy books—it belongs to a different context compared to the Spanish flu... [the] end of the world invokes...myth and dream...novels and movies." Confronted with the end of the world, we simply tune out or enter the realm of fantasy.

9/11 provides examples of both ways of dealing with death. The first is by clinging harder to one's ideology and involves bioethics directly. The second is imagining a death-dealing catastrophe so large that a lesser disaster is facilitated. The first example occurred in the days from August 6 to August 9, 2001. On August 9, President Bush gave a nationally televised speech on what he then believed would be the most important policy decision of his presidency, research on human embryos. He told the country, "We should allow federal funds to be used for research [only] on existing stem cell lines, where the life-and-death decision [for the embryo] has already been made." The Crawford White House had spent almost all of its time the week before this speech thinking about killing human embryos, and this may help explain why, three days prior to the speech, the President and his advisers failed to follow-up on a Presidential Daily Brief entitled: "Bin Ladin Determined to Strike in U.S."

The second example played itself out on 9/11 itself, and involves the failure of the North American Defense Aerospace Command (NORAD) to respond to the hijackings in as timely manner. Prior to 9/11, NORAD had conducted many training exercises to counteract attacks, including attacks in which terrorists use aircraft as weapons. All of the exercises, however, assumed that the planes would originate from outside the United States, which would allow NORAD plenty of time to intercept them. On 9/11, NORAD was scheduled to conduct a major training exercise, Vigilant Guardian, a massive death-dealing scenario involving a bomber attack originating in the former Soviet Union. The 9/11 Commission "investigated whether military preparations for the large-scale exercise compromised the military's response to the real-world terrorist attack on 9/11 . . . . We found that the response, was, if anything, expedited by the increased number of staff at the sectors and at NORAD because of the scheduled exercise." A more reasonable conclusion is that their massive death scenario drills were not helpful at best, and at worst they distracted NORAD from effectively responding to the real attack on 9/11. Consistent with this view is the statement of a nuclear attack preparedness expert before an Institute of Medicine committee that I served on about the reaction of first responders to hearing plans for responding to a nuclear explosion by terrorists in their city. As this expert described it, the first response of these first responders is that their "eyes glaze over."

Writing planning scenarios, or at least imagining them, is the job of government officials, especially those tasked with protecting the country. So, it should not be too surprising that at least some officials have turned to fiction to try to warn the public of dangers and to obtain public support for government action. Bill Clinton's national security adviser, Anthony Lake, for example, wrote *6 Nightmares* after he left the administration, a book that could have been titled *6 Worst Case Scenarios*. Clinton himself said he was influenced to improve counter-bioterrorism activities by reading Richard Preston's *The Cobra Event*. The book is a compelling blend of a fictional response to a biological attack on the United States and nonfiction details of current biotechnology capabilities.

Richard Clarke, in his novel *Breakpoint*, imagines a cyberattack on the world's computer networks by remarkably computer-literate Luddites who object to the direction biotechnology is taking us. A former counterterrorist official, Clarke assures his readers that the 2012 setting of the novel "*is* meant to be predictive." Clarke's musings in his author's note, on the other hand, can be read as everyday bioethics. He notes that abortion, stem cell research, and the teaching of evolution have been politically controversial, but suggests they are just warm-ups to a debate about what is human: "Should humans change the species with human–machine interfaces and genetic alterations?"

Worst case scenarios are usually based on projections of our fears of death into the future, but they can also be imagined for immediate use. The CIA and the FBI, for example, use a daily "threat matrix" that former CIA director George Tenet has said "scared [him] to death." A former Justice Department official has said that his daily reading about plans for a chemical, nuclear, or biological attack on the United States caused him to "imagine a threat so severe that it became an obsession." Terrorism expert Brian Michael Jenkins has identified this phenomenon as a kind of "self-terrorism." In his words, after 9/11 "possible terrorist threats drove vulnerability assessments, which, in turn, made the terrorist threats seem more credible, a circular analysis that gave al Qaeda a nuclear capability without a nuclear bomb."

The military uses a wonderful two-word description of the result of self-stimulation with like-minded people: incestuous amplification. Perhaps the world's expert in applying game theory to nuclear strategy, Thomas Schelling, put it well: "Fear itself may not be the only thing we have to fear, but unless tempered with analytical vision, it can be a burden and a distortion and an obstacle to urgently needed clarity and understanding." Obsessions can be treated with modern pharmacology, but in the absence of treatment can spread to become an epidemic of fear in government circles that predictably produces deformations of legal, ethical, and human rights doctrines.

The bombing of Hiroshima was a real event. Contemporary planning scenarios based on imaginary worst case scenarios are often, if not usually, based on fantasy, and are so extreme as to mostly produce paranoia and counterproductive behaviors, or simple apathy. In his often compelling book, *Terror and Consent*, law professor Phillip Bobbitt, tells readers that he had originally planned to begin each chapter with an excerpt from a play— one way to emphasize his theme of the "theatrical nature" of 21st-century terrorism, a method of seizing the global stage. Bobbitt's own fictional scenarios are themselves worthy of the stage—but not, I think, of many US preparedness resources.

In his first scenario, terrorists hijack a plane at Dulles on the night of the State of the Union address and crash it into the House chambers, killing almost all Members of Congress, as well as most of the cabinet and the Supreme Court. The Secret Service manages to get the president out at the last minute. When the president gets to an evacuation tunnel, however, he is met by a separate band of "suicide bombers" who kill him. Many more things go wrong in trying to establish a post-doomsday government, but to my mind, we were on the verge of unreality with the initial plane attack on the Capitol, and went totally over the edge by positing a separate group of terrorists attacking simultaneously in the tunnels. Why not make it an even worse worst case scenario by adding a third group of terrorists with smallpox hiding in the House gallery?

Lest we think that Bobbitt is out of the preparedness mainstream, it is worth recalling that Bush administration counterterrorism officials invited the Obama transition team to attend a "national-level exercise" the week before the inauguration, to play out a substantially similar scenario: What would happen if the entire top leadership of the nation was wiped out in a single stroke at the inauguration? The head of the Joint Chiefs of Staff,

Admiral Michael Mullen, told the press that in planning for the inauguration he had "run out the worst case scenarios."

One of the most counterintuitive lessons that has been drawn from some of these fictional exercises is that the country needs more laws that give our (endangered) public officials more authority over American citizens. As two prominent public health lawyers have observed: "In tabletop exercises involving biological attacks or naturally occurring disease outbreaks, those players making decisions have repeatedly been plagued by questions about the scope and substance of their legal authorities." Instead of reminding them that it's only a game, the response is usually to try to pass new laws. This action is taken even though past over-reactions, like the USA Patriot Act, should have informed us that the lack of laws has never caused, or prevented, a terrorist attack. In fact, the only effective action taken on 9/11 to thwart attacks was taken by members of the public, the passengers on United flight 93, who made sure the plane crashed in a Pennsylvania field rather than simply watching while it was used to attack Washington.

The most reasonable response to over-the-top fictional worst case scenarios is not law, but comedy. In the first episode of Tracy Ullman's "State of the Union" she impersonates CNN's Campbell Brown, who is reporting from the White House to give "our nation its daily dose of fear:"

> Brian, I can't stress enough how serious this situation could get to be. The Pentagon are using terms like leaked security documents, secret arms caches, escalating out of control, terrorist infiltration, mandatory civilian evacuation, uncontrollable airborne viruses leading to inevitable planetary annihilation. And that, Brian, is the best case scenario . . . .

This daily dose of fear of death, with or without terrorists employing improvised nuclear devices, has also distracted us (or at least our public officials) from much more critical international nuclear problems, including nuclear proliferation (especially in North Korea and Iran), the security of nuclear weapons (especially in Pakistan and the former Soviet Union), and ongoing genocides (such as in Darfur and Congo).

Protecting and maintaining the health of the population and trying to save the lives of the injured has been at the center of national preparedness planning for disaster. Law and public health have been actively, if not always constructively, involved. Bioethics has generally not been involved. This is a missed opportunity. It is not that bioethicists have any special expertise in preparedness planning. They don't. It is because no matter what the disaster, physicians will have the primary role in caring for the sick and injured, including making emergency triage decisions.

Perhaps more importantly, physicians are consistently identified by the public as those professionals most trusted to turn to for advice regarding their health and safety in an emergency. For example, Americans have said they would not get a smallpox vaccine if there was a smallpox attack if a government official recommended it, but they would get vaccinated if their personal physician recommended it. We Americans will need our physicians to get through any major disaster; however, we will not trust our physicians to help us if we do not believe that they will be guided by medical ethics rather than by partisan politics.

The government can also use physicians for its own purposes. In the war on terror, for example, civilian lawyers in the Department of Defense rewrote the rules of medical ethics (and international human rights) for military physicians tasked with caring for prisoners suspected of being terrorists to permit torture and the force-feeding of prison hunger strikers. The ticking time bomb (worst case) scenario, as portrayed in popular culture on the TV series *24*, has been consistently used to justify torture techniques to "save lives." It has also been the main justification for using physicians to certify prisoners as medically fit for torture, to monitor them during torture, and treat them as needed so that the torture can continue. A worst case nuclear scenario even justified our preemptive war with Iraq.

Just as there is, and should be, no special or exceptional medical ethics for military physicians, there is no special hurricane medical ethics, public health emergency medical ethics, or bioterrorism medical ethics. Extreme situations exist in which the ethical practice of medicine may be especially challenging, but ethical standards, like the legal standard of care and nonderogable international human rights, remain constant. The medical ethics lesson of all-hazards preparedness is that there is and should be no special legal or moral immunity for physicians practicing medicine in disasters. Society must be able to trust its physicians. Negligent Samaritans are simply no good, and are not to be trusted.

Medical ethics (and the doctor–patient relationship) is at the core of a discipline that has come to be denoted by the word *bioethics*. Philosopher-bioethicist Peter Singer, was asked by Bill Maher in a March 2009 broadcast of *Real Time*, "What is bioethics?" Singer replied, "Bioethics is looking at ethical issues in the biological sciences. That means in medicine, new developments in the biological sciences like genetics, perhaps new developments in reproduction. Also, at the other end of life, questions when you turn off the machine . . . ." To which Maher responded, "Bio-life-ethics, there you have it. Professors are always trying to make it more complicated." Daniel Callahan, one of the founders of American bioethics, would go further than Singer, saying that bioethics deals with specific problems in medicine and the life sciences, including the "interaction of ethics and human life, and of science and human values."

Bioethics is defined by its subject matter, not by a specific methodology. In this book, I use the term *bioethics* similarly to Callahan's conception. I also accept Al Jonsen's more precise definition of bioethics as "the systematic study of the moral dimensions—including moral vision, decisions, conduct, and policies—of the life sciences and healthcare, employing a variety of ethical methodologies in an interdisciplinary setting," although I would add "and legal" before methodologies, and include public health in "life sciences and healthcare." Bioethics begins with medical ethics, but expands from this core to encompass all medical and scientific research on humans, all life sciences work directed at improving health and lengthening life, and all government activity undertaken to prevent disease and premature death—the field called public health. One can usefully expand the "bio" or life concept to include animals, the environment, and even the solar system and beyond. In this context, worst case scenarios include global warming and species extinction.

I endorse this expansion of bioethics, but in this book I confine myself primarily to the ethics of medicine, the life sciences, and public health. On the other hand, I am not overly enchanted with the movement to add a new prefix to ethics anytime a new technology appears, thereby implying that a new field of ethics is waiting to be explored. Thus, although the development and application of new technologies will always be a core concern of bioethics, readers will not encounter words like genethics, nanoethics, or neuroethics in this book. There is, however, no fighting the epidemic of bio-prefixed words, and I will refer not only to bioethics and biotechnology, but also to biosecurity, bioidentification, and biobanks, as well as to the old favorites, biopower and biopolitics, to identify just a few.

I part company from some traditional philosopher-bioethicists because I see bioethics as not simply ethics per se, but as encompassing ethics as reflected in and sometimes defined by law, especially constitutional law, public policy, and human rights documents. These fields can interact in reinforcing ways as society tackles perplexing ethical problems. Almost no matter what the ethical dilemma, from abortion to euthanasia and cancer research, to protecting civilians in war and torturing terrorists, society has only three basic options: rely on autonomous individual decisions using a market or morality model, rely on government regulation, or use criminal law to ban an activity. The choice of options is always political, and the law is the instrument society uses to embody the choice.

The dynamic interaction of law, bioethics, and human rights convinced me to change the name of my department at Boston University School of Public Health from the Health Law Department to the Department of Health Law, Bioethics & Human Rights. The same dynamics explains why the title of my feature in the *New England Journal of Medicine*, in which the initial versions of most of the chapters in this book (herein expanded, updated, and integrated) were originally published, was changed from "Legal Issues in Medicine" to "Health Law, Ethics, and Human Rights." These three traditionally separate disciplines act like three spiders, each spinning overlapping and intersecting webs. Controversies in US bioethics are often the subject of heated courtroom confrontations, state and federal legislation, and constitutional interpretation, all of which can also be denoted as "American biopolitics."

It is not unusual for Americans to look to the Supreme Court for guidance on, for example, whether "partial-birth" abortion, assisted suicide, or lethal-injection executions are "ethical" practices for American physicians. Each justice has the opportunity to state his or her views, and because many of the most important cases have been decided on a 5 to 4 vote, the public policy arguments of the justices are well articulated. It will probably be of no surprise that worst case scenarios make frequent appearances. Internationally, at least since Nuremberg and the Doctors' Trial, medical ethics has had a direct effect on the formulation of international human rights documents, and international declarations and treaties have in turn directly influenced national legislation around the world.

Bioethics may seem a strange way to confront the mindless terror and over-reaction generated by our fear of death and magnified by worst case scenarios, but it's not. This is partly because, as an intellectual discipline, bioethics has often dealt in worst case scenarios, most notably death itself, usually in the form of slippery-slope arguments. For example, physician-assisted suicide is often opposed on the basis that it will lead to the routine killing of the old, infirm, minorities, and mentally disabled. Abortion is similarly opposed because it is feared that it will lead to infanticide and disrespect for all human life. Human experimentation is likewise condemned because of the fear it that will treat people like animals, human guinea pigs. It has also become a bioethics commonplace to use science fiction cautionary tales, such as Huxley's *Brave New World*, and Mary Shelley's *Frankenstein* as predictive of the society we will create if we let biotechnology run unrestrained in the world. Fiction can and should be used to help us think about problems, to test our systems and our assumptions, and to expand our imaginations. But fantasy is not fact, "what if?" fiction is not a prediction, and (science) fiction stories can, like Frankenstein's monster, take on a destructive life of their own and overwhelm the political process.

American bioethics requires both physicians and lawyers, and these two professions have an inordinate impact on social policy, especially policy related to public health and safety. They are transnational in that both medical and legal ethics are universal, giving these professions a unique opportunity (and responsibility) to articulate and enforce universal norms. Corporations and nongovernmental organizations (NGOs) are also transnational, and their influence on our lives, and our law, is pervasive and should not be ignored.

Although its subject matter is relatively well-defined, the field of bioethics itself is fractured, fragmented, and contentious as political ideology ofen takes the place of rational discourse and analysis. In this regard, bioethics mirrors similar ideological splits in law, most dramatically illustrated by the Supreme Court's series of decisions on abortion and even by the political theater of the Terri Schiavo case. Deep political differences also exist at the national level over the relevance of international human rights law to US law and policy in areas affecting medical practice, including human experimentation, as well as the use of torture and force-feeding of imprisoned terror suspects. Just as physicians have argued that medical ethics rules sometimes must be abandoned for the "good of the patient" or to "save lives," post-9/11 federal officials have argued that laws that seem to restrict government action to protect the country can be violated for "the good of the country," or simply for "national security."

9/11 provides one example. Katrina provides another. The head of Homeland Security, whose job it was to decide if Katrina was an event of national significance warranting federal assistance, was in Atlanta working on preparations for a bird flu epidemic when the levees were breached. The head of FEMA, Michael Brown, later said he didn't think he could have gotten his boss's attention unless he had told him that a terrorist had blown up the levees. Alternative approaches to worst case scenario death and disaster planning deserve much more serious consideration than they have received to date. Some alternatives include taking liberty and human rights more seriously, being more skeptical of government bans and mandates, enabling citizens to help themselves and each other in emergencies, and working more aggressively for international cooperation. In all of these alternative approaches, an understanding of the health law–bioethics–human rights web can be used as a critical analytic tool for public policy development and implementation.

Worst Case Bioethics is divided into three parts. The first, Death and Disaster, deals with America's and Americans' reactions to the prospect of death and disaster generally. It opens with an analysis of what ails the American healthcare system, suggesting that fear of death is at its core and that no real progress can be made in reforming the delivery system or changing the incentives that make it the most expensive system in the world until we confront our overwhelming fear of death. Notably, it is not just that we fear death as we approach the end of life, but that we make "death defying" and death delaying medical decisions all through our lives. Three chapters deal with specific categories of disasters: bioterrorism, medical emergencies, and war. Two chapters are about techniques used to respond to our fear of a worse disaster: torture (and the "ticking time bomb") and force-feeding hunger strikers.

In these last two examples, violations of basic human rights and bioethics have consistently been justified by our magic words: saving lives, national security, and sometimes progress. These terms tend to overwhelm their counterarguments: crimes against humanity, consent, and caution. A special focus is on the use of lawyers and physicians to justify torture and cruel and degrading treatment as part of "enhanced interrogation." The chapter on war focuses on the deaths of civilians in war, the treatment of the bodies of US soldiers killed in combat, and whether there should be exceptions to universal medical ethics precepts for physicians in the US military. This topic also serves as a transition to Part II, Death and the Constitution.

Death and the Constitution examines bioethical controversies that have ended up in court, usually in the Supreme Court, where sharp arguments and counterarguments have been presented before and by the justices. All focus on physicians making decisions involving death—usually in a context in which politicians or judges are arguing that, unless a decision is made one way, the result will be a worst case scenario that imperils lives. The outlines, but not the details, of the illustrative cases will be familiar to most readers, including the continuing arguments for open access by terminally ill cancer patients to investigational drugs and currently illegal substances like marijuana (often called medical marijuana), the use of drugs for physician-assisted suicide, lethal injection as the preferred method to execute condemned prisoners, so-called partial-birth abortion, and the infamous case of Terri Schiavo, which involved all branches of our government in an attempt to overturn her husband's decision to stop tube-feeding her so that she could die.

The use of extreme scenarios can expose the irrationality of a proposition by reductio ad absurdum. The lesson of this section, however, is that worst case scenario logic often, if not always, distorts public policy formation by leading to conclusions that have major unintended negative consequences, conclusions that undercut rather than promote medical ethics. The section ends with a bridge to the final section on Disaster and Public Health: the question of why we haven't taken patient safety seriously in the United States, and what we might be able to do about trying to save some of the one million people who died from preventable medical errors in our hospitals over the past decade. Saving lives usually is a rallying cry, but not in American hospitals. Why is this? A public health, populations approach dedicated to prevention is needed to save lives in our hospitals.

Part III, Disaster and Public Health, focuses on public health, a broad, multidisciplinary field concerned primarily with preventing communicable disease and promoting the health of the public through government regulation and oversight of food, drugs, water, air, medical care, and other necessities of life. This area is a new one for most bioethicists, but has the fastest growing literature in the field; it is sometimes even referred to as its own new field, *health and human rights*. Public health, like the pandemics it seeks to mitigate, knows no national boundaries and is inherently global, making human rights language its natural companion, as I argue in the first chapter of this section, Global Health. Since 9/11, public health has been asked to engage in preparedness for all types of worst case terrorist attacks, most especially a bioterrorism attack involving agents such as anthrax and smallpox. In the Statue of Security and Pandemic Fear, I explore how this new mission has deformed US public health, moving it away from health and toward "security." These two chapters are followed by a third, which provides perhaps the major example of an attempt to merge public health with police and counterterrorism, and the response to this in the area of DNA profiling by the European Court of Human Rights.

These three chapters also suggest how a national prevention agenda can be implemented without government coercion of its citizens or routine government violation of civil rights laws, as well as how fostering rather than frustrating an international human rights agenda focused on health could help defeat terrorism. Finally, I examine the perils of relying on worst case scenarios in preparing for the future by revisiting one I suggested at the UN's Conference on Racism in South Africa the week before 9/11: the prospect of "genetic genocide." This worst case scenario is defended and contrasted with science's seductive promise of posthuman immortality, perhaps the ultimate saving lives rationale.

I conclude the final chapter, and the book, by arguing that only plausible scenarios deserve a place in real world planning. Completely fictional worst case scenarios can be deployed to question implausible best case scenarios (such as justifying genetic engineering experiments to create "better" humans), but their use should be restricted to the academic and theatrical realm; they should not be used to drive political debate or policy decisions, bioethics or otherwise, because they will predictably do more harm than good.

I

. . . .

DEATH AND DISASTER

1

. . . .

American Healthcare

The first thing most Americans think about healthcare is not death and disaster. We're good at denial. Nonetheless, the fragmented non-system we use for healthcare is based primarily on responding to life-threatening events and treating risks of death. It is focused on saving lives and curing or stabilizing diseases, and only secondarily on disease prevention or improving quality of life. Nor is it not just death prevention at the end of life; death, in the form of risks, underlies medicine from the point of view of both patients and physicians from the moment of birth, even from the moment of conception. Death is personal; disasters affect populations. It is not uncommon to portray American healthcare itself as a disaster. At least since World War II, we have sought to reform a system that is itself widely viewed in disaster imagery, perhaps the most popular being that our healthcare system is a "train wreck."

A good example is President Lyndon Johnson's response to what he described as the "bombshell" Medicaid proposal to go along with his

4 Death and Disaster

proposed Medicare plan. He explained his support for both proposals to Wilbur Cohen, the person who would take the lead in drafting them (with Wilber Mills) for his administration. He told Cohen the story about the railroad giving an intelligence test for switchmen. The question was:

> "What would you do if a train was coming east going sixty miles per hour, and you looked over your shoulder and another one was coming from the west going sixty miles an hour?" . . . and the fellow said, "I'd go get my brother." And he said, "Why would you get your brother?" And he said, "Because he hasn't ever seen a train wreck."[1]

The image of a train wreck can be used to mobilize action, but train wreck imagery can be overwhelmed by other metaphors mobilized to resist reform. As I write this chapter, the House and Senate have each reported bills out of committee, but have yet to debate them. President Obama is committed to increasing health insurance access for Americans, but the longer he and his allies delay endorsing a specific plan, the less likely its success becomes, because financial stakeholders in the present system will have time to find ways to frustrate meaningful reform.[2]

Lawrence Brown has suggested that the metaphor blocking health reform to date is the "safety net," which includes emergency departments and community health centers, because this imaginary net is seen as protecting even the uninsured from major health disaster.[3] Similarly, William Sage has observed that we have yet to identify a health systems metaphor with traction.[4] Metaphors referencing two struggling American industries, automobiles ("Do you want Chevrolet or Cadillac coverage?") and airlines (as a metaphor for patient safety), have, for example, failed to capture the public's imagination.

Shortly after the demise of President Bill Clinton's healthcare plan, I suggested that both the military and market metaphors in American medicine had become counterproductive, and that they should be replaced by the ecological metaphor.[5] This has not happened (at least not yet), and the Obama administration has continued to cling to the mast of the Clintons' 1993–94 framing of the healthcare financing reform debate as shipwreck again threatens us. Of course, it is not just a replacement metaphor we need, but one that can help us confront and modify the major characteristics of American healthcare.

The inspiration for American healthcare is perhaps best embodied in Damien Hirst's 2007 diamond-encrusted platinum human skull. The skull was cast from that of an 18th-century man; the original teeth are retained and the skull is coated with 8,600 diamonds. Hirst calls the diamond skull "For the Love of God" and says he was inspired by similarly jeweled Aztec skulls.[6] As a metaphor, the skull displays all four of what I take to be the most enduring and problematic characteristics of American healthcare (and of America itself): it is wasteful, technologically driven, individualistic, and death-denying. Nonetheless, skulls are not inspirational, even diamond-frosted ones, and this one has a strange allure that may subvert rather than promote reform. We need a plan more than we need a metaphor, but a plan without a metaphor is unlikely to be politically (or even economically) viable. What should it be?

Healthcare's Competing Metaphors

American healthcare has historically been dominated by the patriarchal and hierarchical military metaphor. Uniformed physicians aggressively fight invading agents with an increasingly sophisticated and expensive armamentarium designed to destroy the enemy. Patients become brave fighters, and their bodies are the battlefield. As Susan Sontag noted in 1977, when she herself was a cancer patient, the military metaphor has particular salience in the "war on cancer." This seemed like an unwinnable war to her, a war that featured conflicting "bromides" from "the American cancer establishment, tirelessly hailing the imminent victory over cancer, the professional pessimism of a large number of cancer specialists, talking like battle-weary officers mired down in an interminable colonial war . . . twin distortions in this military rhetoric about cancer."[7]

New cancer drugs explicitly adopt the military metaphor. A 2009 headline in the *Wall Street Journal*, for example, touted "New Recruits: Enlisting Genes in the Campaign Against Cancer" and told readers, "Genetic research is making another big advance in the battle against cancer." Sontag expected the military metaphor to recede as its damage, especially to patients, was recognized. This hasn't happened. Instead, the body continues to be viewed as a battlefield, death as the enemy, and there are no limits in terms of either money or weapons that can be used to defeat death. Hospice and even palliative care remain marginalized, viewed by many, if not most, physicians as either retreating from the battle for life or simply surrendering.

It is at least somewhat remarkable that the military metaphor has not been used in the battle to reform healthcare by requiring, as we do with the military, that it be under the control of the government, which sets both its priorities and its budget. A reasonable response might be, following President Dwight Eisenhower, that even in the military most funding goes to private companies and the "military-industrial complex" overwhelms public oversight, thus making control illusory. A parallel complex, sometimes termed simply the "medical-industrial complex," may actually run American healthcare—to the extent anyone does—by, among other things, deploying its own metaphor, the market metaphor. The image of a market in healthcare is equally destructive and deceptive.

Under the market metaphor, healthcare corporations replace healthcare practitioners, patients become consumers, medical care becomes a business, and health insurance is marketed on the basis of cost. Consumer choice becomes the center of market medicine discourse. Physicians are encouraged to "manage care," while risk managers manage them, and a healthy bottom line is seen as more important than a healthy patient population. Advertising and hype become more important than objective measurement of outcomes, especially when new products, such as drugs and devices, are introduced.

The market metaphor is extraordinary. It has even infected the military itself, which has increasingly relied on financial bonuses to recruit and retain soldiers, as well as on outsourcing and privatizing jobs that have historically been performed by soldiers. The market metaphor has had particular salience in medical care since it supports patient choice (and informed consent) and encourages new ideas and methods. The market, of course, generally opposes government regulation and especially "socialized medicine." In relying almost exclusively on corporate structures, the market concentrates power in the unaccountable private sector, breeds conflicts of interest, and encourages medicine to adopt the language of corporations or "corp speak," or perhaps more descriptively, as Christopher Ricks has saliently mused, "corpse speak."[8]

One of the most astute observers of American medicine, surgeon-writer Atul Gawande, has mixed both of these metaphors—and also alluded to one I will discuss later in this chapter, the environmental metaphor—to suggest how difficult changing our nonsystem will be. These comments come after he has described two major competing models of American healthcare: profit-maximizing by physicians who work in a "quantity-driven, untenably fragmented" system, and nonprofit physician groups who work together, as at the Mayo Clinic, "to increase prevention and quality of care, while discouraging overtreatment, undertreatment, and sheer profiteering." In his words, "The result is the most wasteful and least sustainable healthcare system in the world." Gawande continues, arguing that it's even worse than waste: "In the war over the culture of medicine . . . the Mayo model is losing . . . many people in medicine don't see why they should do the hard work of organizing themselves in ways that reduce waste and improve quality if it means sacrificing revenue."[9]

Bill and Hillary Clinton made an attempt to draw the best from these competing metaphors in constructing an argument for healthcare reform based on what they described as six "shining stars" by which to navigate the American healthcare ship: security, savings, choice, simplicity, responsibility, and quality.[10] These six stars or goals can be seen as an attempt to recast and expand the classic three central interrelated challenges of American healthcare: cost, quality, and access. Unfortunately, like the original three, these six goals viciously compete with each other (e.g., security and savings, simplicity and choice, and cost and quality), and thus cannot provide a coherent framework for charting change. To apply the metaphor, you really can guide your healthcare ship only by one star if you don't want to sail in circles.

The Clintons also sought to avoid making the country think about healthcare in the context of the lifecycle ending in death. In a video made for the annual Gridiron Dinner, they played Harry and Louise criticizing their health plan. Hillary says to Bill: "On page 12,743 . . . it says that eventually we are all going to die." Bill eventually responds, "Wow, that is scary! I've never been so frightened in all my life." They then say together, "There's got to be a better way." The sketch was high comedy. Sam Donaldson of ABC, nonetheless, commented the next day that even mentioning death in a political context can only hurt your cause in America. Whatever one's opinion of the Clinton Health Plan, Americans do act as if they believe that, when it comes to death, "There's got to be a better way." The White House never authorized the video to be played again.

The 2008 Presidential Campaign

During the 2008 presidential campaign, three basic views emerged. John McCain was the clearest, as he adopted the market metaphor as a statement of reality. He was also a cost, quality, and access candidate. He saw our major problems as "bringing costs under control," "maintaining quality," and "providing access to healthcare for all of our citizens."[11] He proposed to accomplish these goals by relying on the market to create more competition and on Americans accepting more personal responsibility to take better care of themselves. Other than proposing medical malpractice tort reform, McCain, the candidate with the most personal experience as a patient, said he was pretty happy with the way things are now.

Hillary Clinton and Barack Obama used almost identical reform frames during the campaign. Although rearranged, Clinton essentially retained her original six navigational stars, moving choice up to number one. Her plan was named the American Health Choices Plan, and its major goal is to increase choice ("if you like what you have you can keep it").[12]

Other goals also mirrored the original navigational stars: lower premiums and increase security (savings and security), promote shared responsibility, ensure affordable coverage for all (security), and improve quality. Only simplicity seems to have been jettisoned from the Clinton reform ship.

Obama's Plan for a Healthy America, promised quality, affordability, lower costs, and new initiatives.[13] His seven major goals (which can also be seen as his navigational stars) were to provide guaranteed eligibility, comprehensive benefits, affordable premiums, subsidies, simplified paperwork, choice, and quality. To somewhat oversimplify, Obama adopted the original Clinton navigational framing, omitting only responsibility.

The Massachusetts mandate model (everyone must purchase their own health insurance, with state subsidies for those who can't afford the premiums) is often a reference, and it may prove to be a winning political strategy. But an individual insurance mandate as a key to healthcare reform seems unlikely to be able to garner wide political support—not the least because it undermines the much more powerful of choice. It is also noteworthy that no major candidate discussed a Medicare-for-all plan, most likely because it is seen as too divorced from the market and too close to "socialized medicine" to be politically viable. This even though a Medicare-for-all plan would not involve a Veterans Affairs-like government-owned and operated system, and the Medicare program itself utilizes private hospitals, physicians, suppliers, and pharmaceutical and biotech companies, as well as a wide range of supplementary (and even primary) private insurance plans. Even simply requiring a public option to private health insurance, as suggested by President Obama, has drawn criticism, primarily because it is seen as a possible prototype of a Medicare-for-all plan. Of course, a half-dozen navigational stars don't make one coherent metaphor, and they don't take the inherent difficulty of changing American healthcare, most notably its delivery system, seriously enough. Thus, it should surprise no one that early in the Obama administration, universal insurance coverage was sold with a single goal: cost reduction. It is also unsurprising that a major argument for change is that the cost of healthcare is undermining America's economic growth—at least everywhere except in the healthcare sector itself.

The ecological metaphor, with its emphasis on concepts such as sustainability, natural, limited (resources), quality (of life), community, and even responsibility, could play a more potent role in reframing and reforming American healthcare. Al Gore and others, for example, have finally been successful in moving the environment and climate change to the center of policy debates, in large part by framing the issue in terms of an emergency, in this case a "planetary emergency."[14] Gore has also successfully employed easily understood stories to illustrate the threat, including images of polar bears drowning as a result of the melting of the Arctic icecap. Gawande is also on target to characterize our present healthcare system as "the most wasteful and . . . least sustainable . . . in the world."

Nonetheless, the ecological metaphor, even in its planetary emergency reincarnation, has been overwhelmed by the post-9/11 national security emergency, which has reinforced the old military metaphor in almost all aspects of the public policy debate.[15] Instead of concentrating on health security or even economic security (at least until late 2009), we have spent almost all our political energy since 2001 on national security. Instead of preparing to provide care for our aging citizenry, we spend our preparedness resources developing plans to respond to hypothetical worst case scenarios and fighting a metaphorical global war on terror. Security, one of the goals of all healthcare plans, takes on a life of its own, overwhelming the others like Frankenstein's monster.

George Lakoff is one of the country's most influential political framers. He believes progressives who want to reform our healthcare system must embrace the military metaphor and argue that, just like military and police protection, Americans deserve "healthcare security." During the last presidential campaign, he suggested four framing values to move the country in that direction: empathy, responsibility, protection, and empowerment. Protection is a reframing of security, and empowerment is a reframing of choice. Lakoff would also reframe responsibility to include government responsibility to provide healthcare, and add an entirely new value, empathy.

Lakoff assumes, as I understand him, that Americans really do identify with each other when we are sick or injured, and that we believe that medical care should be available to all Americans who need care. He specifically suggests that progressives base calls to action on stories about "actual flesh and blood people" whom Americans can identify with.[16] This approach was employed during the 2008 campaign most by John Edwards and Hillary Clinton. Clinton's best story was about an uninsured pregnant woman who died shortly after her baby was stillborn. This double tragedy happened, Clinton said she was told, when the woman was denied care by an Ohio hospital because she could not come up with a $100 deposit. It is a good story, but the health reform part of the story turns out not to be true. Trina Bachtel and her baby did both die, but not because she was uninsured (she had insurance through her employer) or because she was turned away from the hospital (she wasn't- she was seen at a different hospital seven times during her pregnancy, hospitalized for childbirth, and spent the last two weeks of her life getting specialty care at three different hospitals).[17]

Clinton said something else on the campaign trail that struck a chord with her audiences—and it is something that is not captured by any of the framing lists or metaphors. She said, "I believe healthcare is a right, not a privilege." This phrase suggests that the rights metaphor may be the one that could break the healthcare reform stalemate. Americans do believe in their rights, including their constitutional rights. Although the "right to health," an internationally recognized right that includes the right to basic healthcare, is not recognized as a general right in the United States, it has been recognized as a limited legal right in the situation Trina Bachtel experienced. Even if Bachtel had been uninsured, she had a legal right to emergency care in a hospital emergency department—and under current federal law, that right includes the right to treatment in labor, whether or not her pregnancy is considered high-risk or an emergency.[18] There is virtually no debate or question that people experiencing a medical emergency should get whatever medical care they need, regardless of insurance or ability to pay, as a matter of right.

American popular culture also supports this right, as illustrated by the longest running medical drama in US television history, *ER*, which premiered the month the Clinton plan was withdrawn from the US Senate, and only ended in the early days of the Obama presidency. The question—and it is not just a framing question—is how to expand the legal and moral right to emergency care, which Americans value so highly, into a more general right to necessary healthcare. In one of the most stirring speeches at the 2008 Democratic National Convention, the father of American healthcare reform, Senator Edward Kennedy, put it simply: "This is the cause of my life—new hope that we will break the old gridlock and guarantee that every American— north, south, east, west, young, old—will have decent, quality healthcare as a fundamental right and not a privilege."

Senator Kennedy repeated this shortly before his death in a letter to the president, portions of which the president read in his September 2009 address to a joint session of Congress. And President Obama himself, asked by Tom Brokaw in the second presidential debate whether he considered healthcare a "privilege, right or responsibility" replied: "Well, I think it should be a right for every American." The now president continued by telling the story about how his mother, who died of cancer at the age of 53, had to spend "the last months of her life in the hospital room arguing with insurance companies" who were saying that her condition may have been "pre-existing" and thus not covered. As the president observed, "there's something fundamentally wrong about that."

Americans, Healthcare, and Death

Two possible frameworks for expanding the right to healthcare are sometimes described as competing, but are I think complementary: the human rights frame, which can also be used as a metaphor, and the social justice frame. Social justice is more at home with Lakoff's insistence on empathy. It is often described in the European context as solidarity, and solidarity was the basis for the United Kingdom's National Health Service, which was founded following World War II. But social justice can also be seen in American terms as a matter of fundamental fairness and equal opportunity.

Human rights, unlike social justice precepts, can become enforceable governmental obligations. Human rights are declared internationally and defined by treaty, but are promulgated nationally by legislation that adopts specific entitlements. In this framework, a national healthcare plan would be a statutory enactment of America's view of the right to healthcare, similar to the statutory guarantee of the right to education (and the statutory guarantee of Medicare), that would also be supported by broad concepts of social justice and equity.

The failure to discover or invent an effective metaphor for reforming our dysfunctional healthcare system suggests that American healthcare has fundamental characteristics that Americans value. One, of course, is money: Every dollar spent on healthcare is someone's income. With one dollar out of every six in the US economy devoted to healthcare financing, that economic fact alone could make major reform unachievable, at least until the doomsday shipwreck disaster occurs.

It may also be that we are searching for metaphors from the wrong perspective, looking at stars when we should be examining the ship itself—as we should have examined the Titanic before it struck an iceberg. It is, for example, plausible that unless we deal directly with the four enduring characteristics of our American healthcare ship—that it is wasteful, technologically driven, individualistic, and death-denying—we will not be able to change American healthcare in more than a superficial way. Each of these characteristics is pervasive and seductive, and can even be thought of as fundamentally American.

We are certainly wasteful. The ongoing Iraq war provides another healthcare story that illustrates both pervasive waste and our enduring fascination with high-tech, high-cost rescue medicine. After the senseless killing of civilians in Haditha[19] by private contractors from Blackwater, US military physicians in Iraq provided heroic care for an infant girl, Amenah, from the town. She was flown to the United States for successful open-heart surgery to repair a congenital heart defect that would have killed her. The

Navy reservist cardiologist who first examined Amenah in Iraq, Captain John Nadeau, put his decision to treat Amenah simply and in a way that could have described our entire healthcare system: "When I look at the money that is wasted here, you know, it's only money. And look at this little girl."[20] Rather than deal with the waste in our system, we are eager to concentrate on individual cases and ignore the healthcare system as a whole.

The second characteristic, technology, does not only drive medicine and the military, it drives virtually all sectors of our economy. It is responsible for most of the increases in cost of American healthcare,[21] including the cost of marginally effective care, and thus of waste. We are infected with what has wonderfully been labeled "gizmo idolatry," the conviction that "a more technological approach is intrinsically better."[22] Cost-effectiveness analysis challenges this view, which is one reason it is so controversial.

The third characteristic, that we are individualistic, is, like technology, not usually seen as a problem at all, but as an American attribute to be encouraged—not least of all by expanding choice. President Obama understands this. This is why he repeats messages that seem at odds with any desire to make meaningful changes in American healthcare, such his statement in September 2009 when he went on every Sunday talk show to promote his healthcare agenda: "The overwhelming part of the American population . . . is trying to figure out, is this going to help me? Is healthcare [reform] going to make me better off?"[23] This individualistic, what's in it for me attitude makes it impossible to even mention the word rationing or the concept of limits, at least outside the context of a hypothetical worst case global pandemic emergency scenario when vaccines, antiviral drugs, and even hospital beds and ventilators are likely to be in short supply.

Finally, and I think most importantly, we are a death-denying culture that cannot accept death as anything but defeat. This means we will prepare for any and every disease and screen for every possible "risk factor," but are utterly unable to prepare for death. Examples are plentiful and the basic problem is illustrated by the prolonged and painful death of the most perceptive writer on medical metaphors, Susan Sontag. Dying from acute myeloid leukemia, she insisted on trying every "experimental therapy" available, ultimately including an extremely long-shot bone marrow transplant. Even after the transplant failed, "she clung to [her doctors] as a shipwrecked sailor to a spar." Her doctors thought they were reframing hope for her, but as her son writes, "I very much doubt that 'hope,' framed or reframed, offers much to someone trying to organize his or her thoughts and feelings in the shadow of extinction." Sontag saw herself as "the exception to every rule." Her son continues: "If, as I believe, she had imagined herself special, my mother's last illness cruelly exposed the frailty of that conceit. It was merciless in the toll of pain and fear that it extracted."[24]

Sontag's death, as horrible as it was, was an altogether American death.[25] We Americans often see ourselves, and our country, as an exception to every rule. And this, I think, is the real point: The American healthcare system is itself a metaphor, a metaphor for America. Metaphors can reflect reality, undermine reality, or transform reality.[26] In this case, our healthcare system is a mirror, reflecting the basic characteristics of America. To the extent this is true, it will take more than a new metaphor or a new frame to change our healthcare system. It will take a fundamental change in America itself, or at least in our perception of ourselves.

President Obama seems to recognize this and, in the context of discussing healthcare reform, has spoken both of the dying experiences of his mother and his grandmother. His grandmother, Madelyn Dunham, had been diagnosed with terminal cancer, and shortly after getting this diagnosis she fell and broke her hip, perhaps because of a mild stroke. In the president's words, she was told by her doctor, "maybe you have three months, maybe you have six months, maybe you have nine months to live." The doctor continued, "Because of the weakness of your heart . . . there are certain risks [to a hip operation] . . . that your heart can't take it. On the other hand, if you just sit there with your hip like this, you're just going to waste away and your quality of life will be terrible." The president's grandmother elected to have the hip replacement surgery, after which she had two good weeks, then went into sudden decline and died the day before the election of her grandson to the presidency. As the president framed the private and public issues raised by his grandmother's experience:

> I don't know how much that hip replacement cost. I would have paid out of pocket for that hip replacement because she's my grandmother. Whether sort of in the aggregate, society making those decisions to give my grandmother, or everybody else's aging grandparents or parents, a hip replacement when they're terminally ill is a *sustainable model,* is a very difficult question. If somebody told me my grandmother couldn't have a hip replacement and she had to lie there in misery in the waning days of her life—that would be pretty upsetting . . . So that's where I think you just get into some very difficult moral issues. But that's also *a huge driver of cost* . . . .[27] (emphasis added)

President Obama was not ready to answer his own questions, but he performs an extremely valuable public service by raising them in the context of his own family. As he went on to say, "I think that there is going to have to be a conversation [with the public] that is guided by doctors, scientists, ethicists. There is going to have to be a very difficult democratic conversation that takes place." Yes, there is, and there is no chance that this conversation, which we have never had, will ever take place without strong and sustained presidential leadership. As for the substance of the hoped-for conversation, I think Ellen Goodman, *Boston Globe* columnist, got it just right: "I think that what our [healthcare] system may need is not more intervention, but more conversation, especially on the delicate subject of dying . . . More expensive care is not always better care. Doing everything can be the wrong thing. The end of life is one place where ethics and economics can still be braided into a single strand of humanity."[28] In the summer of 2009, the national discussion on death planning the president had hoped for focused instead on death denial. Make-believe government "death panels" that would arbitrarily "pull the plug on grandma" were used as a rhetorical device to block any rational discussion of either death generally or end of life care in particular. Ivan Illich seems to have gotten it right in his 1975 *Medical Nemesis*:

> Socially approved death happens when man [sic] has become useless not only as a producer but also as a consumer. It is at this point that [the patient] . . . must be written off as a total loss. Death has become the ultimate form of consumer resistance. [29]

President Obama will have to articulate a compelling rationale for change, and the high cost of caring for not only the terminally and chronically ill, but also for the worried well and the just plain healthy, will not be enough. The American-inspired global recession, and our current disillusion with unfettered capitalism, opens new possibilities to move away from both the military and market metaphors toward government action based on the environmental and the rights metaphors. The financial disaster caused by excesses, mismanagement, and unwarranted faith in a rational market, however, also reinforces cost-containment as a primary concern.

One possibility is for the president to encourage a more reflective America, one in which, for example, we really do put quality of life and care above quantity of life and cure, come to understand that we can learn from the rest of the world as well as teach, and apply cost-effectiveness tools to all new (and existing) drugs and medical technologies, all of which could be contained in an ecological metaphor. But this may be too difficult a course alteration for the passengers of the ship of state to accept—since we have yet to even accept that we are all in the same boat.

It is probably more plausible for the president to speak to Americans in the language of individual rights, and, with the Congress, to declare a new American right, the right to decent healthcare. As Franklin Roosevelt first noted in 1944, just before D-Day, denying healthcare denies equal opportunity and is an assault on human dignity. Concurrently, the language of social justice should be employed, especially by using stories of real Americans denied needed healthcare, to convince Americans—who probably don't need much convincing—that it is simply unfair to deny uninsured and underinsured (and even many insured) Americans decent healthcare, as it is unfair to deny decent education to Americans who cannot afford it. Healthcare is a moral issue and denial of healthcare based on inability to pay is immoral.

The military and market metaphors continue to dominate American medicine, the former primarily in healthcare delivery, and the latter in healthcare financing. The ecological metaphor suggests radical reform of both financing and delivery, but has not, at least yet, gained political traction. The navigational stars for healthcare reform seem set in the cement of political rhetoric, but they are likely to be no more inspirational in promoting change today than they were in 1994.

Damien Hirst's diamond crusted skull is a mirror metaphor for America, but it could also serve as a mutiny metaphor, inciting rebellion. It is, for example, inspired by the Aztecs, who elaborately decorated the skulls of those whom they sacrificed to their gods. As historian Hugh Thomas has noted, a major reason the Spanish were able to defeat the Aztecs was that they used high-tech steel swords designed to kill efficiently. The Aztecs used swords of "sharp stones slotted into wooden shafts intended primarily to wound . . . [because] they hoped for wounded captives, not corpses, for sacrifice at festivals."[30]

To overstate the metaphor somewhat, like the Aztecs, we have a choice. We can continue the festival of American market medicine, which sacrifices the lives and health of large numbers of poor and uninsured Americans, or we can engage in fundamental reform of American healthcare by broadening American values to include the right to decent healthcare for all. Fundamental change in American healthcare will require fundamental change in our culture, and a combination of the ecological and rights metaphors could help us successfully navigate the waters of change.

I have been concerned in this chapter with the ways we use metaphors to shape our perceptions of reality and to incite or prevent changes in healthcare policy. In the next chapter, I continue this theme by examining how art and science affect each other in the realm of bioterrorism, and what ethical stance scientists and physicians working in this arena—filled with worst case biological attack scenarios—should adopt.

2

. . . .

Bioterror and Bioart

Since Hiroshima, the world's worst case scenario has been nuclear war. That is why the WMD (weapons of mass destruction) justification for war with Iraq was framed by the suggestion that Iraq was planning a nuclear attack on the United States, "We don't want the smoking gun to be a mushroom cloud." And a terrorist attack on a US city using an improvised nuclear device (IND) is listed first on the Department of Homeland Security's 15 National Planning Scenarios. Nonetheless, the US Commission on the Prevention of Weapons of Mass Destruction Proliferation and Terrorism, a direct descendent of the 9/11 Commission, concluded in late 2008 that "terrorists are more likely to be able to obtain and use a biological weapon than a nuclear weapon," and that "it is more likely than not that a weapon of mass destruction will be used in a terrorist attack somewhere in the world by the end of 2013."[1]

The Commission is not alone in its assessment. Bioterrorism with a new, lethal disease is now seen by many as the worst case scenario for a terrorist attack. This assessment has also made prevention more imperative and the creation of new ethical and legal rules for biomedical researchers more critical. New laws have been passed, new regulations and oversight of laboratories has been suggested by the Commission, and there have been proposals for new codes of scientific ethics for bioterrorism-related research.

Ethical guidelines for life sciences research that could be related to bioterrorism are critical, and the scientific community should be more actively engaged in setting the standards for such research than it has been. As the National Research Council (NRC) has stated, "biological scientists have an affirmative moral duty to avoid contributing to the advancement of biowarfare or bioterrorism."[2] It is reasonable for society to expect that scientists adopt the equivalent of the physician's "do no harm" principle. Arguing for such an oath well before 9/11, Roger Shattuck noted that it could "help scientists scrutinize the proliferation of research in dubious areas" as well as "renew the confidence of ordinary citizens" in what is now a potentially life-extinguishing endeavor.[3]

As the debate about the role of ethical standards proceeds, some legal standards have already been adopted, and law enforcement has become deeply involved in investigating science. Even with their increased investigative powers, however, the FBI and CIA took almost seven years to identify the person they now believe was responsible for the anthrax attacks in the fall of 2001. Their investigation early focused on Steven J. Hatfill, who worked for the US Army at the Fort Detrick laboratory, and who ultimately was paid $5 million by the US government to settle a lawsuit brought to protest the FBI's aggressive and unjustified actions against him. Among the things that made Hatfill, a physician and virologist, a prime suspect for the FBI was that he had written an unpublished novel about a bioterrorist attack on Washington.[4] In 2008, the FBI announced that it had solved the case, shortly after their new primary suspect, another scientist who also worked at the Army's Fort Detrick laboratory, Bruce Ivins, committed suicide. The FBI may have finally gotten it right, but many people remained unconvinced. There was no confession, and the suggested motive—that he was a "bioevangelist" who had decided to alert the nation to the dangers of a bioterrorist attack by launching one himself—seemed stretched at best.[5]

The botched investigation of the anthrax attacks was not atypical of the post-9/11 FBI as it dealt with scientists and science. It is not surprising therefore that in a survey published in late 2008, 93% of scientists were happy to discuss their work with other scientists, 87% with the public, but only 36% with law enforcement officials. Only 14% thought the FBI should play a role in monitoring their work, and more than two-thirds thought it was illegitimate of the FBI to ask them to monitor the work of another scientist.[6] Much of the distaste for the FBI can be traced to the anthrax case, but other botched cases involving scientists have played a role as well. Two merit detailed attention because of the lessons they suggest about the narrow focus that worst case scenario thinking can induce in criminal investigations involving suspected bioterrorism activities.

Thomas Butler

Thomas Butler was the first, and so far only, physician-scientist to stand trial in the United States on a post-9/11 bioterrorism-related charge. The bioterrorism-related facts are no longer in serious dispute.[7] As described by his colleagues in infectious disease research, Butler has had a long and successful career dating from completion of medical school and residency at Johns Hopkins at the end of the 1960s and his service in Vietnam in the US Naval Medical Research Unit. He was a faculty member at Johns Hopkins and Case Western Reserve before becoming Chief of Infectious Diseases at Texas Tech University's Health Sciences Center in 1987, a post he held until his trial. His work on plague (*Yersinia pestis*) dates from his experiences treating civilians during the Vietnam War, and most recently he was involved in research in Tanzania, where he worked with a local colleague to compare the efficacy of gentamicin versus doxycycline in treating patients with plague infection.[8]

He traveled to Tanzania to help set up the study in 2001, and he returned in 2002 to collect samples of *Y. pestis* taken from the subjects. He returned to the United States with these samples without the required transport permits. In June 2002, he drove to the CDC's Fort Collins, Colorado laboratory to get the samples tested, again without the required government transport permits. In September 2002, he sent a set of plague isolates back to Tanzania in a Federal Express box labeled "laboratory materials" without the required export permits, and in October, he flew from Lubbock to Washington D.C. with plague samples without the required permit.

In November 2002, following a series of confrontations with his institutional review board (IRB) over timely documentation of the morbidity and mortality of subjects in an antibiotic study he was conducting for the biotechnology company Chiron, the IRB suspended him from doing research on human subjects. On January 9, 2003, the IRB reiterated the suspension in an e-mail.[9] The following day, Butler was notified by letter of a formal inquiry into his activities. On January 11, a Saturday morning, Butler noticed that a set of 30 tubes of *Y. pestis* cultures was missing, noting in his journal "Set 5 missing!" The next day he wrote, "Can't explain other than intentional removal, suspect theft."[10] On Monday, January 13, 2003, he reported to the health center's biosafety officer that 30 vials of *Y. pestis* were missing from his laboratory. The following day, senior health center officials met and decided to notify the local police and the health department. The police notified the FBI, and more than 60 FBI agents and local police conducted an immediate investigation.

Butler was questioned by the FBI and waived his right to counsel (almost always a mistake). He first insisted that he did not know what happened to the samples. However, after failing a lie detector test and being told by an FBI agent that if he signed a statement that he had accidentally destroyed them (to reassure the public that there was no danger), that would be the end of the matter, he signed a statement to this effect.[11] But this statement was not the end of the matter. Butler was arrested, spent six days in jail, and was then was put under house arrest. In April 2003, a grand jury returned a 15-count indictment charging him with various crimes relating to his transporting *Y. pestis*, making false statements to the FBI, and tax evasion. Texas Tech also turned against Butler, helping the prosecution reframe the contract disputes the University had with him as crimes. In August 2003, after Butler refused to plead guilty in exchange for a 6-month sentence, 54 additional criminal counts were charged against him, including mail fraud, wire fraud, and embezzlement arising from Butler's research for two companies (Chiron and Pharmacia-Upjohn—now Pfizer), and for concealing two contracts with the Food and Drug Administration (FDA) from the university.

Under Butler's pay structure, a percentage of his income was provided by the State of Texas, and the remainder came from the Medical Practice Income Plan, which included money earned from seeing patients, research grants, and clinical trials. All monies from these sources, with the exception of consulting contracts, were to be remitted to the Health Sciences Center. Butler entered into contracts with both Pharmacia and Chiron in which his fee per subject would be split between the Health Sciences Center and himself. These contracts, the first of which commenced in 1998, continued until August 2001, and did not come to the attention of the Health Sciences Center until July 2002.

Butler voluntarily gave up his medical license prior to trial. After the three week trial, which included testimony from 40 witnesses, a jury found Butler not guilty on almost all of the plague-related charges, including lying to the FBI, and not guilty of tax evasion. It did, however, find him guilty on most of the contract charges related to his split-fee arrangements (44 of the 54 fraud counts), and on 3 of the 18 charges relating to the transportation of plague samples. He was sentenced to 24 months in prison, three years supervised release, $15,000 in fines, and ordered to pay $38,675 restitution to the University. He appealed.

The two most important issues on appeal dealt with the possibly prejudicial effect of combining the plague counts with the contract counts, and whether there was sufficient evidence of criminal intent with regard to the failure to file the required shipping forms for plague samples. As to the first, the appeals court ruled without much discussion (and arguably without much understanding of how medical research is conducted) that all of these counts could be combined because they all had to do with Butler's "research efforts." The appeals court also had little sympathy for Butler's contention that the evidence was insufficient to show that he acted willfully in regard to the only three plague-related charges (of 18 charged) he was convicted of: exporting plague bacteria to Tanzania without a license, describing the bacteria as "laboratory materials" on a Federal Express waybill, and violating federal hazardous materials regulations in shipping plague bacteria to Tanzania.

As to the first and third charge, the court was persuaded that because Butler "had successfully and legally shipped hazardous materials [during the 1990s] at least 30 times before making this particular shipment," there was sufficient evidence that he knew how to ship it properly and that "his infraction could not have been due to a good faith mistake or a misunderstanding of the law." As to Butler's contention that he did not intend to deceive anyone by labeling plague bacteria "laboratory materials," the court accepted the government's argument that he had also certified on the same label that he was "not shipping dangerous goods" and that the jury could reasonably conclude that he knew that plague was a dangerous good requiring proper identification. A further appeal to the US Supreme Court was rejected, and Butler was later released from prison after serving his sentence.

Steve Kurtz

Shortly after Butler's trial, in another part of the country, Buffalo, New York, FBI agents were called in to investigate a suspected act of bioterrorism at the home of SUNY professor and artist Steve Kurtz, who had awoken on May 11, 2004 to find his wife dead beside him. Kurtz and his wife co-founded the Critical Art Ensemble, an artists collective "dedicated to exploring the intersections between art, technology, radical politics, and critical theory." Kurtz distinguishes what he does from the emerging field of "bioart," which is perhaps best known to the public through Alba, the rabbit that glowed green because of the insertion of a jellyfish gene. Kurtz thinks of bioart as consisting of "stunts" and his own art as an exploration of "the political economy of biotechnology." He had previously opposed the introduction of genetically modified food, and had encouraged activists to oppose it by using "fuzzy biological sabotage," such as by releasing genetically mutated and deformed flies at restaurants to stir up paranoia.[12]

When the FBI raided his home in full biohazard gear, he had been studying the history of germ warfare for a new project. In connection with this project, he was growing bacterial cultures that he was planning to use to simulate anthrax and plague attacks. He had obtained the bacteria samples (*Serratia marcescens* and *Bacillus atrophaeus*) from a colleague, Professor Robert Ferrell, a geneticist at the University of Pittsburgh Medical Center, who had ordered them for him from the American Type Culture Collection. He and Ferrell were almost immediately suspected of being involved in a bioterror ring and were massively investigated. Once the department of health determined that the bacteria themselves were harmless, and that Kurtz's wife had died of natural causes, the bioterrorism investigation was appropriately dropped.

The Justice Department nonetheless charged both Ferrell and Kurtz with four counts of wire and mail fraud. The allegation was that Ferrell, at Kurtz's request, defrauded the University of Pittsburgh and the American Type Culture Collection by representing that the bacteria samples he ordered would be used in his University of Pittsburgh lab.[13] Ferrell ultimately pleaded guilty to avoid jail time. When Kurtz's case finally came to trial in mid-2008, the judge summarily dismissed it as alleging actions that were simply not criminal. That the US attorney pursued this case all the way to trial should be a source of extreme embarrassment.

Just exactly what Kurtz was planning to do with the bacteria is unclear, but *Serratia*, which is known for its ability to form bright red colonies, has been used in biowarfare simulations in the past. Perhaps most well-known is a 1950 simulation in which it was used in an aerosol spray by an offshore Naval vessel to blanket a 50-square-mile section of San Francisco to determine what dose could be effectively delivered to the population.[14] Whether using a similar technique as an art exhibit would be bioart, biotechnology, or biohazard (or even bioterrorism) may be in the eye of the beholder even more than in the eye of the artist or scientist.

Bioart is not bioterrorism, but the two are politically related. As bioart curator and commentator Jens Hauser has put it, bioart aims "at the heart of our fears" and is meant to disturb. "These artists expose the gulf between the apologetic official discourse about technoscience on the one hand, and paranoia on the other...."[15] Like defensive and offensive bioweapons research, bioart and biotechnology may be impossible to distinguish by anything other than the researcher/creator's intent. Thus, Alba the bunny with the jellyfish gene (which codes for GFP, green fluorescent protein, which can cause the animal to glow green under blue light) is considered and accepted as bioart, at least in the contemporary art community. Conversely, ANDi, the monkey with the inserted jellyfish gene—as well as

the transgenic marmoset who was able to pass this gene on to his offspring—
is considered science, at least in the biotechnology community. Even "Fat
Man," the bomb dropped on Nagasaki, has been the subject of art. Robert
Wilhite reproduced it in poplar, mahogany, and spruce—a thing of
beauty—to get people to think. In his words, "I wanted something people
could react to. I want people to think about their own values: It's beautiful,
but wait a minute—this is a weapon of mass destruction."[16]

Hauser was referring to paranoia in the face of the "rapid acceleration of
technical prowess." Based on the federal law enforcement reaction to the
actions of Thomas Butler and Steve Kurtz, however, as scary as biotechnolo-
gical advances that have potential applications to bioterrorism and biowarfare
are, the responses of government law enforcement agencies to legitimate
scientists and artists whose actions pose no threat to the public are even scarier.

Butler's arrest came about a year after a simulated bioterrorism event
in Lubbock, Texas using aerosolized ersatz plague bacteria at a civic center.
Simulations have been a centerpiece for bioterror preparation. But, as we
should have learned from our obsession with building bomb shelters during
the Cold War, simulations can promote fear of worst cases and make them
look much more likely than they are. Bioterrorism simulations like Dark
Winter (smallpox) and TOPOFF (plague) are more art than science, and
predictably provoked responses (such as the Bush smallpox vaccination
program described in Chapter 14) based more on fear than logic or
evidence. These simulations should probably be classified as "bioart" in
the sense of performance art, and have their most socially useful outlet not
in federal law enforcement agencies or biosafety laboratories, but in TV
dramas like *24*.

Bioterrorism, Bioethics, and Science

The case of physician-researcher Thomas Butler has been the subject of
many commentaries—most arguing that his prosecution represents a gross
over-reaction on the part of federal authorities. Nonetheless, Margaret
Somerville and Ronald Atlas argued that his prosecution "sent a clear signal
to the research community, especially scientists and university researchers,
that all ethical and legal requirements must be respected when undertaking
research."[17] They continue, "Biosafety regulations are not merely legal technicalities. They constitute some of the terms of the pact between science and
the public that establishes public trust."

Somerville and Atlas are certainly correct to argue that researchers
must take law and ethics seriously, and their call for a new ethics code is

reasonable, as is their echo of Roger Shattuck's call for scientists to adopt the physician's "do no harm" principle. The first entry in their "Code of Ethics for the Life Sciences" is:

> Work to ensure that [your] discoveries and knowledge *do no harm:* (i) *by refusing to engage in any research* that is intended to facilitate or that has a high probability of being used *to facilitate bioterrorism or biowarfare;* and (ii) never knowingly or recklessly contribute to the development, production, or acquisition of microbial or other biological agents or toxins, whatever their origin or method of production, of types or in quantities that cannot be *justified on the basis that they are necessary for prophylactic, protective, therapeutic, or other peaceful purposes.* (emphasis added)

It is nonetheless overbroad to suggest that there are no such things as "legal technicalities," or that all such technicalities are reasonable. Jennifer Gaudioso and Reynolds Salerno, for example, have argued persuasively that not all pathogens and toxins have the same risk, and that risk in the laboratory should "be a function of an agent's weaponization potential and consequences of its use" (rather than current biosafety risk assessment that focuses on "infectious disease dangers and the risk of accidental exposure in the laboratory").[18] They also note that under USA Patriot Act and the Bioterrorism and Response Act regulations, which require entities with select agents to register with the CDC, many fewer of these organizations registered than the CDC had expected. Many research entities simply decided to discontinue their research projects instead of conforming to the new federal administrative and security rules for such research. A National Academy of Sciences report rejected the utility of an agent-specific threat list and recommended instead adopting a "broader perspective...to ensure regular and deliberate reassessments of advances in science and technology and identification of those advances with the greatest potential for changing the nature of the threat spectrum."[19]

Ethics and law are related, but they are not the same. Law provides the floor below which we cannot go without becoming "outlaws"; if we don't like it, of course, we must nonetheless follow it (while working to change it) or risk, as Butler did, being prosecuted as an outlaw. And all Americans, including scientists and artists, should recognize that when the FBI wants to talk to you about your role in a possible bioterrorist event, you should not talk to them until you talk to your lawyer. We can go to jail for violating the law, but not for violating ethics codes. Ethics is aspirational—we deserve praise (at least some) for behaving "ethically"; we deserve none for simply following the law, some of which is made up of "legal technicalities."

Because the differences between research on offensive and defensive biological weapons is a matter of degree, not kind, and because biotechnology research is an international activity, any evidence that such research is doing more to put the public at risk than to protect the public will be damaging to the entire enterprise. This is one reason why Butler's report of missing plague bacteria (still unaccounted for) could not be tolerated by federal officials supportive of expanding research on countermeasures. It is the reason why the US Army decided to ban one of its premier biodefense labs, part of the Armed Forces Institute of Pathology, from doing any more work with dangerous pathogens (the lab did not report the discovery of four broken vials of "select agents").[20] It is also what makes the "bioart" of Kurtz so disturbing—it confronts the public with the dark side of bioterrorism-related research and provokes a response. The inherent dual nature of biodefense research has been dubbed "the Persephone effect," referring to Demeter's daughter, who was forced to spend half a year with Pluto in hell so she could live the other half of the year on earth.[21]

One possible response to both the disputes between Butler and the Justice Department, and that between Kurtz and the Justice Department could be Mercutio's in *Romeo and Juliet,* "A plague on both your houses." This is because the public is currently more victim and bystander than participant, and seems much more likely to be harmed than helped by much of the research. The public recognizes this, and its skepticism of federal authorities, the effectiveness of countermeasures, the proliferation of biosafety laboratories, and the entire bioterrorism scare is well illustrated by the tiny numbers of people who took the offered anthrax vaccine after the anthrax attacks. This same skepticism, combined with lack of evidence of Iraqi stockpiles of smallpox and the certainty of side effects, also explains the small number of health professionals who volunteered to take the smallpox vaccine immediately before and shortly after the commencement of the Iraq war.[22]

Research directed at creating new pathogens or toxins that have direct bioterror or biowarfare applications deserves condemnation. The NRC, for example, has identified seven classes of microbial experiments that should "require review and discussion by informed members of the scientific and medical community before they are undertaken." If such experiments are undertaken at all, I believe there should also be a requirement for prior publication and public input into the decision as well. There should be no secret or classified biological research. As Laura Donohue has persuasively argued, censorship of science hurts our ability not only to respond to a bioterrorist event, but to respond to natural disease outbreaks as well (and these are likely to be much more deadly).[23] The seven categories of experiments that the NRC's committee would require prior review of are those that seek to:

1. Demonstrate how to render a vaccine ineffective
2. Confer resistance to therapeutically useful antibiotics or antiviral agents
3. Enhance the virulence of a pathogen or render a nonpathogen virulent
4. Increase transmissibility of a pathogen
5. Alter the host range of a pathogen
6. Enable the evasion of diagnostic/detection modalities
7. Enable the weaponization of a biological agent or toxin[24]

Research directed at individual pathogens and their weaponization potential also risks diverting scientific resources from much more important public health concerns,[25] the way in which it has seemed to divert FBI attention from much higher-priority criminals. A consensus seems to exist in the scientific community that the free and open exchange of information is ultimately the best defense to both naturally occurring pandemics and purposeful biological attacks.[26] There is also a growing recognition of the importance of developing an international code of ethics for scientists, as well as a recognition that such a code must "become part of the lived culture" of scientists.[27] Like bioart and the concept of biosecurity itself, the development and implementation of this code of ethics remains a work in progress.

This chapter has concentrated mostly on how scientific research has been affected by national security concerns and how bioartists have attempted to use art to draw the public into debates about the limits of national security as an excuse for secrecy in science. In the next chapter, I discuss another all-purpose excuse for doing whatever one believes is right, whether government official, practicing physician, or simply a person wanting to help: the state of emergency.

3

. . . .

State of Emergency

Emergencies have their own logic and their own rules. In medicine, for example, the working rule in a medical emergency (in or out of the emergency department) is, "treat first and ask legal questions later."[1] And "saving lives" always justifies action, so much so that cardiopulmonary resuscitation (CPR) is automatic—virtually the only action a physician does not need consent to perform on a patient. Instead, the patient must prospectively refuse it by issuing a DNR ("do not resuscitate" or more accurately, a DNAR order, "do not attempt resuscitation") to prevent what would otherwise be treated as a medical "emergency" justifying immediate intervention. Because it always produces a "life or death" crisis, hospital-based bioethics committees spent most of their early lives working out rules for DNR orders, only later adding living wills and healthcare proxies to their agendas. But, of course, emergencies don't occur only in medicine.

In airline emergencies, such as the January 15, 2009 crash landing of US Airways flight 1549 in the Hudson River, pilots and crew had been trained in simulators for crashes in the expectation that, in a real emergency, they would revert to their training.[2] Likewise, as mentioned in the introduction, the Department of Homeland Security's 15 National Planning Scenarios represent a variety of worst case scenarios of natural and humanmade disasters.

These scenarios were designed with one purpose in mind: to help federal, state, and local preparedness officials plan for disaster responses.[3] Emergencies are seen as both so unusual and so threatening to society that many internationally recognized human rights can be suspended "in time of public emergency which threatens the life of the nation . . . to the extent strictly required by the exigencies of the situation."[4] The primary goal of almost all emergency responses is to save lives, and in the case of a national emergency—sometimes called a national security emergency—to ensure the survival of the state as well.

Although law plays a limited role in emergency responses, a recurring question for at least the past 50 years has been whether certain individuals or professions should be granted prospective legal immunity for helping their fellow humans in an emergency situation. In medicine, the Good Samaritan rule provides that licensed physicians who provide emergency medical assistance outside the scope of their employment and in "good faith" cannot be sued for negligence. The idea is that physicians might be reluctant to provide aid if they felt that they were at risk for a malpractice suit should they further injure the victim. And in our post-9/11 world, there have been persistent calls for granting immunity to healthcare professionals, and even to lay volunteers, who respond to a "public health emergency." The rationale for these proposals is that, faced with a massive emergency, health professionals will not be able to provide their usual standard of care and should operate instead under a reduced "catastrophic standard of care."[5]

My own view has long been that neither action is necessary or desirable. As to the run-of-the-mill lay would-be rescuer, I believe that it is reasonable to assume that "negligent Samaritans are no good," and that lay people should not be encouraged to act unreasonably or without careful thought, especially in emergencies.[6] Likewise, it is simply a legal mistake to think that healthcare professionals need new or different legal standards of care for different emergency situations: There really is only one standard of care, and it covers all contingencies by its own terms. Healthcare professionals are obligated to act in a manner consistent with what a reasonably prudent healthcare professional (of their same specialty) would do in the same or similar circumstances.[7] This standard takes into consideration the emergency conditions themselves, as well as the resources available to render assistance. For example, a reasonably prudent healthcare practitioner would engage in triage if this was medically reasonable and necessary under the circumstances.[8]

It is also worth noting that the standard of care for lay people is even lower: what would a reasonably prudent lay person do in the same or similar circumstances? Members of the public seem at home with this. For example, when US Airways 1549 crash-landed in the Hudson River, ferry boats from around the area immediately converged on the downed plane to help in the rescue. In all of the ensuing publicity and aftermath of the successful rescue, not one lay responder said he or she thought about personal liability even for a second, and certainly no one wondered whether he or she was covered by any of New York's Good Samaritan statutes. Immunity statutes were, and likely always will be, simply irrelevant to the emergency task at hand.

Whether or not it is worth trying to persuade healthcare professionals with free-floating anxiety and a firm desire not to be sued that statutory protection in the form of prospective legal immunity for emergency care is neither necessary nor helpful to them is debatable. But the fact that the law grants physicians tremendous latitude in addressing emergencies is not debatable. This is probably because even worse than an emergency itself is the thought that physicians and other healthcare professionals would not do the best they could to respond to people whose lives were in danger.

The extreme deference the law affords physicians, even physicians in training, to act to save a life in an emergency situation is illustrated by a famous case in which the parents of the child "saved" by physicians did not want the child "saved." The parents had rejected treatment for their daughter, Sidney Miller, an extremely premature neonate, because her medical condition was so devastating that further treatment was deemed useless.[9] Even though her birth occurred in 1990 and the legal case was decided in 2003, nothing has changed in the practice of neonatal or emergency medicine since then that would prevent repetition of either the unwanted rescue or the legal review of it today.

The Case of Sidney Miller

Karla Miller, the mother of the infant Sidney, went into premature labor at approximately 23 weeks gestation. On ultrasonography, her fetus was found to weigh about 629 grams, and attempts were made to stop labor by using drugs. Subsequently, an infection developed that Miller's medical team thought could endanger her life if delivery were further postponed. Her obstetrician, Mark Jacobs, and a neonatologist, Donald Kelley, informed her and her husband, Mark Miller, that the fetus had little chance of being born alive and that if it did survive, it would probably suffer severe impairments, including brain hemorrhage, blindness, lung disease, and mental retardation. Mark Miller later testified that the physicians also told him that they had "never had such a premature infant live and that anything they did to sustain the infant's life would be guesswork."

Jacobs and Kelley then asked the Millers to decide whether the infant should be treated at birth. The Millers told the physicians that they wanted no heroic measures performed. Kelley recorded this decision in the medical record of Karla Miller, and Jacobs informed the medical staff of the hospital that no neonatologist would be needed at the delivery. Mark Miller then left the hospital to make funeral arrangements. While Miller was away, the nursing staff informed other medical personnel about the instruction not to have a neonatologist present at the birth. Meetings were held with various hospital administrators and physicians, who then met with Miller on his return to the hospital. Miller later testified that a hospital administrator in charge of the neonatal intensive care unit, Anna Summerfield, told him that the hospital had a policy that required the resuscitation of any baby who was born weighing more than 500 grams. Jacobs recalls the decision then made in this way:

> What we finally decided that everyone wanted to do was not to make the call prior to the time we actually saw the baby. Deliver the baby, because you see there was this [question,] is the baby really 23 weeks, or is the baby further along, how big is the baby, what are we dealing with. *We decided to let the neonatologist make the call by looking directly at the baby at birth.* (emphasis added)

The neonatologist in training who attended the birth, Eduardo Otero, was not at the meeting, but he agreed with Jacobs that he would have to see the newborn to decide what treatment, if any, was appropriate. Mark Miller testified that, after the meeting, the hospital administrators asked him to sign a consent form that would allow resuscitation, but he refused. When Miller asked the administrators how he could prevent resuscitation, he was told that he would have to remove his wife from the hospital.

Later that evening, Karla Miller's condition worsened, and it was determined that labor should be augmented (rather than stopped as it had been) before further complications developed. When Sidney was born, she weighed 615 grams and had a heartbeat. Otero noted that she gasped for air, cried spontaneously, and had no unusual dysmorphic features. Accordingly, he immediately manually ventilated and intubated her and placed her on a ventilator. He did this, in his words, "because this baby is alive and this is a baby that has a reasonable chance of living . . . [and] is not necessarily going to have problems later on. There are babies that survive at this gestational age—with this weight—that later on go on and do well."

Neither parent objected to the treatment of Sidney after her birth, and therefore, treatment decisions in the neonatal intensive care unit (NICU) were not explored at trial. Sidney seemed to do well at first—the score on her Apgar test, which, on a scale of 1 to 10 reflects the condition of a newborn immediately after birth, improved from a 3 at one minute to a 6 at five minutes—but a few days later, she suffered a brain hemorrhage that caused severe physical and mental impairment. At the time of the trial, she was seven years old and "could not walk, talk, feed herself, or sit up on her own ... [,] was legally blind, suffered from severe mental retardation, cerebral palsy, seizures, and spastic quadriparesis in her limbs ... [,] could not be toilet-trained, required a shunt in her brain to drain fluids, and needed care twenty-four hours a day." No improvement in her condition was expected.

The parents did not sue any of the physicians involved but, instead, sued Women's Hospital of Texas in Houston and its parent company, HCA, for battery and negligence. Mark Miller explained to the press that he did not blame the physicians, because he and his wife "thought the doctors just did what they were told" to do by hospital officials.[10] The physicians were involved in the trial because the lawsuit alleged that they acted as the agents of the hospital, and so the hospital was legally responsible for their actions. The jury concluded that the resuscitation had been performed without consent and that the negligence of the hospital and HCA "proximately caused the occurrence in question." Moreover, the jury concluded that both HCA and the hospital were grossly negligent, that the hospital itself acted with malice, and that Otero was the hospital's agent in the resuscitation of Sidney. The jury awarded the Millers $29,400,000 for medical expenses, $17,503,066 in interest on these expenses, and $13,500,000 in punitive damages.

In a very strange ruling, the Texas Court of Appeals reversed the jury verdict and ordered that the Millers get nothing.[11] The court reasoned that, in Texas, parents could withhold medical treatment from a child only after the child's medical condition had been certified as "terminal" under the Texas Natural Death Act. The appeals court also noted that a court order is usually required to override a parental refusal of treatment, but it ruled that if the need for treatment of a child who is not terminally ill is urgent, a court order is unnecessary. The court thus agreed with HCA that it owed no duty to the Millers to refrain from resuscitating Sidney or to have a policy prohibiting resuscitation of patients like Sidney without parental consent.

The Texas Supreme Court essentially ignored the reasoning of the appeals court and instead summarized the case very narrowly as requiring it "to determine the respective roles that parents and healthcare providers play in deciding whether to treat an infant who is born alive but in distress and is so premature that, despite advancements in neonatal intensive care, [he or she] has a largely uncertain prognosis." This was the first time a case that raised this question had come to the Texas Supreme Court, and the court began by summarizing existing law: "Generally speaking, the custody, care, and nurture of an infant resides in the first instance with the parents." This includes, the court stated, the presumption that the parents have the right to consent to their infant's medical treatment as well as to refuse such treatment. The real question relates to the limits of the parents' right to refuse. In this regard, the court noted that the state punishes parents only for what amounts to child abuse or child neglect and that "as long as parents choose from professionally accepted treatment options, the choice is rarely reviewed in court." In other words, in the absence of child neglect, parents have the right to give or withhold consent for medical treatment for their children.

The ultimate question the court confronted was this: Is there an emergency exception to this general rule that permits physicians to treat neonates without parental consent? The court relied exclusively on dicta from a 1920 case that involved a tonsillectomy in a child, to which an older sister had consented. The child died as a result of the anesthesia, and the father sued the surgeon for failure to obtain his consent for the surgery. In that case, the court determined that parental consent was legally required, because although "there was an absolute necessity for a prompt operation," the situation was "not emergent in the sense that death would likely result immediately upon failure to perform it."[12] The 1920 case, according to the court, "implicitly acknowledges" that a physician may perform an operation "under emergent circumstances—i.e., when death is likely to result immediately upon failure to perform it." In its application of the reasoning of this pre-NICU case, the court ruled, "We hold that *a physician, who is confronted with emergent circumstances and provides life-sustaining treatment to a minor child, is not liable for first obtaining consent from the parents.*" (emphasis added)

Rules for Emergencies

This is a reasonable rule when parents are not available for consultation and consent, but what if the parents are present and refuse? The court concludes that parental presence (and refusal to give consent) simply does not matter in extreme cases, because the exception that allows treatment in emergency circumstances is not based on the concept of implied

consent. The physician is privileged by law to treat in emergency circumstances because the physician is trying to prevent a harm (death) that
outweighs any harm from treatment. Other courts have ruled that consent
is "implied" in emergencies; however, the Texas court correctly saw this
formulation as wrong (no one implies anything simply by having a medical
emergency, and if this were the correct rule, contemporaneous explicit
refusal of treatment by the Millers would have to have been honored).

The court's conclusion is another way of saying that physicians in
emergencies are permitted to err on the side of the preservation of life (to
avoid the worst case scenario of death). This is a perfectly reasonable
general rule, but may not be so reasonable in the case of an extremely
premature newborn. This is because the choice is never so clear-cut. It is not
life or death alone, but the chance of survival in a severely disabled condition such as Sidney's, that makes neonatal treatment decisions so difficult.
Nonetheless, after the determination that treatment was necessary to save
the child's life had been reached, the only remaining issue for the court was
procedural: Is a physician obligated to seek court approval before proceeding with emergency treatment when the parents object to it?

The Millers contended that there was plenty of time to seek a court
order because they had objected to treatment 11 hours before the birth and
that physicians should not be permitted to delay a decision in such a case
until the situation becomes an emergency. The court agreed that the
"physician cannot create emergent circumstances from his or her own
delay or inaction and escape liability for proceeding without consent."
Nonetheless, the court concluded that the circumstances of extreme prematurity were unique because a decision about resuscitation could not
reasonably be made before birth. In the court's words:

> The evidence established that *Sidney could only be properly evaluated when
> she was born. Any decision the Millers made before Sidney's birth* concerning
> her treatment at or after her birth would necessarily be based on
> speculation. [A decision made before the birth] could not control
> whether the circumstances facing Dr. Otero were emergent because
> it *would not have been a fully informed one* according to the evidence in this
> case. (emphasis added)

But was Otero himself negligent in making the decision to resuscitate
Sidney without either parental consent or a court order? The court decided
that he was not negligent because of the nature of the decision itself: "Dr. Otero
had to make a split-second decision and [even though] the Millers were both
present in the delivery room, there was simply no time to obtain their consent to

treatment or to institute legal proceedings ... without jeopardizing Sidney's life." Moreover, since the circumstances that required this "split-second decision" resulted from the inability to evaluate Sidney until she was born, not from any delay or inaction on the part of the hospital or physicians, neither the hospital nor the physician could be held responsible for the emergency situation.

The court stressed that the best practice is to obtain parental consent before birth to make an evaluation and render "warranted medical treatment." Nonetheless, the court concluded, "We decline to impose liability [for either battery or negligence] on a physician solely for providing life-sustaining treatment under emergent circumstances to a new-born infant without that consent."

The conclusion of the court—that an informed decision about resuscitating an extremely premature infant can be made only by actually examining the infant at birth—is reasonable and in accord with good medical practice. No clinical test or objective indicator can accurately predict outcome (the hospital denied that it had a rule about the resuscitation of infants who weigh at least 500 grams and, even if it had such an arbitrary rule, this would have been no substitute for a more comprehensive evaluation of the infant at birth).

The court did not have to say more to decide the case in front of it, but more can and probably should be said. Many observers had hoped that this case would help to clarify the legal rules for treatment decisions involving extremely premature infants and help physicians and hospitals to develop better procedures for making decisions in this area of great and inherent medical uncertainty.[13] More specific guidelines were probably too much to hope for, and the court's decision was a narrow one. For example, although the ruling permits a neonatologist to make decisions about resuscitation immediately after birth in the case of extreme prematurity, nothing in the decision requires the presence of a neonatologist at the delivery.

Life and Death Decisions

More troubling, the court implies that life is always preferable to death for a newborn, and the decision thus could be interpreted in the future to support the neonatologist who always resuscitates newborns, no matter how premature or how unlikely their survival without severe disabilities will be. This interpretation, however, is problematic, because such a neonatologist is not exercising any medical judgment or making a "split-second" decision. In these circumstances, the decision to attempt resuscitation has been made at a time when the court believes it cannot reasonably be made: before the birth. All-or-nothing responses, nonetheless, seem to be common in neonatology. As F. S. Cole has observed, "In the absence of biologically reliable predictors of outcome, decisions on care for extremely premature infants have historically fallen between the inflexible extremes of mandated nontreatment and mandated full treatment by relying on individual evaluation by parents and physicians."[14]

Given the inherent uncertainty in outcomes, trials of therapy that can be ended when reasonable clinical goals cannot be achieved seem more consistent with legal principles and good medical practice. More data are unlikely to provide a yes-or-no answer to whether resuscitation should be attempted at birth. In one major prospective study of extremely premature infants, about half of the survivors had substantial disability, with approximately one-quarter having severe disability, and no clear predictors of outcome were identified. The authors concluded, "The prevention or amelioration of disability in survivors of extreme prematurity remains one of the most important challenges in medicine."[15] Life is not always preferable to death, as is illustrated by the exceptions to the old Baby Doe regulations (which pertained to refusals of treatment for newborns with serious disabilities, not premature newborns) and by the entire series of so-called right-to-die cases, especially the case of Terri Schiavo.[16]

The decision to resuscitate Sidney triggered a new series of decisions about her continued treatment. Although these decisions were not the subject of the lawsuit, the Texas Supreme Court made it clear that the parents had the legal authority to make all of these subsequent decisions. If the parents disagreed with the physicians about, for example, whether to continue ventilation, the obligation of the physicians was either to follow the wishes of the parents nonetheless or to seek court authorization to ignore them. It seems unlikely, for instance, that anyone would have questioned the Millers' decision to cease the provision of aggressive care after Sidney had the intracranial bleeding that drastically decreased her chances of living anything but a severely disabled life. A DNR order, for example, would not have been challenged—although most observers would agree that we spend far too much time on all-or-nothing decisions like DNR.[17] The special difficulty with the DNR order is that it seems to be an order for death and thus is often treated like the last, and most important, decision to be made, whereas it applies only to cardiac and respiratory resuscitation and is just one of a number of equally important medical care decisions.

This confusion about the meaning of a DNR order is not confined to the NICU. It is now well-known that at Memorial Medical Center in New Orleans, in the midst of Katrina, a triage decision was made regarding the patients in the hospital that was largely based on a profound misunderstanding of the meaning of a DNR order by the doctors and nurses involved. As physician-journalist Sheri Fink, who interviewed almost everyone involved, has written, about two dozen doctors and a few nurse managers met to decide how to evacuate the hospital's 180 patients. They quickly agreed, she writes, babies in the NICU, pregnant women, and critically-ill adults in the ICU – those who it was believed would suffer the most from the heat – should get first priority. Then a leading physician at the hospital suggested that all patients with DNR orders should go last. Other doctors agreed, and the plan was adopted, even though it is now clear that many of the physicians did not understand the meaning of a DNR order, thinking it meant not only "do not attempt resuscitation" if the patient's heart stops, but that such patients had "the least to lose" by dying.[18] It is also worth noting that for competent patients a DNR requires informed consent, and that consent to a DNR can be withdrawn at any time.

Likewise, giving parents the right to make treatment decisions for their extremely premature newborns in the NICU is not only consistent with basic legal principles but also accords with good medical practice. Treatment in the high-technology NICU, however, takes on a life of its own. For example, although there is no ethical or legal difference between starting and stopping an intervention such as ventilation, stopping it is much more emotionally and psychologically difficult for both parents and physicians. This is just one reason why trials of therapy should be discussed before they are initiated and why such trials should be evaluated at regular intervals, to reevaluate the child's condition to see if the therapeutic goals remain reasonable or achievable.

Reasonable people may disagree about what the therapeutic goals should be for a particular patient. Defining a therapeutic goal depends on a combination of the medical prognosis, the family's circumstances, and the quality of life of the child, and no one-size-fits-all legal or medical rule is possible. Even the standard of the best interests of the child raises questions. The phrase "best interests" is often translated into the unhelpful slogan "better off dead"—that is, the infant should be treated aggressively unless all agree that the infant would be better off dead. A standard of comparing benefits to burdens is preferable, but of course such a standard cannot definitively resolve difficult cases.

The President's Commission for the Study of Ethical Problems in Medicine and Biomedical and Behavioral Research observed in 1983: "Permanent disabilities justify a decision not to provide life-sustaining treatment only when they are so severe that continued existence would not be a net benefit to the infant. Though inevitably somewhat subjective and imprecise in actual application...net benefit is absent only if the burdens imposed on the patient by the disability or its treatment would lead a competent decision maker to choose to forgo the treatment."[19] The application of a benefit–burden standard would not have prevented Sidney from being resuscitated in the first place, but it could have led to a more thoughtful examination of the aggressiveness of continued treatment after her cranial hemorrhage. The decision to treat at this point would have remained with the parents.

When I began working in health law and bioethics in 1972, making treatment decisions about neonates with intracranial bleeding was seen as so difficult, and the outcomes so uncertain, that it was believed there could be no substantive rules, just procedural rules. The basic procedural rule was that it is acceptable to withdraw treatment if both the physician and the parents agree. Implementing this rule led to a backlash, which gave rise to the Baby Doe regulations. These regulations were drafted in response to a 1981 case in which parents refused to consent to a surgical repair of a tracheal-esophageal fistula that would have enabled the child to eat. The baby died during the court proceedings. The Baby Doe regulations were based on the assumption (never demonstrated, and almost certainly wrong) that many physicians were terminating treatment on newborns because of "quality-of-life" assessments that devalued disability.[20] After the Baby Doe rules were rescinded, the standard of the best interests of the child returned to prominence, and child neglect became a relevant factor in treatment decisions for neonates.[21]

When asked about the Miller case, C. Everett Koop, the former surgeon general of the United States and main promoter of the Baby Doe regulations, was quoted as saying, "I don't think parents should have the discretion to kill their children. I'm a great believer in the slippery slope. You get into the terrible quagmire of having only perfect children, and nobody can guarantee that."[22] Koop is, of course, correct about guarantees, but it is the very inability of physicians to predict outcomes that leads most commentators to insist that parents, with physicians' input, be the ones to make the ultimate decisions about treatment for their children, at least when there exists a range of reasonable medical options, including termination of treatment. In addition, although the court did not deal with the issue, many of the interventions in the NICU, including resuscitation, can reasonably be classified as experimental.[23]

The Texas Supreme Court's decision limits physicians' life and death discretionary decisions to the moments immediately after birth. The court does not require the neonatologist or obstetrician to treat or resuscitate a newborn, only to use medical judgment to decide whether or not to treat or resuscitate at birth. The standard to be applied in making this determination is never well articulated, since both the best interests of the child and the contention that the treatment is "warranted" are vague and can often be used to justify a decision either to treat or not to treat.

The Texas Supreme Court has also made it clear that after the initial "emergency" assessment, when many more treatment decisions must be made in the NICU, parental consent is legally required. If parental consent is not forthcoming, a court order must be obtained before treatment proceeds or the parent's wishes must be respected. More important are the ethical issues that pertain to making decisions in the NICU. These require, at the least, clear, regular, and honest discussions with the parents about the health of and prognosis for their child, as well as trials of therapy that have realistic stopping points. Because clear rules seem to be impossible to formulate in this arena, adherence to reasonable procedures in making treatment decisions may still be the best we can do.

The narrow decision of the Texas Supreme Court was reasonable in the emergency context, but nonetheless unfortunate and devastating for the Millers. The medical result for Sidney was not entirely predictable, but the financial consequences of a lifetime of medical care—the cost will total in the tens of millions of dollars—were foreseeable. Public funding of Sidney's care would certainly help the Millers, and such funding—for example through a national healthcare insurance plan, as discussed in Chapter 1— could have made this lawsuit unnecessary. To the extent that society insists on treatment, public support seems morally obligatory, so that, as the President's Commission noted more than 25 years ago, "these children, once rescued [in NICUs], are not then left to drown in a sea of indifference and unresponsiveness."[24]

The resuscitation of extremely premature newborns is an extreme case of emergency medicine. Nonetheless, the lessons of the Miller case are generalizable: In life and death emergencies, courts will give physicians very wide discretion in using their clinical judgment to "save lives." There is no need for new "altered" or "catastrophic" standards of care to encourage physician (or nonphysician) involvement in emergency situations. The law and public policy both support physicians (and others) who respond to emergencies with a helping hand, and will judge them harshly only in the rare situation in which their actions amount to "gross" negligence. Worst case scenarios justify flexible rescue rules, but do not require abandonment of accountability which is likely to make a bad situation worse.

In the next two chapters, I explore why professionals, especially physicians and lawyers, should be held accountable for their actions— even, perhaps especially—those taken under extreme situations that we might even classify as worst case scenarios, like ticking time bombs and terrorists organizing to attack us. At issue are torture of suspected terrorists and force-feeding of hunger strikers at Guantanamo, and how lawyers and physicians conspired to justify war crimes in the first instant and violations of international standards of medical ethics in the second. Our post-9/11 state of emergency elevated national security justifications, but did not displace reliance on the standard saving lives justification.

4

. . . .

Licensed to Torture

F ictional British secret agent James Bond was "licensed to kill." Real-
life American physicians and lawyers were "licensed to torture"
during the post-9/11 era of the Bush administration. This chapter
explores how it came to be that physicians (and other CIA employees)
refused to torture unless they were granted legal immunity by government
lawyers, and how government lawyers concluded that only the complicity of
physicians could permit them to grant legal immunity in the face of international and national laws that prohibit torture under all circumstances.[1]

International human rights law was born from the ashes of World War II.
The most notable post-World War II products are the United Nations, the
Nuremberg Trials, the Universal Declaration of Human Rights (UDHR), and
the Geneva Conventions of 1949. International human rights law continued to
develop and expand right up to 9/11, including most notably the International
Covenant on Civil and Political Rights (ICCPR), the Convention Against
Torture (CAT), and the establishment of the International Criminal Court.
With the exception of the criminal court, the United States has consistently
seen itself as the leader of the international human rights movement.

The terrorist attacks on New York City and the Pentagon stopped
our nation's human rights momentum and caused our leaders to believe

that we could and should barter our human rights for security. Our leaders also adopted measures, like torture, that the United States had insisted are always immoral and illegal. In his inaugural address, President Obama rejected the post-9/11 tradeoff paradigm saying "we reject as false the choice between our safety and our ideals." He continued:

> Our Founding Fathers, faced with perils we can scarcely imagine, drafted a charter to assure the rule of law and the rights of man, a charter expanded by the blood of generations. Those ideals still light the world, and we will not give them up for expediency's sake.

The president, of course, has more power than any other government official, and as president is also commander-in-chief of the military. Nonetheless, as President Obama insists, we are a country of laws, including international human rights laws. That is why, two days after he became president, he reaffirmed our country's support of both the Geneva Conventions and the CAT, and vowed to close Guantanamo within a year. How did we get to the point that a new American president had to take these steps? How did America become a human rights outlaw?

There are many possible explanations. There is no longer any doubt, however, that it would have been impossible for the administration of George W. Bush to embrace torture (under the rubric of "harsh" or "enhanced" interrogation—which Jeffrey Toobin has noted is like calling death "enhanced sleep"), or to establish and operate Guantanamo, without the active cooperation of lawyers and physicians, and arguably the silence of bioethicists as well. The lawyers and physicians who counseled or cooperated in using torture, ignoring the Geneva Conventions and disregarding the Nuremberg principles, can reasonably be labeled as human rights outlaws. Understanding their role is critical to preventing similar derelictions of professional duty in the future.

A "New Kind of War"

In *State of Denial*, Bob Woodward describes a January 18, 2002 meeting at the White House during which the decision not to follow the Geneva Conventions with respect to al Qaeda or the Taliban was made. Secretary of State Colin Powell asked the president to honor our commitments to Geneva, and he was backed up by General Richard Myers who said:

Mr. President, you may notice *I'm the only guy here without any backup. I don't have a lawyer.* [The other principals on the National Security Council present had their legal advisers with them.] *I don't think this is a legal issue.* And I understand technically why the Geneva Conventions do not apply to these combatants [regarding POW status]. I got that. But I think there is another issue we need to think about that maybe hasn't gotten enough light. *You have to remember that as we treat them, probably so we're going to be treated.* We may be treated worse, but we should not give them an opening. Terrorists or other future enemies could easily use the U.S. policy against the Taliban as an argument that they too could ignore the Geneva Conventions.[2] (emphasis added)

Perhaps the most disastrous mistake in the "global war on terror" has been to designate it as a war at all, instead of a police action. War metaphors not only immediately give credibility to the "enemy," they also call for absolute solutions, such as "unconditional surrender," and suggest that the country is in a constant state of emergency, with representatives of the good challenged by "evil-doers."[3] And there is more to our metaphorical declaration of war against terror: This was a "new kind of war," a war of good versus evil, that requires the good guys to adopt, at least temporarily, the methods of the savage evil-doers.[4]

Two weeks after the White House meeting the president signed a memorandum on the "Humane Treatment of al Qaeda and Taliban Detainees" that specifically determined that the Geneva Conventions of 1949 would not be applied to al Qaeda and Taliban detainees. The rationale presented in the memorandum, which had been prepared by White House Counsel Alberto Gonzales, was: "the war against terrorism ushers in a new paradigm, one in which groups with broad, international reach commit horrific acts against innocent civilians, sometimes with the direct support of States. Our Nation recognizes that this new paradigm—ushered in not by us, but by terrorists—requires new thinking in the law of war." The memo concludes, specifically that the administration would "accept the legal conclusion of the Department of Justice and determine that common Article 3 of Geneva does not apply to either al Qaeda or Taliban detainees . . . ."[5]

The White House meeting and the wording of this memorandum provide support for the musings of the then General Counsel of the Navy, Alberto Mora, who said that his dealings with White House, Justice Department, and even Department of Defense civilian lawyers made him wonder "if they were even familiar with the Nuremberg trials—or with the laws of war, or with the Geneva conventions." In retrospect, it is safe to conclude that they were not.

Had they even a rudimentary knowledge of history, for example, they would have known that the United States was not the first government to use the excuse that engagement in a "new kind of war" justified suspension of international humanitarian treaties like the Geneva Conventions, and its precursor, the Hague Convention. Winston Churchill provides another example in the third volume of his memoirs of World War II. Churchill refers to what he characterizes as a "terrible decision of policy" adopted by Hitler on June 14, 1941, at the outset of the war between Germany and the Soviet Union, which led to "many ruthless and barbarous deeds."[6] Churchill quotes directly from the evidence produced at the Nuremberg Trial from the two generals who were at the meeting with Hitler, Generals Franz Halder and Wilhelm Keitel. Keitel's testimony at Nuremberg includes the following:

> The main theme [of Hitler's instructions] was that this was the decisive battle between two ideologies and that this fact made it impossible to use in this war methods as we soldiers knew them and which were considered to be the only correct ones under International Law. The war could not be carried on by these means. In this case completely different standards had to be applied. This was an entirely *new kind of war*, based on completely different arguments and principles.[7] (emphasis added)

The statement of General Halder was similar:

> At this conference the Fuhrer stated that the methods used in the war against the Russians will have to be different from those used in the war against the West . . . He said that the struggle between Russia and Germany is a Russian struggle. *He stated that since the Russians were not signatories to The Hague Convention the treatment of their prisoners of war does not have to follow the Articles of the Convention.*[8] (emphasis added)

The point is not that President Bush was acting like Hitler. The point is that the president's advisers seemingly knew nothing of the history of World War II or the opinion of Winston Churchill (who the president often referred to as his model of a wartime leader) on the specific subject of their legal advice to ignore the Geneva Conventions.[9] It is unimaginable that President Bush would have modeled his actions on Hitler rather than Churchill, so ignorance of history must be the explanation.

Among other specific items, Common Article 3 of the Geneva Conventions prohibits "cruel treatment and torture" as well as "humiliating and degrading treatment."[10] The issuance of the president's Geneva memorandum began the process of institutionalizing torture. The president could not institutionalize torture by himself. Elaine Scarry is surely correct in noting that the institutionalization of torture in a society requires the active cooperation of doctors and lawyers. In her words:

> *[I]t is in the nature of torture that the two ubiquitously present* [institutions] *should be medicine and law,* health and justice, *for they are the institutional elaborations of body and state.* These two were also the institutions most consistently inverted in the concentrations camps, though they were slightly differently defined in accordance with Germany's position as a modern, industrialized mass society: the "body" occurring not in medicine, but in its variant, the scientific laboratory; the "state" occurring not in the process of law, the trial, but in the process of production, the factory.[11] (emphasis added)

Torture is a particularly horrible crime and any role of physicians (or lawyers) in conducting or enabling it has always been difficult to comprehend. As General Telford Taylor, the prosecutor, explained to the US judges at the trial of the Nazi doctors in Nuremberg (the "Doctors' Trial"), "To kill, to maim, and to torture is criminal under all modern systems of law . . . these [physician] defendants, all of whom were fully able to comprehend the nature of their acts . . . are responsible for wholesale murder and unspeakably cruel tortures."[12]

Taylor told the judges that it was the obligation of the United States "to all peoples of the world to show why and how these things happened" so that they might be prevented in the future. The Nazi doctors defended themselves primarily by arguing that they were engaged in necessary wartime medical research (designed to save lives), and were following the orders of their superiors. These defenses were rejected because they are at odds with the "Nuremberg Principles." These principles were articulated at the International Military Tribunal at Nuremberg: there are crimes against humanity (like torture), individuals can be criminally responsible for committing them, and obeying orders is no defense.[13]

Sixty years later, the question of torture during wartime, and the role of physicians and lawyers in it, is once again a source of consternation and controversy. Physician-bioethicist Steven Miles, for example, relying primarily on government documents, has noted that at Abu Ghraib and Guantanamo, "at the operational level, medical personnel evaluated detainees for interrogation, and monitored coercive interrogation, allowed interrogators to use medical records to develop interrogation approaches, falsified medical records and death certificates, and failed to provide basic medical care."[14] The Red Cross, based on an inspection of Guantanamo in June 2004, alleged that the physical and mental coercion of prisoners at Guantanamo is "tantamount to torture," and specifically labeled the active role of physicians in interrogations "a flagrant violation of medical ethics."[15] Physician-lawyer Gregg Bloche and lawyer Jonathan Marks have reported, based on their interviews with some of the physicians involved in interrogations at Guantanamo and in Iraq, that the physicians believed "that physicians serving in these roles do not act as physicians and are therefore not bound by patient-oriented ethics."[16] Psychiatrist Robert Jay Lifton has suggested that the reports of US physician involvement in torture from Iraq, Afghanistan, and Guantanamo have echoes of the Nazi doctors who were "the most extreme example of doctors becoming socialized to atrocity."[17] And the muting of criticism of torture following the release of the torture photos from Abu Ghraib prompted Elie Wiesel to ask why the "shameful torture to which Muslim prisoners were subjected by American soldiers [has not] been condemned by legal professionals and military doctors alike."[18]

Since World War II, the United States has grown accustomed to setting the world standard in condemning torture as always criminal and always an inexcusable human rights violation. Nuremberg, for example, was quickly followed by the drafting and adoption of the UDHR in 1948. Article 5 of the UDHR is unequivocal, "No one shall be subjected to torture or to cruel, inhuman, or degrading treatment or punishment." The UDHR is a declaration, but it was followed 20 years later by a treaty that the United States has always supported, the ICCPR. Article 7 adopts the language of Article 5 and adds a sentence, inspired by the Doctors' Trial, to it: "No one shall be subjected to torture or to cruel, inhuman, or degrading treatment or punishment. In particular, no one shall be subjected without his free consent to medical or scientific experimentation."

Many of the provisions of the ICCPR can be suspended in a national emergency under Article 4 that provides in part, "In time of public emergency which threatens the life of the nation and the existence of which is officially proclaimed, the States Parties to the present Covenant may take measures derogating from their obligations under the present Covenant to the extent strictly required by the exigencies of the situation...." Nonetheless, Article 4 also provides that there are some obligations under the treaty from which no derogation can be taken. These obligations include protection of the "inherent right to life," the prohibition of slavery, the application of ex post facto criminal laws, the recognition of legal personhood, freedom of thought and religion, and, most centrally for this discussion, honoring the absolute prohibition against the use of torture and "cruel, inhuman, or degrading treatment or punishment."[19]

Given this legal history, it was especially disturbing to watch Alberto Gonzales being questioned about the administration's policy on torture at a hearing on his nomination to Attorney General in January 2005. The first question he was asked by Chairman Arlen Specter was, "Do you approve of torture?" Gonzales replied, "Absolutely not, Senator."[20] Two weeks later, Secretary of State designee Condoleezza Rice, at her nomination hearing, pointedly refused to characterize forced nudity and waterboarding as torture techniques, instead insisting that "the determination of whether interrogation techniques are consistent with international obligations and American law are made by the Justice Department."[21] Her comment, and her deferring to lawyers, mirrored a strategy that had been used by Secretary of Defense Donald Rumsfeld, and she may have taken her lead from him.

At a White House meeting to discuss the rules to be used in setting up military tribunals at Guantanamo, the president brushed off suggestions from Attorney General John Ashcroft and National Security Adviser Rice. As reported by Bob Woodward, he interrupted Rice to ask Rumsfeld, "Don, what do you think about this?" Rumsfeld replied, "They are bad guys" who we have to keep off the battlefield. Bush, Woodward writes, agreed, but asked how. "I'm not a lawyer," Rumsfeld replied.[22] Rice and Rumsfeld had no legal training, and, of course, neither had the president or the vice-president. Even though ignorance of the law is no excuse to violate it, the Rumsfeld-Rice "I'm not a lawyer" strategy greatly increased the influence of the legal advice they were given, and, I think, increased the obligation of the administration lawyers who gave it to faithfully and fairly interpret the law. Rumsfeld understood this, and consistently took steps to get his generals to rely on his civilian lawyers in the Pentagon rather than on the military Judge Advocate Generals (JAGs). The JAGs, among other things, strongly opposed marginalizing the Geneva Conventions and argued for following the *Army Field Manual*, which itself followed Geneva.[23]

Any knowledgeable lawyer should have given the president a legal opinion that torture was absolutely prohibited by US law. This is not only because of Nuremberg and the ICCPR, but also because of the US ratification of a specific treaty, the CAT, and the subsequent enactment of a US criminal law against torture. "Torture" is defined in the CAT, as:

> *any act,* directed against an individual in the offender's custody or physical control, *by which severe pain or suffering . . . whether physical or*

mental, is intentionally inflicted [for the purposes of obtaining] information
or a confession, punishing that individual for an act that individual
or third person has committed or is suspected of having committed,
intimidating or coercing that individual or a third person or for any
reason based on discrimination of any kind.[24] (emphasis added)

Torture is prohibited in the United States by the Fifth (whose
prohibition against self-incrimination was adopted specifically to prohibit torture to extract confessions), Eighth (which prohibits "cruel and
unusual   punishment"),   and   Fourteenth   Amendments   to   the
Constitution. Torture is a crime under state criminal statutes prohibiting
assault and battery as well. The federal statute that followed ratification
of the CAT makes it a crime for any person "outside the United States"
(including, of course, Guantanamo and Abu Ghraib) to commit or
attempt to commit torture, defined for this purpose as "an act committed
by a person acting under the color of law specifically intended to inflict
severe physical or mental pain or suffering ... upon another person
within his custody or physical control."[25] It is primarily this federal
statute that has been the subject of conflicting interpretations from the
Justice Department. After 9/11, Justice Department lawyers argued that
the president as commander-in-chief had the authority to order the
torture of prisoners, and that, contrary to the Nuremberg Principles,
obeying such an order would be a valid defense to a war crime or crime-
against-humanity charge.[26]

The August 1, 2002 memorandum from the Justice Department to
Alberto Gonzales also concluded that to constitute torture under the statute, the intensity of the pain inflicted "must be equivalent in intensity to the
pain accompanying serious physical injury, such as organ failure, impairment of bodily function, or even death." This memorandum, in which the
Justice Department lawyers acted more like mafia attorneys by advising
their clients how they might avoid prosecution under the antitorture
statute rather than on how to follow the law, has been widely and rightly
criticized—and the Justice Department withdrew it shortly after it became
public in June 2004.

One week before the hearing on the nomination of Alberto Gonzales
to be Attorney General, on December 30, 2004, the Justice Department
issued a replacement memorandum setting forth its new interpretation of
the antitorture law, which is much more consistent with both the language
of the law and US policy.[27] This memo begins by expressing the overriding
theme of US law on torture: "Torture is abhorrent both to American law
and values and to international norms. This universal repudiation of torture

is reflected in our criminal law ... international agreements ... customary international law, centuries of Anglo-American law, and the longstanding policy of the United States, repeatedly and recently affirmed by the President." Unfortunately, the memorandum also raises significant problems of hypocrisy and secrecy, stating as it does in footnote 8 that prior opinions—released only after the inauguration of President Obama—that approved various interrogation techniques "for detainees" in the custody of the CIA were not affected by the new memorandum.[28] Although much of the history of this period remains hidden, from what we know in mid-2009, it appears that Bush administration policy regarding torture was turning away from at least some techniques, like waterboarding, at this time.

In contrast to its own continued equivocation, the new Justice Department memorandum quoted statements of the President on June 30, 2003, "Torture anywhere is an affront to human dignity everywhere," and July 5, 2004, "America stands against and will not tolerate torture ... torture is wrong no matter where it occurs, and the United States will continue to lead the fight to eliminate it everywhere." Few people believed the president, perhaps because he was never clear on what he meant by torture. President Bush was forced to repeatedly declare that the United States "does not torture," including just before the 2006 November elections when he repudiated a statement by the vice president that seemed to approve the use of waterboarding, or at least approved of using a "dunk in the water" to prevent a second 9/11.[29]

The Ticking Time Bomb

Aside from his fascination with waterboarding, the ticking time bomb—perhaps everyone's worst case scenario—has been Dick Cheney's favorite rhetorical device to promote the use of torture.[30] He is not alone. In the immediate aftermath of 9/11, Americans seemed to abandon their post-World War II absolute rejection of torture, causing David Luban to observe, "American abhorrence to torture now appears to have extraordinarily shallow roots."[31] Luban attributed this to a primal urge to be cruel to our enemies.

Luban also noted that, paradoxically, "liberalism's insistence on limited governments that exercise their powers only for instrumental and pragmatic purposes creates the possibility of seeing torture as a civilized, not an atavistic, practice, provided that its sole purpose is preventing future harms." Put another way, saving lives is an all-purpose justification that ends in rationalizing almost anything. It is in this context that the power of the ticking time bomb scenario can be understood. In Luban's words, and I rely heavily on Luban because I believe that his analysis of the ticking time bomb case is the best to date, "this jejune example has become the alpha and omega of our thinking about torture."

Luban raises five questions concerning the ticking time bomb hypothetical to demonstrate why we should not base public policy on torture on it, which I summarize:

1. How sure do you have to be that you have captured a man who actually knows about the bomb plot? With what likelihood (1%) will you justify torturing him until he talks?
2. Do you make your decision by the numbers, i.e. Does a 1% chance of saving 1,000 lives mean you can torture 10 people with a 1% chance of discovering information?
3. If you think 1 person of 50 at Guantanamo knows where Osama bin Laden is hiding, can you torture them all to find out?
4. What if there was no certainty that capturing bin Laden would save any lives? Does the war on terror itself justify torture? Can't we torture "in pursuit of any worthwhile goal?"
5. Finally, if you are willing to torture 49 innocent persons to identify one guilty suspect, why stop there? Why not torture the loved ones, especially the spouse and children, in front of the suspects? They are, after all, no more innocent than the 49.

Luban continues,

The point of the examples is that in a world of uncertainty and imperfect knowledge, the ticking time-bomb scenario...is the picture that bewitches us...*Once you accept that only the numbers count, then anything, no matter how gruesome, becomes possible*...As [Bernard] Williams says, "there are certain situations so monstrous that the idea that the processes of moral rationality could yield an answer to them is insane," and "to spend time thinking what one would decide if one were in such a situation is also insane, if not merely frivolous." (emphasis added)

Mark Danner makes a similar point, referring to the enchantment of many Americans with superheroes who break the law to save us. We have, Danner believes, "sacralized," in TV dramas like *24* and movies like *Dirty Harry*, the myth of the ticking time bomb and "the ruthless U.S. agent who will do anything to stop its detonation." This is because, Danner continues, "The story of the ticking bomb and the torturing hero who defuses it offers a calming message to combat pervasive anxiety and fear—no matter what horrible threats loom, there are those who will make use of untrammeled government power to protect the country." Is it any wonder that torture proponents consistently refer to Jack Bauer as if he were a real person?

I find Luban's arguments completely persuasive, but I recognize that many people do not. Alan Dershowitz, for example, has not changed his post-9/11 position that we should establish an official government system to sanction torture, complete with the requirement to get a "torture warrant" signed by a high, responsible government official (most likely the president), in the same way we seem to sanction a presidential order to shoot down a commercial airline if it is endangering others.[32] Aside from being a complete abrogation of our treaty obligations, and turning torture from a prohibited criminal activity into an officially sanctioned one, Dershowitz, I think, unravels his own argument by attempting to place strict limits on the torturer—limits that would be impossible to sustain in a real-life situation.

Dershowitz would limit the torturer to using a "sterilized needle" placed under the fingernails. The sterilized needle requirement seems designed to make sure no lasting physical harm is caused. But the sterilized needle method begs the question: Is it true that as atavistic as we may be, Americans need the active involvement of both lawyers and physicians to justify torture? Dershowitz certainly seems to believe this, and his adjective "sterilized" harkens back to an old saying of the Nazis, who used physicians on submarines to administer the death penalty by lethal injection: "the needle belongs in the hands of the physician."[33] As I will discuss later, in Chapters 9 and 10, a majority of justices on the Supreme Court also approve of killing with lethal injection in certain circumstances—capital punishment and late-term abortions.

There are other objections to making policy based solely on the ticking time bomb hypothetical, including:

- You can't get by with just one trained torturer—you will need enough to span the globe so they will be readily available when you capture the suspect (since time is of the essence, you will need many places of torture as well). You will become a torture society.
- *24* and its hero Jack Bauer are entertainment, and we should not make policy based solely on fictional heroes or antiheros. For Jack, torture often works, but even for him it becomes completely corrupting, leading to treason on the part of a US president who conspires to kill large numbers of innocent Americans. Whether

you like Jack Bauer or not, there is no such person in the real world who is always on the scene and can move from city to city and even country to country in minutes.

- From a purely pragmatic perspective, no scientific evidence demonstrates that torture works, and evidence suggests that other methods are effective.[34]

Physicians and Torture

Almost overshadowing the US government's public views on US torture law has been its view on international law, specifically the Geneva Conventions.[35] It seems to have been assumed that if neither the US Constitution nor international law applied in Guantanamo, the administration could write its own rules of conduct for the prison, and it did. Secretary of Defense Donald Rumsfeld, for example, specifically approved types of torture that could be used in the interrogations there.[36] He also specifically involved physicians in torture by requiring that prisoners obtain "medical clearance" prior to having these techniques applied to them. In the words of his directive, the new techniques can only be used after, among other things, "the detainee is medically and operationally evaluated as suitable (considering all techniques to be used in combination)." These torture techniques made their way to Abu Ghraib when the commander of Guantanamo, General Geoffrey Miller, was transferred to Iraq.[37]

The Geneva Conventions were to apply in Iraq, according to the administration. Had they been followed, the torture and abuse of prisoners at Abu Ghraib would not have occurred. Even if the administration sincerely believed that there was some emergency exception to the prohibition of torture and cruel and degrading treatment, a pure pragmatist would have known that public knowledge of the treatment of prisoners, like those photographed at Abu Ghraib, would have done more to injure the cause of America in the war on terrorism than any terrorist organization could do itself.

Physicians also had the opportunity to stop what the lawyers had promoted by acting as human rights monitors. Not only do the Geneva Conventions prohibit torture and abusive and humiliating treatment of prisoners, they also specifically protect physicians who follow medical ethics by reporting and refusing to participate in torture and abuse of prisoners.[38] The Department of Defense's Independent Panel highlighted professional ethics as the core consideration in torture and abuse prevention, recommending that "All personnel who may be engaged in detention operations, from point of capture to final disposition, should participate in a professional ethics program that would equip them with a sharp moral compass for guidance in situations often riven with conflicting moral obligations."[39] As to physicians, "The Panel notes that the Fay investigation cited some medical personnel for failure to report detainee abuse. As noted in that investigation, training should include the obligation to report any detainee abuse."

In the early days of the Obama administration, three closely related events occurred. First, former Vice President Cheney reaffirmed—on numerous occasions—both his support of torture if required to prevent another terrorist attack, and his total reliance on law and lawyers for his belief. His position initially came in response to John King's question of whether he thought President Obama's stance on waterboarding and his plan to close Guantanamo had made Americans "less safe":

> Cheney: I do. I think *those programs were absolutely essential to* the success we enjoyed of being able to collect the intelligence that let us *defeat all further attempts to launch attacks against the United States* since 9/11. I think that's a great success story. *It was done legally. It was done in accordance with our constitutional practices and principles.*
>
> President Obama campaigned against it all across the country. And now he is making some choices that, in my mind, will, in fact, raise the risk to the American people of another attack.[40] (emphasis added)

The second event was the release by writer Mark Danner of the secret (and meant to be secret) report of the International Committee of the Red Cross on the torture of the 14 "high-value" detainees who were kept in CIA "black sites" until their transfer to Guantanamo. The report was based on interviews with the 14, and was sent to the acting general counsel of the CIA, John Rizzo, on February 14, 2007. The conclusion of the report was, as properly described by Danner, "stark and unmistakable":

> The allegations of ill-treatment of the detainees indicate that, in many cases, the ill-treatment to which they were subjected while held in the CIA program, either singly or in combination, constituted torture. In addition, many other elements of the ill-treatment, either singly or in combination, constituted cruel, inhuman, or degrading treatment.[41]

The report details the specific torture techniques applied to individuals, including Abu Zubaydah, and chillingly makes references to physicians involved at almost every step along the way—including treatment to prepare the prisoner for prolonged torture sessions and monitoring the sessions themselves to make sure that the prisoner was not actually killed.[42] In short, the CIA program relied on lawyers for its justification and on physicians for its implementation.

Just how much the physicians relied on the lawyers and the lawyers on the physicians was not clear until the third event: the release of four Justice Department memos done at the request of the CIA. One of them, dated May 10, 2005, attempts to explain why torture is not really torture under US law if it is supervised by a physician who has the authority to stop it if it is causing "severe physical or mental pain or suffering . . . ." Two portions of the memo (signed by Steven G. Bradbury) are worth emphasizing—the first an overview of physician responsibilities, the second a detailed application of medical knowledge to waterboarding. First the overview:

> *We also assume that there will be active and ongoing monitoring by medical and psychological personnel of each detainee who is undergoing a regimen of interrogation, and active intervention* by a member of the team or medical staff as necessary, so as to avoid the possibility of severe physical or mental pain or suffering within the meaning of [US anti-torture law] . . . . (emphasis added)

The memo goes on to describe how, upon arrival at the interrogation site, the detainee is "given a medical examination" and is subjected to "'precise, quiet, and almost clinical' procedures . . . [and] is given medical and psychological interviews to assess his condition and to make sure there are no contraindications to the use of any particular interrogation techniques." Then individual "techniques" are described in some detail, as is the active participation of physicians. The "waterboard" is described in the memo as a "technique" in which the detainee is "lying on a gurney that is inclined at an angle of 10 to 15 degrees to the horizontal, with the detainee on his back and head toward the lower end of the gurney." A cloth is then placed over his face, "and cold water is poured on the cloth from a height of approximately 6 to 18 inches. The wet cloth creates a barrier though which it is difficult—or in some cases not possible—to breathe." The critical and active role of the physician includes not only prior approval, but also monitoring and intervention:

> *During the use of the waterboard, a physician and a psychologist are present at all times. The detainee is monitored* to ensure that he does not develop respiratory distress. If the detainee is not breathing freely after the cloth is removed from his face, he is immediately moved to a vertical

position in order to clear the water from his mouth, nose, and nasopharynx. The gurney used for administering this technique is specially designed so that this can be accomplished very quickly if necessary. *Your medical personnel have explained* that the use of the waterboard does pose a small risk of certain potentially significant medical problems and that certain measures are taken to avoid or address such problems. First, a detainee might vomit and then aspirate the emesis. To reduce this risk, any detainee on whom this technique will be used is first placed on a liquid diet. Second, the detainee might aspirate some of the water, and the resulting water in the lungs might lead to pneumonia. To mitigate this risk, *a potable saline solution is used in the procedure.* (emphasis added)

The memo continues by describing what the CIA seems to believe is the major risk of waterboarding, and how physicians will intervene to treat the prisoner:

Third, it is conceivable (though, we understand . . . highly unlikely) that *a detainee could suffer spasms of the larynx that would prevent him from breathing* even when the application of water is stopped and the detainee is returned to an upright position. *In the event of such spasms, a qualified physician would immediately intervene to address the problem,* and, if necessary, the intervening physician would perform a tracheotomy. Although the risk of such spasms is considered remote (it apparently has never occurred in thousands of instances of SERE training), we are informed that *the necessary emergency equipment is always present— although not visible to the detainee—during any application of the waterboard.* (emphasis added)

Two of the four memos released were dated May 10, 2005; a third May 30, 2005; and a fourth, signed by Jay Bybee, was dated August 1, 2002. The latter addressed techniques to be used on Abu Zubaydah and, like the later memos, relied on physicians to make a "legal" determination that the torture techniques described by the CIA were not torture: "We understand that a medical expert with SERE [Survival, Evasion, Resistance, and Escape] experience will be present throughout . . . and that the procedures will be stopped if deemed medically necessary to prevent severe mental or physical harm to Zubaydah."

The memo paints a picture of clinical care, noting that Zubaydah had suffered an injury when captured, and that "steps will be taken to ensure that this injury is not in any way exacerbated by the use of these methods and that adequate medical attention will be given to ensure that it will heal properly." The memo, as endorsed by Dick Cheney and imagined by a public saturated with Jack Bauer, implies that waterboarding will only have to be used once and the prisoner will talk. In the case of Zubaydah, it has since been disclosed that he was waterboarded at least 83 times in August 2002. Khalid Shaikh Mohammed, known as the mastermind of 9/11, was waterboarded 183 times in March 2003. Even Jack Bauer, I suspect, would not find this torture method particularly effective in the ticking time bomb scenario.[43]

The conclusion (again, but worth repeating) is that the physicians would not engage in torture unless the Justice Department lawyers granted them legal immunity for their actions, and the Justice Department lawyers would not grant them (or, as importantly, their CIA colleagues) immunity unless the physicians agreed to actively participate in the torture and be on hand to stop it if "medically necessary," so that everyone could argue that no one intended to actually inflict "severe pain or suffering," a necessary element of torture.

The Supreme Court ultimately decided that prisoners at Guantanamo could challenge their imprisonment in US courts, as well as bring civil claims for injury and abuse under the Alien Tort Statute.[44] The Court thus rejected the position of the Bush administration as stated in oral argument before the Ninth Circuit that, even if the United States was engaged in "murder and torture" at Guantanamo, US courts could not interfere.[45] In another case decided that same day, the Supreme Court ruled that a US citizen captured on the battlefield and originally held at Guantanamo had a right to a fair hearing under the Constitution to contest his status as an "enemy combatant."[46] In dicta, the Supreme Court cited provisions of Geneva Convention III (relative to prisoners of war) as authoritative on the "law of war." In all of these cases, the judicial branch of government has been much more articulate than the executive in condemning torture and upholding both US and international law.

Telford Taylor argued persuasively at Nuremberg that prevention of war crimes and crimes against humanity, such as torture, must be our primary goal. Torture remains widely practiced around the world, even though universally condemned. Amnesty International, for example, estimates that as many as 100 countries may condone torture. Torture is wrong under all circumstances because it is cruel and degrading to humans, and an extreme violation of human rights under international law. Jean-Paul Sartre's description of torture almost 50 years ago during the French-Algerian War, echoes in post-9/11 America: "Torture is senseless violence, born in fear. The purpose of it is to force from one tongue, amid its screams and its vomiting up of blood, the secret of everything. Senseless violence: whether the victim talks or whether he dies under his agony, the secret that he cannot tell is always somewhere else and out of reach. It is the executioner who becomes Sisyphus. If he puts the question at all, he will have to continue forever."[47] In other words, torture primarily begets more torture.

Abu Ghraib and the torture debate gained worldwide attention primarily because of the photographs of cruel and inhuman treatment of prisoners by American soldiers.[48] This documentation made denial impossible. In Guantanamo, the only emblematic photograph was taken on the first day that prisoners arrived there: unable to see because of goggles, and dressed in orange jumpsuits, they were all made to kneel before their American guards.[49] Since that day, however, information from Guantanamo has been carefully guarded, only the names of a few physicians serving there are known, only a handful of incomplete medical records have become available, and few prisoners have been able to obtain either a physical or psychiatric examination by an independent physician.

President Bush said in mid-2006 that he would like to see Guantanamo "closed," but took no steps to do so.[50] President Obama has credibly pledged to close Guantanamo before February 2010, although he has encountered fierce political opposition to bringing any prisoners currently held at Guantanamo to the United States. While Guantanamo remains in operation, prisoners there who protest their continued detention in this legal black hole by going on hunger strikes continue to be force-fed by military physicians, with the blessing of lawyers. All the facts are not known, but from what is known, it seems reasonable to conclude that the US military, including military physicians, continue to react in a cruel and inhuman manner against prisoners on hunger strikes there. I turn to this worst case scenario in the next chapter.

5

. . . .

Hunger Strikes

I n his "Account of Torture," former Soviet dissident Vladimir Bukovsky
describes how, while a political prisoner, he went on a hunger strike in
1971 to protest the treatment of one of his fellow prisoners who was being
denied a lawyer for an approaching trial. His jailers decided to force-feed him
in a "medical unit" in a particularly brutal way. As Bukovsky describes it:

> They started feeding me forcibly through the nostril. By a rather thick
> tube with a metal end on it . . . *The procedure will be that four or five KGB
> guys will come to my cell, take me to a medical unit, put a straightjacket on me, tie
> me up to a table,* and somebody will be still holding, even so I was tied
> down, holding my shoulders and head and legs, and one will be *pushing
> this thing through my nostril.* And of course it doesn't go . . . and its painful
> like hell I must tell you . . . *then they would pour down some liquid food through
> this rubber tube* . . . and the next day, when it [the nose] will start
> healing . . . they will take you again and it will be even narrower
> than it used to be and they will force it through again and so I went
> in and out for twelve days.[1] (emphasis added)

Bukovsky's story was reprinted by President George Bush's Council on
Bioethics. The Council described the force-feeding as "violent and brutal"

and as "torture," asking readers to consider: "Bukovsky's torturers assaulted and injured his body. Did they assault and injury Bukovsky?"[2] Americans want to believe that only totalitarian dictatorships force-feed hunger strikers in brutal, tortuous manners. In this chapter, I consider whether it is possible that substantially similar abusive force-feeding of hunger strikers continues to occur at Guantanamo, even post-Obama, and if—like torture—Americans need the blessing of lawyers and the participation of physicians to justify it.

On September 11, 2005, 131 prisoners at Guantanamo were on hunger strikes. At the end of 2005, that number had dropped to 84.[3] Then a new technique was introduced into the prison camp to break the hunger strike: use of an "emergency restraint chair." The chair is described by its inventor, a former sheriff who had one of his jailers injured by a prisoner, as a "padded cell on wheels."[4] His company, E.R.C., Inc., supplied 25 such transportation chairs to Guantanamo. The prisoner can be strapped into one of them using 8-point restraints, including not just hands and feet, but also shoulders, head and torso, and safely transported to a medical care facility. The chair was designed for transportation, not for either treatment or punishment. Nonetheless, at Guantanamo, since early 2006, these chairs have been used to immobilize prisoners on hunger strikes to force-feed them as a strategy to break the strikes. And, to a large extent, this strategy has succeeded. As of late February 2006, reportedly only three prisoners were still being force-fed in the restraint chairs, and by November 2006 that number had been reduced to two.[5] Since then the record has been less spectacular, with the number of prisoners on hunger strikes rising to as many as 50 by the week after President Obama's inauguration, and remaining at about that level thereafter.

Medical records of the Guantanamo prisoners who have been force-fed in the restraint chairs, some of which were introduced into evidence in lawsuits seeking to prohibit further use of the chairs, contain what appears to be a preprinted "medical officer note" that reflects the use of a medical practice not as treatment of a physical condition, but as punishment for undesirable behavior:

> Despite being advised that *hunger striking is detrimental to his health*, the detainee refuses to eat. *Restraints were ordered for medical necessity* to facilitate feeding the detainee. There is no evidence that medications or a medical process is causing this detainee's refusal to eat. Detainee does not have any medical condition/disability that would place him at greater risk during feeding using medical restraints. Detainee was told that *he will remain in restraints until feed and post feed observation time (60–120 minutes) is completed.* Detainee

understands that if he eats, that involuntary feeding in medical restraints will no longer be required.

GITMO Dr _____ (emphasis added)

Then-20-year-old prisoner Yousif Al-Shehri's medical records, for example, contain this identical entry twice a day for eight consecutive days from January 18 to January 25, 2006, after which the records indicate he ended his hunger strike and became "compliant."[6] He has since been released from Guantanamo. The name of the physician had been redacted. Records of another prisoner at Guantanamo who was being force-fed (and who has also been released) indicate that his restraints "may be removed early if detainee meets behavioral standards" and that during his "tube feeding . . . detainee will be observed continuously and encouraged to express his frustration. He will be reminded of how his behavior must change if he is to be allowed out of restraints." The medical record continues with the following checklist:

Detainee was told that he will remain in restraints until he:

Demonstrates control of his behavior with no attempts to harm self, staff, or others

Ceases profanity and threatening language

Listens to and follows directions

Makes no attempts to loosen or pull at restraints (except to discuss with medical staff that he is uncomfortable)

Makes no attempt to resist placement or remove medical devices such as IV/NGT

GITMO Doc [signature redacted]

Medical Ethics of Force-Feeding

The use of force-feeding by physicians of competent prisoners on hunger strikes is widely condemned as both illegal and unethical.[7] But some controversies persist, most related to assessment of the prisoner's competence and motivation, as well as the likely impact of a successful hunger strike on prison security. How does medical ethics counsel physicians employed by the state, whether prison or military physicians, about the appropriateness of treating competent hunger strikers against their will? Guantanamo provides a case study that can help answer this question.

Various types of hunger strikes have been occurring at Guantanamo almost since it opened in early 2002.[8] As many as 200 prisoners have been on hunger strikes at once, and there were probably about 100 on hunger strikes in November 2005, when Secretary of Defense Rumsfeld was asked, "Do you approve of the force-feeding of detainees [at Guantanamo] who are on hunger strike?" He replied (reprising his "I'm not a lawyer" torture position),

> *I'm not a doctor* and I'm not the kind of a person who would be in a position to approve or disapprove. It seems to me, looking at it from this distance, is that *the responsible people are the combatant commanders* of the Army as the executive agent for detainees. *They make—have expert medical people who make decisions of that type.* And they've made a decision that they think it's appropriate for them to provide nourishment to people who, for whatever reason, at various points in their detention decide they want to not provide normal nourishment to themselves.
>
> There are a number of things that one can glean from the way it's being done. *I don't think there's a serious risk of people—well I shouldn't say that, I'm not in a position to know that.* But there are *a number of people who go on a diet* where they don't eat for a period and then go off of it at some point, and then they rotate and other people do that. So it's clearly a technique to try to get the attention of you folks [the press], and they're successful.[9] (emphasis added)

In short, the decision whether to force-feed a prisoner at Guantanamo seems to be a military decision to be made by the base commander; the decision about the technique used to actually do the force-feeding is a medical one to be made by military physicians. Rumsfeld also attempts to trivialize the issue, characterizing hunger strikers as people who are assigned to "go on a diet" temporarily by their superiors. This notion of free choice to make trifling decisions is one I have also found pervasive from those who defend Guantanamo. Four food examples are illustrative. The first dates from 2004, in which I was told that the cuisine at Guantanamo was exceptionally good, and that for fish meals the prisoners had their choice of three different sauces with their fish. The second, from two years later, was that those being force-fed had their choice of colors of the nasogastric tube, and that blue or yellow seemed to be the favorites. The third, is from early in 2009, when I was told that those being force-fed now had their choice of lubricants to apply to the nasogastric tube before it was inserted, and that "most preferred olive oil." The final one is from mid-2009, when a Guantanamo physician told reporters that they used three "delicious flavors" (strawberry, butter pecan, and chocolate Ensure) to entice the hunger strikers to eat. These "choices," of course, trivialize both the brutality inherent in force-feeding and the concept of choice itself.

The use of physicians to aggressively break a prison hunger strike raises complex medical ethics and legal issues that have been the subject of international debate for decades. US courts have occasionally been asked to rule on the legality of force feeding prisoners, and have usually permitted it if done by a physician in a medically reasonable manner for the primary purpose of either preventing suicide or maintaining order in the prison.[10]

I have written about hunger strikes a number of times over the past three decades, once concluding, in 1982, "We restrict the rights of prisoners in many ways. Force-feeding them rather than permitting them to starve themselves to death is probably one of the most benign."[11] This is also the position the US Department of Defense has taken on the Guantanamo hunger strikes. As the most senior civilian physician in the Pentagon until 2007, William Winkenwerder, put it in response to questions about breaking a Guantanamo hunger strike: "There is a moral question. Do you allow a person to commit suicide? Or do you take steps to protect their health and preserve their life?"[12] But both my 1982 position and Winkenwerder's 2006 position seem overly simplistic and mechanistic in the context of Guantanamo, and I grossly underestimated the pain and medical complications force-feeding can impose on a competent prisoner. Physicians must answer three interrelated questions to determine their legal and ethical obligations to prison hunger strikers: Is the prisoner on a hunger strike? When is it ethical for a physician to force-feed a hunger striker? And what means can be used by a physician to force-feed a hunger striker?

Hernan Reyes of the International Committee of the Red Cross (ICRC) has written the most authoritative article on hunger strikes, which he also terms voluntary total fasting.[13] Fasting, voluntariness, and a stated purpose are all needed before a prisoner can be said to be on a hunger strike. Simply refusing to eat as a reaction to a specific situation, whether in frustration or anger, for example, qualifies one as a food refuser, but not as a hunger striker. Thus, the initial rounds of food refusals at Guantanamo, which occurred in early 2002 in response to specific actions of the guards toward individual prisoners, would not count. Nor do mentally incompetent prisoners who refuse to eat out of severe depression or other mental illness, and with no goal in mind other than their own death, qualify as legitimate hunger strikers.

The determination of a hunger striker to fast until either political demands are met or death occurs may vary from person to person. This is especially true when fasting occurs in groups, as Secretary Rumsfeld seems to have believed was happening. This is because members of the group may be less free to discontinue a hunger strike, a fact that must be taken into

account by physicians when deciding whether the prisoner-patient is voluntarily continuing to refuse food. The usual advice for physicians in this
circumstance is to separate the possibly coerced hunger striker in a secure
environment where the prisoner can discontinue the hunger strike without
the knowledge of his fellow hunger strikers. The determination of the
hunger striker will also suggest the likely medical consequences of continuing the hunger strike. Most hunger strikers, for example, have taken some
water, salt, sugar, and vitamin B_1 at least for a time before asserting an
intention to fast to death.[14] These nutrients significantly decrease the
chances of permanent disability should the strike end prior to death
(which is never the desired end point of a true hunger striker).

The World Medical Association (WMA) in its Tokyo Declaration
ruled out physician participation in prisoner force-feeding. The WMA's
more specific Malta Declaration on Hunger Strikers, nonetheless, permits
physicians to attend a prison hunger striker in the context of a traditional
physician–patient relationship if consent and confidentiality can be maintained. The WMA's definition of a hunger strike is much broader than that
of the ICRC, in that it does not require a specific goal: "A hunger striker is a
mentally competent person who has indicated that he has decided to
embark on a hunger strike and has refused to take food and/or fluids for
a significant interval."[15]

It had been the position of the United States that the Geneva
Conventions do not apply to the prisoners at Guantanamo and that military
commanders can lawfully order physicians to force-feed prisoners held there
for political purposes. As I discussed in the last chapter, both positions are
wrong as a matter of human rights law and medical ethics, and Common
Article 3 of the Geneva Conventions has been ruled to apply to all prisoners
held at Guantanamo by the Supreme Court, as well as by executive directive
of President Obama. The hunger strike policy, however, remains as of this
writing. Whether force-feeding competent hunger strikers is a violation of
Common Article 3 (as I will argue it is), it is certainly a violation of medical
ethics for physicians to treat their competent patients against their will solely
for military or political purposes. The Department of Defense seems to
understand this, and so has publicly relied on two basic rationales for
ordering military physicians to force-feed prisoners: it is in the best medical
interest of prisoners; and it is done in accordance with US Bureau of
Prisons hunger strike regulations that apply to prisoners in federal prisons.[16]

Both arguments seem reasonable, but neither fits the facts at
Guantanamo. The first is acceptable if it applies only to prisoners who are
not actually on hunger strikes (as defined by the ICRC), but who have
stopped eating because of a mental illness, such as depression. These

prisoners can reasonably be declared incompetent to refuse treatment, including forced feeding, if and when such feeding is necessary to sustain their lives or health. So, to the extent that a competency assessment has been properly conducted and the prisoner is determined incompetent to refuse, forced feeding is medically indicated. This category is not likely to apply to many prisoners at Guantanamo, however. As commanding general Jay W. Hood told a group of visiting physicians in the fall of 2005, the prisoners at Guantanamo are protesting their confinement, they are not suicidal.[17] Moreover, only a few independent civilian physicians have been allowed to evaluate the prisoners at Guantanamo for either competency or health status, and in a review done in February 2009 for President Obama, physicians at Guantanamo classified only 8% of the prisoners as having a mental illness (although this number seems very low, since it is lower than that in the general US nonprison population). The second argument requires a closer examination of the Bureau of Prisons hunger strike regulations.[18] These regulations are triggered when the hunger striker "communicates that fact to staff and is observed by staff to be refraining from eating for a period of time, ordinarily in excess of 72 hours." Upon referral for medical evaluation, the inmate shall have a medical and psychiatric exam, and be placed "in a medically appropriate locked room for close monitoring" (if necessary to accurately measure food and fluid intake and output), where weight and vital signs are monitored at least every 24 hours. If and when the physician determines "that the inmate's life or health will be threatened if treatment is not initiated immediately," the physician shall make "reasonable efforts to convince the inmate to voluntarily accept treatment," including explaining the risks of refusing, and document these efforts. After such efforts (or in an emergency), if "a medical necessity for immediate treatment of a life- or health-threatening situation exists, the physician may order that treatment be administered without the consent of the inmate."

Whether or not one thinks these are reasonable regulations, only a physician is permitted to make treatment decisions under them (not the warden), and then only after reasonable attempts to get voluntary compliance. To the extent that military commanders are making the decisions about force-feeding, the federal Bureau of Prison rules are not being followed at Guantanamo. This may be the reason why a past commander of the medical group responsible for prisoner health care, Navy Captain John S. Edmondson, said that military healthcare personnel are screened before they are deployed to Guantanamo "to ensure that they do not have ethical objections to assisted feeding."[19] In addition, under the Bureau of Prison rules, 72 hours of fasting triggers a medical evaluation—it does not trigger emergency force-feeding, which generally requires weeks, if not months, of continuous fasting.

US courts have generally upheld actions like those authorized by the Bureau of Prisons regulations, at least as long as the actual force-feeding (misleadingly described as "assisted feeding") is performed by a physician in accordance with good and accepted medical procedures, and the prisoner is either suicidal or the treatment refusal presents a significant security problem for the entire prison. In terms of American constitutional law, competent prisoners have a constitutional right to refuse treatment, but prison officials may overrule it when they have a "legitimate penological interest," which includes preventing suicide in prisoners and maintaining order in the prison itself. It should be underlined, however, that the standard in US prisons is set by the Eighth Amendment of the Constitution, which prohibits "cruel and unusual" punishments, and requires only that wardens not be "deliberately indifferent" to the health of their prisoners. The Constitution does not apply to Guantanamo—but Common Article 3 of the Geneva Conventions does, and its prohibitions, which include "inhuman and degrading treatment," are more stringent than those of the Constitution.

The much more complex medical ethics question is what a physician should do after the competent hunger striker becomes incompetent, it reasonably appears the hunger striker will die or sustain permanent injury if he continues to refuse food, and there is no reasonable possibility that his demands will be met. Three medical ethics positions have been articulated over the past decades, the first two of which, I believe, are not helpful or persuasive. The WMA concluded in 1991 that "when the hunger striker has become confused and is therefore unable to make an unimpaired decision or has lapsed into a coma, the doctor shall be free to make the decision for his patient as to further treatment which he considers to be in the best interest of that patient . . . ." The WMA nonetheless required the physician to honor the patient-prisoner's prior decision to fast to the death unless he had informed the prisoner of his inability to honor this wish and provided the prisoner with the chance to obtain another attending physician.

The 1995 position of the Royal Dutch Medical Association, drafted in response to hunger strikes by Vietnamese asylum seekers, is more specific and is designed to try to fill in some of the ambiguity of the WMA statement. Specifically, it suggests that each hunger striker have access to a "doctor of confidence" who will act as their physician, keeping them fully informed of the medical consequences of the hunger strike, but also follow their wishes of nontreatment in the event of incompetence or coma.[20] To reduce uncertainty in the event of incompetence, the Dutch guidelines call for hunger strikers to sign a specific "statement of non-intervention" (similar to a living will) that directs their care and refuses artificial or forced feeding in the event of incompetence. This written statement is not to be made public unless and until the prisoner-patient actually becomes incompetent. Of course it would be nice if all prisoners had access to independent physicians, whether called doctors of confidence or not. The major problem at Guantanamo, however, is precisely that the only physicians prisoners have access to are the military physicians at the base. Moreover, the living will solution is no solution at all, since it suggests that the prisoner might have made arrangements with his physician to "save" him before he suffers death or serious harm, and so undercuts the power of the hunger strike itself.[21]

The third, current, and most persuasive medical ethics position was set forth in October 2006, when the WMA met in South Africa to clarify further its Declaration on Hunger Strikers. The clarified declaration continues to give physicians the ethical authority to act in the incompetent hunger striker's "best interests" in the absence of an advance directive from the hunger striker, and to even go against such a directive if the refusal is thought to have been made under duress. On the other hand, the right of competent hunger strikers to refuse forced feeding is strengthened in article 21:

> *Forcible feeding is never ethically acceptable.* Even if intended to benefit, feeding accompanied by threats, coercion, force, or use of physical restraints is a form of inhuman and degrading treatment. Equally unacceptable is the forced feeding of some detainees in order to intimidate or coerce other hunger strikers to stop fasting. (emphasis added)

Saving Lives

US military officials at Guantanamo have refused to follow the WMA's medical ethics position. Their position has been that they will not permit anyone at Guantanamo to "fast to death" because of an envisioned worst case scenario in which the dead hunger striker becomes an international cause célèbre, in the mold of Irish hunger striker Bobbie Sands and his colleagues. Because of this potential, hunger striking at Guantanamo has been dealt with as a global security risk. After the first three suicides by hanging at Guantanamo in June 2006, however, this rationale no longer seems persuasive. All three dead prisoners had been on hunger strikes at one time or another, and at least one of them, Ali Abdullah Ahmed, had been repeatedly subjected to force-feeding in a restraint chair.

Winkenwerder's position that the military can rewrite the WMA's Malta Declaration to permit earlier intervention because it "only makes good sense" to force-feed a hunger striker before he becomes incompetent or "near death" is also not persuasive. "Preventive treatment" can be seen as reasonable in some settings, and with the patient's consent, but when the real prevention is simple eating, and when the prisoner is on a hunger strike (i.e., not eating), force-feeding is not treatment but simply punishment for an undesirable behavior. Preventing the deaths of incompetent prisoners is a laudable medical goal. Use of the restraint chairs for force-feeding competent prisoners, however, can never be ethically, legally, or medically justified. And, even in the case of an incompetent suicidal prisoner whose incompetence to refuse treatment is determined by an independent qualified psychiatrist, the use of the restraint chair would be unethical and illegal. This is because any prisoner who needs to be forcibly restrained in this device for force-feeding is almost certainly strong enough that the prisoner is in little or no health danger from continuing to fast. The primary justification for use of the restraint chair for force-feeding seems to be punishment and intimidation rather than medical care. The use of any medical intervention as punishment is prohibited by all relevant international treaties, medical ethics principles, and even US constitutional law.

The military physicians might reply that their sole motivation is medical treatment, not punishment, and that, like the Justice Department torture memos discussed in the previous chapter, their intent alone should govern the characterization of their actions. Even if this rather bizarre argument were accepted, however, it would raise another fundamental human rights violation, one also specifically prohibited by the holding of the Nuremberg Doctors' Trial and the second sentence of Article 7 of the ICCPR: "In particular, no one shall be subjected without his free consent to medical or scientific experimentation." Because the emergency restraint chairs had never been used for medical treatment before (and were, of course, not designed for this purpose), and they were being used in this context to test the hypothesis that their use on prisoner-subjects would be more successful in breaking the hunger strike than the use of medically accepted means, it is reasonable to consider this a medical experiment. Looked at in this way, the experiment has many of the characteristics of those conducted by the Nazi physicians, including its primary rationale—military necessity—and its total lack of "free consent."[22]

The experimentation model may seem off-point to those who believe that the military is simply trying to make the best of a bad situation at Guantanamo—and that is certainly a reasonable position to take. Nonetheless, the more we learn about Guantanamo, the more we have discovered that those who run it see it as a big experiment. A Senate investigation, for example, found that the term "America's Battle Lab" was often used to describe Guantanamo by its military commanders. The context was, according to Colonel Britt Mallow, a former commander of the Criminal Investigative Task Force there, "that interrogations and other procedures there were to some degree experimental, and their lessons would benefit DOD in other places." Mallow told Senator Carl Levin, "I personally objected to the implied philosophy that interrogators should experiment with untested methods, particularly those in which they were not trained." In a similar vein, President Obama, in May 2009, referred to Guantanamo as "quite simply a mess, a misguided experiment."

I have had the opportunity to speak about force-feeding at Guantanamo to a number of physician audiences, and I have been repeatedly impressed with how many physicians identify so closely with the military physicians at Guantanamo that they see the nasogastric feeding done there as routine and beneficent. Because of this experience, I hope I will be forgiven for underlining that the primary ethical problem with force-feeding at Guantanamo does not lie in the technique of using a nasogastric tube (at least if the proper size tube is used in a medically appropriate manner; not, for example, with a Soviet-style steel tip), but rather in its forced use on a competent prisoner who is put in a restraint chair with eight-point restraints (any restraints would be objectionable). It is also ethically unacceptable that the hunger striker is maintained in restraints for up to 2 hours of "post-feed observation" during which time the prisoner must urinate and defecate on himself. This is punishment, not treatment, and seems to be motivated by military commanders for humiliation and subjugation, not by physicians for a health benefit. More generously, as one of the former physicians at Guantanamo put it to me, "We were told we had to do it [force-feed hunger strikers] for the good of the country."

There seems to be real tension between the physicians at Guantanamo (in the Joint Medical Group) and the base's overall commander (Commander, Joint Task-Force Guantanamo), who also commands not just the medical group, but the separate Joint Detention Group (in charge of the prisoners) and the Joint Intelligence Group (in charge of interrogations) as well. It is often argued that seldom, if ever, must a physician in the military choose between being a military officer first and a physician second, or being a physician first and a military officer second.[23] At Guantanamo, however, the choice is stark. Military physicians cannot follow military orders to force-feed competent prisoners without violating basic precepts of medical ethics never to harm them by using their medical knowledge.

Revised Department of Defense medical instructions, dated June 6, 2006, acknowledge some of this (requiring, for example, that involuntary treatment be preceded by "a thorough medical and mental health evaluation of the detainee and counseling concerning the risks of refusing treatment" and that any treatment be "carried out in a medically appropriate manner"), but nonetheless continue to permit force-feeding of mentally competent prisoners.[24] This is, to my knowledge, the first time the US military has explicitly instructed its physicians that they cannot follow internationally recognized medical ethics standards, as spelled out, for example, by the WMA. This radical medical ethics policy change could only have been possible, it seems to me, if force-feeding hunger strikers at Guantanamo was viewed at the Pentagon or the White House as essential for national security.

Geneva at Guantanamo

Guantanamo has been called a "gulag," an "anomaly," and a "legal black hole."[25] The Supreme Court's 2006 ruling in *Hamdan* that the Geneva Conventions have full force in Guantanamo as a matter of both US and international law was widely hailed, especially by military attorneys.[26] The Court also ruled that Geneva's Common Article 3 applies to all prisoners in US military custody. It prevents not only the use of tribunals that are not "regularly constituted," but also requires all prisoners to be "treated humanely" and explicitly prohibits "cruel treatment and torture," as well as "outrages upon personal dignity, in particular, humiliating and degrading treatment."[27] Any reasonable reading of Common Article 3 would prohibit use of the restraint chairs to force-feed prisoners, competent or not, and I hope it's not too much to expect that the Obama administration will arrive at this conclusion long before this book is published.[28]

Four of the justices in *Hamdan* also ruled that the protocols to the Geneva Conventions, although not ratified by the United States, are binding international law.[29] This is significant, since the protocols specifically prohibit interference with actions by physicians that are consistent with medical ethics. This means that the use of the restraint chairs to break a hunger strike by a competent prisoner would be prohibited two ways: as "cruel treatment" and "humiliating and degrading treatment," and also as a violation of medical ethics.

The force-feeding debacle and the *Hamdan* opinion provided an opportunity for the US military to adopt as formal military doctrine the rule that a physician in the military is always a physician first and a military officer second. That it did not take this opportunity is disappointing. American military physicians have a justifiably proud record. They have always had the obligation to disobey an unlawful order and the option to disobey an order contrary to medical ethics. Nonetheless, as I will discuss in more detail in the next chapter, the "physician first, last, and always" doctrine would make it much less likely that any such orders would be issued in the first place.

Although unfamiliar with or contemptuous of the Nuremberg Principles and the Geneva Conventions, Bush administration lawyers nonetheless almost immediately understood that they and those who took their advice to disregard the Geneva Conventions could be prosecuted criminally for war crimes under the US War Crimes Act. As Alberto Gonzales put it in a memorandum to the president dated January 25, 2002, one advantage of determining that the Geneva Conventions did not apply to the Taliban is that such a presidential determination "substantially reduces the threat of domestic criminal prosecution under the War Crimes Act (18 U.S.C. 2441) . . . [because] your determination would create a reasonable basis in law that Section 2441 does not apply, which would provide a solid defense to any future prosecution."[30]

This ultimately was not protection enough for the Bush administration officials who, at least after the disclosures at Abu Ghraib and Guantanamo, began to see themselves as human rights outlaws who might be brought to justice in their own country. As historian Arthur Schlesinger, Jr. concluded in regard to the administration's legal defense of torture: "No position taken has done more damage to the American reputation in the world—ever."[31] Administration lawyers worried that they could come to be seen as traitors to American values; that more than any other action, the Abu Ghraib disclosures undercut the power and legitimacy of American forces abroad; and that a future administration would hold them accountable.

Thus, it came as little surprise that after *Hamdan* and just before the presidential election of 2006, the administration pushed the Military Commissions Act through Congress. Mostly, the Act was a direct response to *Hamdan*. But it also explicitly provided administration officials and those who followed their advice on torture with immunity from prosecution under the War Crimes Act by granting the President the authority "to interpret the meaning and application of the Geneva Conventions." The act also redefined torture and other grave breaches of the Geneva Conventions, making these new definitions (which, for example, would not cover the sexual humiliation at Abu Ghraib or much of the force-feeding at Guantanamo) retroactive to November 26, 1997, the date of the War Crimes Act.[32]

During the brief debate on the War Commissions Act, Senators John McCain, Lindsey Graham, and John Warner took the position that the law should not change the obligations of the US armed forces under the Geneva Conventions. In this position, they were strongly supported by both current and former JAGs, as well as by former chairmen of the Joint Chiefs of Staff.[33] Both General Jack Vessey and General Colin Powell wrote letters to McCain citing *The Armed Forces Officer*, a book commissioned after World War II by General George C. Marshall, which, Powell wrote, is "used to tell the world and to remind our soldiers of our moral obligations with respect to those in our custody."[34] Among other things, the text lists "strong belief in human rights" as the first desired characteristic of "every military officer" and specifically instructs:

> *The United States abides by the laws of war. Its Armed Forces, in their dealings with all other peoples, are expected to comply with the laws of war in the spirit and to the letter.* In waging war, we do not terrorize helpless non-combatants if it is in our power to avoid so doing. Wanton killing, torture, cruelty, or the working of unusual and unnecessary hardship on enemy prisoners or populations is not justified under any circumstances.[35] (emphasis added)

Actual prosecution in the United States seems unlikely, although unpredictable. It has nonetheless proven embarrassing for our country to have US and German citizens seek to prosecute Donald Rumsfeld and others for war crimes involving torture at Abu Ghraib and Guantanamo in a German court under the theory of universal jurisdiction.[36] An earlier attempt to get the German prosecutor to act was rejected on the grounds that the United States might take appropriate action itself.[37] Since retro-active immunity has been granted to US officials, however, a war crimes trial of an American official in another country no longer seems improb-able. Unlike the initial request in 2004, the November 2006 request included not just those DOD officials and military officers in charge of Abu Ghraib and Guantanamo, but also many of the lawyers who wrote the memos justifying the use of torture and cruel and inhuman treatment in these prison camps, including now former Department of Justice lawyers Jay Bybee and John Yoo, former Department of Defense General Counsel William James Haynes II, and former Vice President Cheney's Chief of Staff, David S. Addington, as well as former White House counsel and Attorney General, Alberto Gonzales.[38] This is substantially identical to lists drawn up in 2009, although some critics would add Bush and Cheney themselves.

The German court ultimately refused jurisdiction again. But, in the human rights world, "naming and shaming" is a revered tactic, and the spectacle of a German prosecutor even considering war crimes and crimes against humanity charges against American officials is incredible, and certainly nothing the US prosecutors at Nuremberg could ever have envisioned. Nonetheless, it is well worth recalling that it was not just the physicians who were prosecuted for actions during World War II, but also German jurists. As General Taylor put it in his opening statement for the prosecution in the Justice Case:

> *The defendants and their colleagues distorted, perverted, and finally accomplished the complete overthrow of justice and law in Germany* . . . But the defendants are not now called to account for violating constitutional guaranties or withholding due process of law. On the contrary, the defendants are accused of participation in and responsibility for the killings, tortures, and other atrocities which resulted from, and which the defendants know were an inevitable consequence of, the conduct of their offices as judges, prosecutors, and ministry officials. These men share with all the leaders of the Third Reich—diplomats, generals, party officials, industrialists, and others—responsibility for the holocaust of death and misery which the Third Reich visited on the world and on Germany herself. *They can no more escape that responsibility by virtue of their judicial robes than the general by his uniform.*[39] (emphasis added)

This prosecution of German lawyers and judges seemed exactly right to the United States at Nuremberg, and many, if not most, Americans would see a similar prosecution of the lawyers who distorted the Nuremberg Principles, the Geneva Conventions, the ICCPR and the CAT, among other laws, as reasonable as well. As Jose Alvarez concluded after an examination of the torture memos, "when government lawyers torture the rule of law as gravely as they have done here, international as well as national crimes may have been committed, including by the lawyers themselves."[40]

Other actions short of criminal prosecution can be taken against the lawyers and physicians involved in torture and force-feeding. For lawyers who perverted the law at the behest of their superiors, it seems reasonable and just to disbar them. Removing the licenses to practice from physicians involved in torture and unethical force-feeding is also reasonable and responsible. In 1993, my colleagues Michael Grodin, Leonard Glantz, and I proposed the establishment of an International Medical Tribunal that could hear cases, develop an international code, and publicly condemn the actions of individual physicians who violate international standards of medical conduct.[41] Even though such a tribunal would not be able to punish with criminal sanctions, its decisions could result in the professional isolation of physicians and be a powerful deterrent to grossly unethical conduct.[42] It would seem equally worthwhile to have an International Legal Tribunal to hear cases brought against attorneys and judges who misuse their profession to encourage the commission of war crimes and crimes against humanity.

In the absence of such international forums, the other primary avenue available is the licensing board responsible for granting the medical or legal license. In the case of physicians, for example, an action seeking the revocation of the physician's license could be brought before the medical board that issued the physician's license. As with lawyers, these are all state-level entities. The few times that this tactic has been tried to date have not been successful, but this is primarily because the board has seen the action as primarily political rather than ethical.[43] In the case of a military physician who was responsible for treatment of prisoners at Guantanamo, the California medical licensing board, for example, has refused to hear the case because it believes it should be heard, if at all, by the military itself.[44] I think they are wrong about this. Physicians cannot practice medicine in the military unless they are licensed. Retention of a license to practice medicine requires conformance with the precepts of medical ethics—it is not a license to torture or to commit war crimes. When medical ethics precepts are violated, even—or perhaps especially—in compliance with the wishes of the state, revocation or suspension of the physician's medical license is fitting.[45]

Preventing torture and cruel and inhuman treatment is everyone's business—but three professions seem especially well-suited to prevent torture: physicians, lawyers, and military officers. Each also has special obligations. Physicians have special obligations because of their universally recognized and respected role as healers. Lawyers also have special obligations to respect and uphold the law, including international humanitarian law. And military officers have special obligations to follow the international laws of war, including the Geneva Conventions. Any violation of international human rights or humanitarian law, especially a grave violation of the Geneva Conventions, or aiding and abetting the violation thereof, should be sufficient grounds for a licensing authority to question the person's fitness to be a physician or lawyer, and those found to be human rights outlaws should lose their privilege to practice their professions.

In the next chapter, modestly titled "War," I discuss whether it makes any sense to rely on "the law of war" in actual wars, or whether national security, and even saving lives, will always overwhelm ethical and legal precepts.

6

. . . .

War

War is always a public health and medical disaster. As historian John Keegan has put it, because of its inherent cruelty and savagery "it is scarcely possible anywhere in the world today to raise a body of reasoned support for the opinion that war is a justifiable activity."[1] Human rights are seldom associated with war, except in commentaries about their routine violation. But the relationship between war and human rights is complicated and even paradoxical: The worse the scale of human rights violations in warfare, the more likely it is that international human rights law will be strengthened in an attempt to prevent similar human rights violations in the future. The human rights paradox is well-framed by physician and human rights activist Jack Geiger, speaking of the second half of the 20th century: No period of human history has produced "human rights documents of such sweeping scope and rigorous specificity," nor have human rights ever been "violated on so massive a scale, nor with such efficacy and savagery."[2]

But even this paradox contains yet another: Is it possible that the existence of laws of war that seek to limit death, pain, and suffering of civilians can actually make war appear more benign than it is, and thus encourage brutal wars that would not otherwise have been fought? This question raises a related one: Is it ever justified to go to war to protect civilians from human rights abuses, as has recently been attempted in Kosovo, Bosnia, East Timor, Liberia, and Haiti, and proposed in Darfur?[3] The issue is complex, and requires much more attention than it has received. This is because war, even one waged for "good" purposes, always terrorizes civilians.

This chapter continues the discussion of human rights abuses involving torture and force-feeding hunger strikers by looking more generally at human rights and bioethics in war. In it, I will give a brief overview of the law of war, especially as it relates to the protection of the lives and health of civilians, the treatment of the bodies of soldiers killed while fighting America's wars, and the ethical standards that should be followed by physician members of the American military. War is itself a worst case scenario, and like other worst cases, the "worst" case scenario can always be made even worse.

War and Human Rights

World War I, with its horrors of trench warfare and chemical weapons, was known as the "war to end all wars." The failure of the League of Nations to prevent World War II, a global disaster, led to what was hoped were much stronger tools to prevent war, including the United Nations and specific international human rights laws. The most important human rights documents, including the Universal Declaration of Human Rights, the International Covenant of Civil and Political Rights, and the International Covenant on Economic, Social, and Cultural Rights, were all direct products of World War II. Although they have a longer pedigree, dating from the mid 19th century, the same can be said about the most important humanitarian treaty, the 1949 Geneva Conventions. And, of course, the Nuremberg Principles were established at the war crimes trials of Nazis after World War II. These principles are that there are such things as war crimes and crimes against humanity (including murder, torture, and slavery), that individuals (not just states) can be held criminally responsible for committing them, and that it is no defense to prove that one was "just obeying orders" or following the law of one's country.[4] The rapid growth of international human rights laws following World War II has been profound, and at least some familiarity with what preceded their development can help us understand their roles and contemporary usefulness.

Humanitarian law is the unlikely term for the law of war, especially that part of the law of war devoted to rules designed to restrain the actions of the warring parties. The law of war is generally divided into two parts: the law relating to primary prevention by discouraging going to war in the first place (*jus ad bellum*), and the law relating to what may be thought of as secondary prevention—the conduct of war, especially to the protection of civilians (*jus in bellum*).[5]

Because war is so terrible, it has, at least since Roman times, required justification, perhaps best set forth in various versions of the just war doctrine. This doctrine requires that the war be waged under a public authority, be either for self-defense or to punish a grievous injury, and only be pursued to achieve just ends, and not for vengeance. What constitutes self-defense is open to some interpretation, but the Bush preemption doctrine that permits "preemptive" war when a future threat, even one involving weapons of mass destruction, is thought to exist has no just war pedigree. Nations need not wait to defend themselves until they are actually attacked, but an attack must be imminent and unstoppable by other means to justify a self-defense war response.

Secondary prevention or damage control is the goal of *jus in bellum*, the attempt to produce rules that limit the destructiveness of an inherently destructive activity. It is reasonable to view rules for mass killings as strange and even macabre, and it is even possible that such rules could make going to war easier to justify. Nonetheless, the wholesale slaughter of civilians, at least of those from nations denoted as being part of the "civilized world," has only been viewed as unacceptable since the Thirty Years War (1618–48) and the work of Dutch jurist Hugo Grotius. Prior to this time, humanitarian rules simply did not exist. Shakespeare's rendition of Henry V's threat to the mayor of a French city from whom he demanded unconditional surrender or he would loose his troops to murder, rape, and pillage, reflects the custom of the Middle Ages:

> Take pity of your town and of your people
> Whiles yet my soldiers are in my command . . . .
> If not, why, in a moment look to see
> The blind and bloody soldier with foul hand
> Defile the locks of your shrill-shrieking daughters;
> Your fathers taken by the silver beards,
> And their most reverend heads dashed to the walls;
> Your naked infants spitted upon pikes,
> Whiles the mad mothers with their howls confus'd
> Do break the clouds, as did the wives of Jewry
> At Herod's bloody-hunting slaughtermen.

What say you? Will you yield, and this avoid?
Or, guilty in defense, be thus destroy'd?
(Henry V, III, 2)

This savagery has become unacceptable. The pre-World War I Hague Conventions, for example, apply to land warfare and prohibit, among other things, "the attack or bombardment of towns, villages, habitations, or buildings which are not defended," as well as "the pillage of a town or place, even when taken by assault."

Following the horrors of World War I, provisions were added for the treatment of prisoners, as well as separate rules prohibiting the use of chemical and biological weapons. The League of Nations was singularly ineffective in preventing World War II, and the Hague rules designed to protect civilians were systemically ignored not only by Germany and the Soviet Union, but also by Britain in its firebombing of German cities, especially Dresden, Hamburg, and Berlin. The Dresden firebombing was immortalized by one of its survivors, prisoner-of-war Kurt Vonnegut, in his *Slaughterhouse-Five*.

Nor could the United States resist fire-bombing more than two dozen Japanese cities in 1945, and ultimately using two atomic weapons on the Japanese cities of Hiroshima and Nagasaki in August 1945. To this day, public discussion of the Hiroshima and Nagasaki bombings is muted in the United States. It remains impossible, for example, to even have an exhibit on the atomic bomb attacks on Japan that includes the victims in the US Air and Space Museum. Nonetheless, there was an almost immediate recognition in the United States that the Hague rules provided no protection in practice to civilians from indiscriminate bombings. In the words of a *Life* magazine editorial dated August 20, 1945:

> The Japanese Christian, old Kagawa, made a broadcast after the Hiroshima holocaust. He said that American cruelty, expressed in this horrible weapon, exceeded that of Genghis Khan and contrasted especially with the "careful and thoughtful" Japanese air raids on Shanghai and Nanking against which we protested so piously in 1937. Strange as this sounds, it is not untrue. Every step in bomber's progress since 1937 has been more cruel than the last. From the very concept of strategic bombing, all the developments—night, pattern, saturation, area, indiscriminate—have led straight to Hiroshima .... It is bootless to argue at what stage of modern warfare, or by whom, the old Hague rules of war were violated. The point is that Americans, no less than

Germans, have emerged from the tunnel with radically different practices and standards of permissible behavior toward others.[6]

Two basic justifications were given for dropping the first atomic bomb on a city. The first was (as it had been, at least up to the post-World War II recognition that *all* human beings had dignity and rights) that the laws of warfare applied only to the "civilized nations" and that uncivilized peoples could be killed with impunity.[7] As President Harry Truman himself put it on August 9, the day Nagasaki was bombed: "I know that Japan is a terribly cruel and uncivilized nation in warfare ...."[8] His position has a long pedigree, including the Crusades, the conquest of the New World, and global colonization. The second, and still the most prevalent, is that it "saved [American] lives" by making an invasion of Japan unnecessary.

World War II was followed by the first international war crimes trial in history, conducted at Nuremberg. In his opening statement to the international tribunal, made up of judges from the United States, England, France, and the Soviet Union, Justice Robert Jackson made it clear to all that he understood the critique that the tribunal was designed to render a "victor's justice" based on vengeance "which arises from the anguish of war," rather than justice based on international law. In his words:

> We must never forget that the record on which we judge these [Nazi] defendants today is the record on which history will judge us tomorrow. *To pass these defendants a poisoned chalice is to put it to our lips as well.* We must summon such detachment and intellectual integrity to our task that this trial will commend itself to posterity as fulfilling humanity's aspirations to do justice. (emphasis added)

The final judgment not only labeled the waging of aggressive war as a crime against humanity, but also cataloged specific acts, including murder, torture, and slavery, as war crimes and crimes against humanity. It was hoped that holding individuals accountable for committing such crimes would help prevent them in the future. It was also hoped, at least by the prosecution team, that the world would establish what was described as a "permanent Nuremberg" court to be on hand to hold individuals in the future accountable for war crimes and crimes against humanity. In 2000, the International Criminal Court was finally established based on this model, but the major military powers, including the United States, have so far refused to agree to its jurisdiction, primarily because they fear being judged unfairly and arbitrarily by the community of nations.

In short, the legacy of Nuremberg is mixed—perhaps inherently so since the primary sponsor of Nuremberg, the United States, continues to oppose a "permanent Nuremberg" tribunal, has never publicly acknowledged any doubts about the justice of using atomic weapons on civilian targets, and opposes treaties that would explicitly make first-strike use of nuclear weapons a war crime and a crime against humanity. Nonetheless, we have recognized that use of an improvised nuclear device by terrorists is perhaps the major risk we face from terrorism and that the world would be much better off with far fewer, and even better off with no, nuclear weapons.

Protecting Civilians in War

The killing of millions of civilians during World War II, as well as the deaths of millions of prisoners of war, led to an expansion of the Geneva Conventions, first with the Geneva Conventions of 1949 (especially IV, regarding the protection of civilians), and the two protocols of 1977 (especially protocol l, related to the protection of victims of international armed conflicts). The most specific requirements for protecting civilians appear in Article 51 of protocol l, Protection of the Civilian Population:

1. The civilian population and individual civilians shall enjoy general protection against dangers arising from military operations.
2. The civilian population as such, as well as individual civilians, shall not be the object of attack. Acts or threats of violence the primary purpose of which is to spread terror among the civilian population are prohibited.
3. Civilians shall enjoy the protection afforded by this section, unless and for such time as they take a direct part in hostilities.
4. Indiscriminate attacks [with no military objective] are prohibited . . . .

An occupying power is also responsible under the Geneva Conventions and the protocols to ensure that the civilian population is provided with food and medical supplies, and "to the fullest extent of the means available to it" with "clothing, bedding, means of shelter, [and] other supplies essential to the survival of the civilian population. . . . "

Civilian populations nonetheless continue to bear the brunt of modern warfare. Until the United States adopted its new counterinsurgency strategy in Iraq in 2007, civilian deaths were said to have been viewed with relative indifference. Thomas Ricks, for example, begins his book on the Iraq surge, entitled *The Gamble*, by describing the indiscriminate killing of women and children by Marines at Haditha on November 19, 2005. Following an attack on a Marine squad that killed one of their members and wounded two others, Marines attacked two nearby houses, kicking in the doors and killing everyone in the families that were home. Altogether, 24 Iraqis were killed, including women and children. As Ricks describes the failure of the Marine command even to investigate the incident (in words that parallel those of the *Life* editorial on Hiroshima):

> What happened that day in Haditha was the disturbing but logical culmination of the shortsighted and misguided approach the US military took in invading and occupying Iraq from 2003 through 2006: Protect yourself at all costs, focus on attacking the enemy, and treat the Iraqi civilians as the playing field on which the contest occurs.[9]

This is why General David Petraeus' counterinsurgency plan seemed so radical and novel for Iraq: Instead of treating civilians as the playing field, his plan called for protecting civilians, and isolating (but not necessarily killing) the enemy insurgents. Limiting civilian deaths also became part of the new strategy in Afghanistan in 2009 when the United States determined to send more troops there to counter a Taliban resurgence. When the presidents of Afghanistan and Pakistan visited Washington in May 2009, for example, the most contentious issue was the deaths caused by US airstrikes on a village in Farah province on May 4, 2009. Secretary of State Hillary Clinton personally expressed deep regret over this incident in which an unknown number, perhaps dozens, of innocent civilians were killed. She told Afghan President Hamid Karzai that even though all the circumstances were not known and that there would be an investigation of the airstrikes, "We deeply regret it . . . any loss of life, any loss of innocent life, is particularly painful. And I want to convey to the people of both Afghanistan and Pakistan that we will work very hard . . . to avoid the loss of innocent civilian life. And we deeply, deeply regret that loss."[10]

Similarly, the primary criticism of Israel for its late 2008 invasion of Gaza has been the loss of civilian lives and the reported indifference of at least some Israeli soldiers to killing civilians. Some complained that the war was being described as a "religious war" by the army's rabbi. The killing of civilians in Gaza led philosophers Avishai Margalit and Michael Walzer to suggest, consistent with the Geneva Conventions, that in future wars, Israeli soldiers should "Conduct your war in the presence of noncombatants on the other side with the same care as if your citizens were the noncombatants."[11] This high standard would seem to make any war in Gaza unjustifiable.

Perhaps because of this, not everyone was convinced that the killing of civilians in Gaza was either unjustified or out of proportion. Defense Minister Ehud Barak, for example, told Israel Radio that reported incidents of direct and intentional killing of civilians were the exception. In his words, "The Israeli Army is the most moral in the world, and I know what I'm talking about because I know what took place in the former Yugoslavia, [and] in Iraq."[12] In this instance, the defense minister sounded a lot like President Truman after Hiroshima—ready to not only justify the killing of civilians, but also to simultaneously claim the moral high ground in so doing. A United Nations fact-finding mission, led by Judge Richard Goldstone, later determined that Isreal's military had committed war crimes in the attack, including deliberate attacks against the civilian population, such as using Palestinians as human shields, attacking a mosque, and targeting food and water facilities.

As traumatic as killing "innocent civilians" is in wartime, it has seemed to be even more unacceptable to have one's own soldiers killed. The inability to deal with the deaths of one's own soldiers may lead Britain to withdraw its troops from Afghanistan, and had led the United States to adopt a policy, only recently changed, of denying the press access to casket arrival ceremonies at Dover Air Force Base, raising questions of war politics and family privacy.

American Military Casualties

The "Dover test" is shorthand for how many casualties the American public can tolerate before a war becomes politically unsustainable. The policy of banning the filming of the flag-draped coffins was first put into place by then Secretary of Defense Dick Cheney after President George H.W. Bush was televised laughing during an unrelated press conference on one half of a split TV screen while coffins of American soldiers returning from Panama at Dover were shown on the other half of the screen. The ban was retained during Operation Desert Storm, generally not followed during President Bill Clinton's administration, and reinstated at the outset of war in Iraq.

It was not changed until the beginning of the Obama administration, when it was modified so that the families of dead soldiers, whose expenses the government now pays to travel to Dover, are given the option of excluding the press. In the first month of the new policy, almost all of the 27 families of the dead soldiers made the trip to Dover to witness the casket arrival, and 19 permitted the news media access.[13] The original Bush press exclusion policy had been challenged in court, and the Court of Appeals for the District of Columbia upheld it.[14] The court concluded that the First Amendment did not give the press unlimited access to government installations and that family interests supported the policy. These family interests included the interest in reducing the hardship of the families who would feel under pressure to travel to Dover if public arrival ceremonies were held there (ceremonies were instead held at the soldier's home base), and "the interest in protecting the privacy of families and friends of the dead, who may not want media coverage of the unloading of caskets at Dover." The court noted that the family's privacy interest depends on the ability of outsiders to identify the particular soldier in the closed casket, but nonetheless concluded, "We do not think the government [is] hypersensitive in thinking that the bereaved may be upset at public display of the caskets of their loved ones."

But if there is really no way to identify the soldier in the casket (and even families are not permitted to open the casket to view the body), publication of a photograph does not implicate family privacy. In April 2004, for example, the Air Force responded to a request based on the Freedom of Information Act by releasing hundreds of photographs of flag-covered coffins at Dover. In the cover letter, Colonel Laurel A. Warish wrote, "We removed all personally identifying information of the remains as release could rekindle grief, anguish, pain, embarrassment, or disrupt the peace of mind of surviving family members, invading their privacy."[15] The photographs were posted on a Web site[16] and published by all the major media. Subsequently, the administration of President George W. Bush indicated that the official photos were provided in error and that the no-press policy would continue.[16] On the one hand, of course, any wartime administration may not want the official photos published for political reasons. On the other hand, it is plausible to argue that even though specific individual soldiers cannot be identified as occupying specific coffins, the family members of recently killed soldiers may nonetheless feel that their privacy is being violated by the publication of these photos.

There is no consensus among military families on the issue. The National Military Family Association has taken the position that "the privacy of families of the departed service members" is important and that "sensitivity to the grief of surviving families should be paramount [so that] how much the press is able to intrude at this very difficult time should be at the discretion of the individual family."[17] This permits families, rather than the government or the press, to determine whether photos of identifiable caskets can be taken, and even whether the press may be present when the caskets arrive at Dover. This is the new DOD policy, which was in place when President Obama did something no contemporary president has done: he went to Dover in the middle of the night in late October 2009 to witness the arrival of

18 flag-draped caskets. Because the family of Army Sergeant Dale R. Griffin agreed to allow the press to film the ceremonial transfer of his casket from the plane to the mortuary, the president's dignified participation in the casket arrival and transfer was seen around the world.

It is worth noting, nonetheless, that the family has no authority over the body at Dover. Since 2004, for example, every soldier killed in Iraq or Afghanistan has been given a whole body computed axial tomography scan, and since 2001 pathologists in the Armed Forces Medical Examiner System have performed autopsies on them. Both procedures are done at the Dover facility. Families are informed about the autopsy and can obtain a copy of the report. Journalists are not permitted inside the pathology lab.[18]

Military Medical Ethics

The continuing wars in Afghanistan and Iraq have brought renewed attention not only to civilian and military deaths, but also to the role of military physicians. Are physicians in the US military physicians first, soldiers first, or physician-soldiers—or does some other formulation best describe their medical–ethical obligations? Physician-bioethicist (and World War II veteran) Edmund Pellegrino, arguably the world's leading expert on military medical ethics, has insisted that medical ethics are and must be the same for civilian and military physicians "except in the most extreme exigencies."[19] Pellegrino argues that there are no special medical ethics for active-duty military physicians, any more than there are for Veterans Affairs physicians, National Guard physicians, public health physicians, prison physicians, or managed-care physicians.

The only real question is whether "extreme exigencies" exist that justify physicians' suspension of their medical-ethical obligations. It is not surprising that wars have produced battlefield situations in which suspending patient-centered medical ethics has seemed reasonable, at least to military commanders. Perhaps the best-known example from World War II is the decision during the North African campaign to provide penicillin first to troops with sexually transmitted diseases, rather than to seriously wounded troops, because the former could be quickly returned to combat.

In the first Gulf War, the primary medical-ethical problem was whether military necessity justified physicians prescribing investigational drugs without the informed consent of troops. More recently, controversy has also arisen about the use of psychotropic medications to retain soldiers in combat areas or to return them for another tour of duty. What role can ethical military physicians play in such situations?

The editors of the textbook *Military Medical Ethics* conclude that a military physician is a "physician first, officer second" and that "instances of significant conflict" between civilian and military medical ethics are "very rare."[20] This formulation states the problem rather than the solution, since it is only these "rare" cases (which could be labeled "worst case bioethics scenarios") involving "military necessity" that could require military physicians to betray medical ethics in favor of military or national security concerns. The use of the investigational drug pyridostigmine bromide as a chemical warfare "pretreatment" during the first Gulf War illustrates this point. In seeking a Food and Drug Administration (FDA) "waiver of informed consent" for use of the drug, the Department of Defense (DOD) confused military necessity with medical ethics.[21] In that case, the DOD thought that the FDA had granted permission to use an investigational drug without informed consent because the FDA had concluded that the drug was safe. The FDA, on the other hand, thought that DOD had sought permission to use the drug without informed consent because the DOD had concluded that use of the drug was required by military necessity.

In the war on terror, military physicians have faced at least three major challenges to medical ethics: orders that they help to interrogate terrorist suspects using "enhanced interrogation" methods; force-feeding prisoner hunger strikers at Guantanamo; and certifying soldiers as fit to be redeployed to Iraq or Afghanistan. As discussed at length in the last two chapters, the medical ethics rule in the first two instances is clear and is reinforced by international human rights standards: No physician can take part in any action involving torture or cruel or inhuman treatment, or use medical knowledge or skills for punishment.

The third example of ethical conflict is provided by military psychiatry. The durations of the wars in Iraq and Afghanistan and the shortage of troops have required that more troops receive mental health treatment for serious mental disorders than in previous wars, and suicide rates of both enlisted personnel and veterans is at an all-time high. Increasingly, soldiers' depression, posttraumatic stress disorder and anxiety are being treated with newer psychotropic medications, especially selective serotonin reuptake inhibitors (SSRIs). There is no military doctrine on the use of SSRIs in combat situations, but some military psychiatrists have recommended that their colleagues in Iraq "should consider having one SSRI in large quantities to be used for both depressive disorders and anxiety disorders" to, in the words of the motto of the Army medical corps, "conserve the fighting strength."[22] This goal is consistent with medical ethics only if the treatment is part of an overall personalized medical plan, is medically indicated, and is provided with the voluntary and informed consent of the soldier-patient.

At a 2006 press conference called to announce the DOD's new policies regarding the treatment of military prisoners, then Assistant Secretary of Defense for Health Affairs William Winkenwerder said:

> We operate under principles of medical ethics. There is no conflict medically, ethically speaking, in our view, between what we are doing and what's laid out in a variety of ethical documents in the medical world.... [As for hunger strikes,] we view what we are doing as largely consistent with that [Malta] declaration.[23]

Of course, "largely consistent" means that there must be parts that are inconsistent. As Winkenwerder went on to say, the new policy specifically authorizes physicians to violate the World Medical Association's Malta Declaration on torture and hunger strikes when ordered to do so. It may be understandable that the DOD does not want an international organization to set standards for the US military. Nonetheless, because medical ethics standards are universal, the DOD position should not be acceptable to the medical profession, and the American Medical Association (AMA) appropriately objected to it. The force feeding of hunger strikers in military custody is dealt with in detail in Chapter 5.

The DOD's new position that its physicians need not follow nationally and internationally accepted medical ethics represents a major policy change. Until 2006, and at least since Nuremberg, the US military has consistently operated under the assumption that its physicians are required to follow not only US medical ethics but also internationally recognized medical ethics. At Nuremberg, the US military went even further, asking the AMA to select an expert witness (the AMA selected Andrew Ivy) to explain the standards of medical ethics to the judges at the Nazi doctors' trial. Under existing military practice, ethics enforcement seems to have been left primarily to state medical licensing boards, which have tried to avoid investigating ethics complaints against active-duty military physicians. Until there is a special federal medical license for the military (not, I believe, a good idea), state licensing boards should take their responsibility to uphold ethical principles much more seriously.

Pellegrino has emphasized that "medical ethics begins and ends in the patient–physician relationship" and that there is no military exception to this rule. Thus, in the case of using SSRIs to prepare troops for redeployment, the military psychiatrist's loyalty must be to the patient-soldier's mental health and the prevention of further psychological injury. This conclusion does not mean that physicians can or should purposely under-mine the military mission by always recommending that their patients not be returned to combat. Rather, it is based on another judgment: that the US military is likely to be healthier, physically, mentally, and ethically, when its physicians can consistently follow medical ethics by treating their soldier-patients with dignity and honor. Thus it is wrong, I think, to argue that the military mission must take precedence over medical ethics. This position makes no more sense than saying that the soldier's pledge, to "never leave a fallen comrade on the battlefield" must not be honored if it could compro-mise the military mission.[24] In some instances it might, but in all instances the fighting force is likely to be stronger if soldiers know they will be cared for by both their comrades in arms and their physicians.

There are battlefield and prison conflicts that military physicians must resolve, but these conflicts are not captured by oversimplified expressions such as "mixed agency" or "dual loyalty." These frames set up a classic false choice. Basic human rights violations, including torture, inhumane treatment, and experimentation without consent, can never be justified. Other conflicts should be analyzed as possible exceptions in extremis to the rule that medical ethics are universal. What really seems to be happening in the US military is captured better under the rubric of "dual use" rather than dual loyalty. Specifically, it is not that the military physician has loyalty both to the patient and the military mission; it is that the military has learned that it can use physicians in two distinct ways (one of which is ethical, and the other of which is not): as physicians for care and treatment of patients, and as military officers for interrogation and punishment of prisoners. In short, the "physician first" guidance is only half the story; the other half is "last and always."

Finally, it is worth acknowledging another paradox of war, this time a bioethics paradox. Simply put, in war, healing becomes an integral part of killing. No matter how dedicated military physicians are to their patient-soldiers, war itself should never be romanticized: "There is no heroic tale to tell about war and medicine . . . in wartime, physicians minister to men's bodies in order that other men's bodies can be destroyed."[25]

It is not just in war, when civilians and soldiers are surrounded by death and disaster, that patients need physicians whose only loyalty is to them. In the next section, Death and the constitution, I deal with bioethics issues as they have been seen by judges, most especially by the Justices of the US Supreme Court, as well as by the members of the US Congress, notably dealing with worst case scenarios involving death. I begin the section with the death Americans fear more than any other: death from cancer.

II

....

DEATH AND THE CONSTITUTION

7

. . . .

Cancer

J.M. Coetzee's violent, antiapartheid *Age of Iron* is written as a letter by a retired South African classics professor to her daughter, who lives in the United States. Mrs. Curren is dying of cancer, and her daughter advises her to come to the United States for treatment. She replies, "I can't afford to die in America. . . . No one can, except Americans."[1] Dying of cancer has been considered a "hard death," a worst case scenario, for at least a century. Unproven and even quack remedies have been common, and cost has been a secondary consideration. Efforts sponsored by the federal government to find cures for cancer date from the establishment of the National Cancer Institute (NCI) in 1937. Cancer research was intensified after President Richard Nixon's declaration of a "war on cancer" and passage of the National Cancer Act of 1971, and again in 2009 when President Obama announced he would double the amount of money the NCI could spend on cancer research.

Frustration with the methods and the slow progress of mainstream medical research has helped fuel a resistance movement that distrusts both conventional medicine and government and that has called for the recognition of a right for terminally ill patients with cancer to have access to any drugs they want to take. Prominent examples include the popularity of krebiozen in the 1950s and of laetrile in the 1970s. As an NCI spokesperson put it more than 20 years ago, when thousands of people were calling the NCI hotline pleading for access to interleukin-2, "What the callers are saying is, 'Our mother, our brother, our sister is dying at this very moment. We have nothing to lose.'"[2] Today, families search the Internet for clinical trials; and even untested chemicals such as dichloroacetate seem to offer them some hope. In addition, basing advocacy on their personal experiences with cancer, many families have focused their frustrations on the Food and Drug Administration (FDA), which they see as a government agency denying them access to treatments they need.

In 2006, these families won an apparent major victory when the Court of Appeals for the District of Columbia, in the case of *Abigail Alliance v. Von Eschenbach*[3] agreed with their argument that patients with cancer have a constitutional right of access to investigational cancer drugs. In reaction, the FDA began rewriting its own regulations to make it easier for terminally ill patients not enrolled in clinical trials to have access to investigational drugs.[4] In late 2006, the full bench of the Court of Appeals vacated the three judge opinion, and the case was reheard by the full bench in March 2007.[5] The subsequent decision of the full bench hinged on the answer to the central question: Do terminally ill adult patients with cancer for whom there are no effective treatments have a constitutional right of access to investigational drugs that their physicians think might be beneficial? In this chapter, I concentrate on the now-reversed three judge opinion because its cancer-death-as-the-worst-case-scenario justification for authorizing the use of unproven medications is both legally novel and psychologically seductive.

Self-Defense and Saving Lives

The Abigail Alliance for Better Access to Developmental Drugs (the Abigail Alliance) sued the FDA to prevent it from enforcing its policy of prohibiting the sale of drugs that had not been proven safe and effective to competent adult patients who are terminally ill and have no alternative treatment options. The Abigail Alliance is named after Abigail Burroughs, whose squamous cell carcinoma of the head and neck was diagnosed when she was only 19 years old. Two years later, in 2001, she died. Before her death, she had tried unsuccessfully to obtain investigational drugs on a compassionate use basis from ImClone and AstraZeneca and was accepted for a clinical trial only shortly before her death. Her father founded the Abigail Alliance in her memory.[6]

The district court dismissed the Abigail Alliance lawsuit. The appeals court, in a 2-to-1 opinion written by Judge Judith Rogers, who was joined by Judge Douglas Ginsburg, reversed the decision. It concluded that competent, terminally ill adult patients have a constitutional "right to access to potentially life-saving post-Phase I investigational new drugs, upon a doctor's advice, even where that medicine carries risks for the patient," and remanded the case to the district court to determine whether the FDA's current policy violated that right.

The appeals court found that the relevant constitutional right was determined by the due process clause of the Fifth Amendment: "No person shall be . . . deprived of life, liberty, or property without due process of law." In the court's words, the narrow question presented by *Abigail Alliance* is whether the due process clause "protects the right of terminally ill patients to make an informed decision that may prolong life, specifically by use of potentially life-saving new drugs that the FDA has yet to approve for commercial marketing but that the FDA has determined, after Phase I clinical human trials, are safe enough for further testing on a substantial number of human beings."

The court answered yes, finding that this right has deep legal roots in the right to self-defense, and that "Barring a terminally ill patient from the use of a potentially life-saving treatment impinges on this right of self-preservation." In a footnote, the court restated this proposition: "The fundamental right to take action, even risky action, free from government interference, in order to save one's own life undergirds the court's decision." The court relied primarily on the *Cruzan* case,[7] in which the Supreme Court recognized the right of a competent adult to refuse life-sustaining treatment, including a feeding tube:

> *The logical corollary is that an individual must also be free to decide for herself whether to assume any known or unknown risks of taking a medication that might prolong her life.* Like the right claimed in *Cruzan*, the right claimed by the [Abigail] Alliance to be free of FDA imposition does not involve treatment by the government or a government subsidy. Rather, much as the guardians of the comatose [sic] patient in *Cruzan* did, the Alliance seeks to have the government step aside by changing its policy so the individual right of self-determination is not violated. (emphasis added)

The appeals court concluded that the Supreme Court's 1979 unanimous decision on laetrile,[8] in which the Court concluded that Congress had made no exceptions in the FDA law for terminally ill cancer patients, was not relevant because laetrile had never been studied in a Phase I trial and because the Court did not address the question of whether terminally ill cancer patients have a constitutional right to take whatever drugs their physicians prescribe.

Judge Thomas Griffith, the dissenting judge, argued that the suggested constitutional right simply does not exist. He noted, for example, that the self-defense cases relied on are examples of "abstract concepts of personal autonomy" and cannot be used to craft new rights. He concluded that the FDA's drug-regulatory efforts have been reasonable responses "to new risks as they are presented." Accepting his arguments leaves the majority resting squarely on *Cruzan* and the laetrile case. Regarding *Cruzan,* the dissent argued that "A tradition of protecting individual *freedom* from life-saving, but forced, medical treatment does not evidence a constitutional tradition of providing affirmative *access* to a potentially harmful, even fatal, commercial good." As to the laetrile case, the dissenting judge noted simply that the Supreme Court had agreed with the FDA that, "For the terminally ill, as for anyone else, a drug is unsafe if its potential for inflicting death or physical injury is not offset by the possibility of therapeutic benefit."

Finally, the dissenting judge argued that if the new constitutional right were accepted, it was too vague to be applied only to terminally ill patients seeking drugs that had been tested in Phase I trials. Specifically, the judge asked, must the right also apply to patients with "serious medical conditions," to patients who "cannot afford potentially life-saving treatment," or to patients whose physicians believe "marijuana for medicinal purposes . . . is potentially life saving?" In other words, there is no principled reason to restrict the constitutional right the majority created to either terminally ill patients or to post–Phase I drugs.

The facts, as illustrated by stories of patients dying of cancer while trying unsuccessfully to enroll in clinical trials, are compelling, and our current system of ad hoc exceptions to FDA rules is deeply flawed. The central constitutional issue, however, rests primarily on determining whether this case is or is not like the right-to-refuse-treatment case of Nancy Cruzan, a woman in a permanent vegetative state whose family wanted tube feeding discontinued because they believed that discontinuation was what she would have wanted. I do not think *Abigail Alliance* is like *Cruzan*. Rather, it is substantially identical to cases involving physician-assisted suicide, in which a terminally ill patient claims a constitutional right of access to physician-prescribed drugs to commit suicide.

The Supreme Court has decided, unanimously, that no right to access to physician-prescribed drugs for suicide exists.[9] There is no historical tradition of support for this right. And although the right seems to be narrowly defined, it is unclear to whom it should apply—Why only to terminally ill patients? Don't patients in chronic pain have even a stronger interest in suicide? Why is the physician necessary, and why are physician-prescribed drugs the only acceptable method of suicide? None of these questions can be answered by examining the Constitution.[10]

Similarly, in *Abigail Alliance*, the new constitutional right proposed has no tradition in the United States, and it cannot be narrowly applied. For example, why should a constitutional right apply only to people who have a particular diagnosis or medical status? And why should a physician be involved at all? If patients have a right to autonomy, why isn't the requirement of a government-licensed physician's recommendation at least as burdensome as the requirement of the FDA's approval of the investigational drug? And why would the Constitution apply only to investigational drugs for which Phase I trials have been completed? Why not include access to investigational medical devices, like the artificial heart, or even to Schedule I controlled substances, like marijuana or LSD? If it is a constitutional right, these interventions should be available too, at least unless the state can demonstrate a "compelling interest" in regulating them.

I predicted (not a terribly difficult prediction) that after rehearing this case en banc, the full Circuit Court would reject the position of the Abigail Alliance for the same reasons that the Supreme Court rejected the "right" of terminally ill patients to have access to physician-prescribed drugs they could use to end their lives. This is in fact what happened. The majority opinion for the full bench was written by the original dissenter, Judge Griffith, for himself and 8 of his colleagues. Only Judges Rogers and Ginsburg dissented.[11] For the Circuit Court to have decided otherwise would have entirely undermined the legitimacy of the FDA. Patients in the United States have always had a right to refuse any medical treatment, but we have never had a right to demand mistreatment, inappropriate treatment, or investigational or experimental interventions.

This will not, however, be the end of the matter. After the physician-assisted suicide cases, the fight appropriately shifted to the states, although so far only two, Oregon and Washington, have provided physicians with immunity for prescribing life-ending drugs to their competent, terminally ill patients. The debate begun with *Abigail Alliance* will continue in Congress and in the FDA itself.

Stories of Death in Congress and the FDA

Congressional action also had its birth with the story of one patient with cancer and was also heavily influenced by another individual patient involved in a controversy over removal of a feeding tube, discussed in detail in Chapter 11. "Terri's Law" was enacted in Florida in 2003 to try to prevent the removal of a feeding tube from Terri Schiavo. The case was substantially similar to *Cruzan*. Terri's case gained national attention two years later. In the midst of its media-driven frenzy, in March 2005, the *Wall Street Journal* asked, in an editorial titled "How About a 'Kianna's Law'?," "If Terri Schiavo deserves emergency federal intervention to save her life, people like Kianna Karnes deserve it even more." At the time, Kianna Karnes was a 44-year-old mother of four who was dying of kidney cancer. Her only hope of survival, according to the editorial, was to gain access to one of two experimental drugs in clinical trials, but neither of the two companies running the trials (Bayer and Pfizer) would make the drugs available to her on a compassionate use basis. This was because, according to the *Wall Street Journal*, the FDA "makes it all but impossible" for the manufacturers "to provide [drugs] to terminal patients on a 'compassionate use' basis."[12]

Almost immediately after the editorial was published, both drug man-ufacturers contacted Kianna's physicians to discuss releasing the drugs to her. But within two days after publication of the editorial, she was dead. The *Wall Street Journal* editorialized about Kianna again, "Isn't it a national scandal that cancer sufferers should have to be written about in the *Wall Street Journal* to be offered legal access to emerging therapies once they've run out of other options?"[13] It noted that Mrs. Karnes' father, John Rowe—himself a survivor of leukemia—was working with the Abigail Alliance on a Kianna's Law. That law, formally titled the Access, Compassion, Care, and Ethics for Seriously Ill Patients Act or the ACCESS Act, was introduced later in 2005 and was an attempt to make it much easier for seriously ill patients to gain access to experimental drugs.[14]

The act begins with a series of congressional findings, including that "Seriously ill patients have a right to access available investigational drugs, biological products, and devices." The act permits the sponsor to apply for approval to make an investigational drug, biologic product, or device available on the basis of data from a completed Phase I trial, "preliminary evidence that the product may be effective against a serious or life-threatening condition or disease," and an assurance that the clinical trial will continue. The patient, who must have exhausted all approved treatments, must provide written informed consent and must also sign "a written waiver of the right to sue the manufacturer or sponsor of the drug, biological product, or device, or the physicians who prescribed the product or the institution where it was administered, for an adverse event caused by the product, which shall be binding in every State and Federal court."

Congress is the proper forum to address this issue. Nonetheless, this initial attempt has some of the same problems as the three judge *Abigail Alliance* decision: The patients to whom it applies are ambiguously classified, and clinical research seems to be equated with clinical care. Also troubling is that the patients (and would-be subjects) are asked to assume all of the risks of the uncontrolled experiments, and current rules of research—which protect subjects by prohibiting mandatory waivers of rights—are jettisoned, with the requirement of such waivers becoming the price of obtaining the investigational agent from an otherwise reluctant drug company.

In direct response to the *Abigail Alliance* litigation, the FDA proposed amending its rules to encourage more drug companies to offer their investigational drugs through compassionate use programs. These programs first came into prominence during the early days of AIDS, when there were no effective treatments and AIDS activists insisted that they have early access to investigational drugs because, in the words of their inaccurate slogan, "A Research Trial Is Treatment Too."[15] Because the FDA could not stand the political pressure generated by the activists, the compassionate use program was developed as a kind of political safety valve to provide enough exceptions to save their basic research rules. In late 2006, the FDA continued this political safety valve approach by issuing new proposed regulations (which were adopted in 2009) with a title that could have been taken directly from the AIDS Coalition to Unleash Power (ACT-UP): "Expanded Access to Investigational Drugs for Treatment Use."[16]

As adopted in 2009, the FDA's new expanded-access regulations apply to patients who have "an immediately life-threatening disease or condition" or a "serious" disease or condition ("a disease or condition associated with morbidity that has substantial impact on day-to-day functioning"), where potential benefits justify potential risks, and providing the investigational drug "will not interfere with the initiation, conduct, or completion of clinical investigations . . ." Manufacturers are required to file an "expanded access submission," and the product must be administered or dispensed by a licensed physician who will be considered an "investigator," with the informed consent and reporting requirements that role entails.

These new FDA regulations may expand access to investigational drugs, but it seems unlikely. The major bottleneck in the compassionate use program has never been the FDA. The drug manufacturers have no incentives to make their investigational products available outside clinical trials. This is because direct access to investigational drugs by individuals may make it more difficult to recruit research subjects, and thus to conduct the clinical trials necessary for drug approval. Direct access to investigational drugs could also subject the drug manufacturer to liability for serious adverse reactions. Even without a lawsuit, a serious reaction to a drug outside a trial could adversely affect the trial itself.[17] The drug companies are right to worry that the approaches of the judiciary, Congress, and the FDA could make clinical trials more difficult to conduct, because few seriously ill patients who have exhausted conventional treatments would rather be randomly assigned to an investigational drug than have a guarantee that they will receive the investigational drug their physician recommends for them. This could result in significant delays in the approval and overall availability of drugs that demonstrate effectiveness—a result no one favors. Even if patients with cancer are willing buyers, drug manufacturers are not willing sellers.

Physicians and Death

The cover story for the proposed changes is patients' choice. But without scientific evidence of the risks and benefits of a drug, choice cannot be informed, and for seriously ill patients, fear of death will predictably overcome fear of unknown risks. This is understandable. As the late psychiatrist Jay Katz, the world's leading scholar on informed consent, noted, when medical science seems impotent to fight nature, "all kinds of senseless interventions are tried in an unconscious effort to cure the incurable magically through a 'wonder drug,' a novel surgical procedure, or a penetrating psychological interpretation."[18]

Another *Wall Street Journal* article, entitled "Saying No to Penelope," illustrates the impossibility of limiting access to unproven cancer drugs to competent adults. The article tells the story of 4-year-old Penelope, who is dying from neuroblastoma that was resistant to all conventional treatments. Her parents seek "anything [that] has a prayer of saving her." In her father's words, "The chance of anything bringing her back from the abyss now is very low. But the only thing I know for sure is if we don't treat her, she will die." With Penelope hospitalized and in pain, her parents continue "searching Penelope's big brown eyes for clues as to how long she wants to continue to battle for life."[19] It is suggested that the requirement of a physician's recommendation can safeguard against "magical thinking" and help make informed consent real.[20] But as Katz has noted, although physicians (and, he could have added, drug companies) often justify such last-ditch interventions as simply being responsive to patient needs, the interventions "may turn out to be a projection of their own needs onto patients."

Another recurrent theme in the drug-access-for-terminally-ill-patients movement is the belief that government regulation is evil, a central tenet of the laetrile litigation of the 1970s. The three judge panel in *Abigail Alliance* was correct to note that laetrile never underwent a Phase I trial, but every indication was that the drug, also known as vitamin B_{17}, was harmless, albeit also ineffective against cancer. Laetrile became a legal cause celebre in 1972, when California physician John A. Richardson was prosecuted for promoting laetrile. Richardson was a member of the John Birch Society, which quickly formed the Committee for Freedom of Choice in Cancer Therapy, with more than 100 committees nationwide.[21] It took another seven years before the FDA prevailed in its case against laetrile in the Supreme Court. The basic arguments against FDA regulation remain the same today: The FDA follows a "paternalistic public policy that prevents individuals from exercising their own judgment about risks and benefits. If the FDA must err, it should be on the side of patients' freedom to choose."[22]

The FDA would prevail again today, not only because there is no constitutional right of access to unapproved drugs, but also because, even if there were, the state has the same compelling interest in approving drugs as it has in licensing physicians. From a public policy view, the three judge *Abigail Alliance* court, the Congress, and the FDA all seem to have been suffering from the "therapeutic illusion" in which research, designed to test a hypothesis for society, is confused with treatment, administered in the best interests of an individual patient.[23] Of course there is a continuum, and it is perfectly understandable that many patients with cancer, told that there is nothing conventional medicine can do for them, will want access to whatever is available in or outside the context of clinical trials. But this is a problem for patients, physicians, the FDA, and drug manufacturers—not a solution. It is a problem for two fundamental reasons. First, terminally ill patients can be harmed and exploited—there are better and worse ways to die, and there really are fates worse than death. Second, it is only through research, not "treatment," that cancer may become a chronic illness that is treated with a complex array of drugs, given either together or in a progression.[24] The right to choose in medicine is a central right of patients, but the choices can and should be limited to reasonable medical alternatives, which themselves are based on available evidence.

This is, I believe, good public policy. But it is also much easier said than done.[25] Death really is our worst case scenario, and death is feared and even dreaded in our culture. Few Americans are able to die at home, at peace, with loved ones in attendance, without seeking the "latest new treatment." There always seems to be something new to try, and there is almost always anecdotal evidence that it could help. This is one reason why even extremely high prices do not affect demand for cancer drugs, even those that add little or no survival time, and why Medicare continues to pay for such drugs.[26] It is also why, as I reviewed in Chapter 1, rationing cannot even be discussed in the context of healthcare reform.

When does caring for the patient demand primary attention to palliation rather than to long-shot, high-risk, investigational interventions? Coetzee's Mrs. Curren, who rejected new medical treatment for her cancer and insisted on dying at home, told her physician, whom she saw as "withdrawing" from her after giving her a terminal prognosis: "His allegiance to the living, not the dying ... I have no illusions about my condition, doctor. It is not [experimental] care I need, just help with the pain."

Like Mrs. Curren, many cancer patients can face death, but would like drugs either to ease their pain or to end their lives. In the next chapter, I examine how the US Supreme Court has adjudicated the question of what power states have to enact laws permitting these actions: California's medical marijuana act and Oregon's death with dignity act.

8

. . . .

Drug Dealing

T here are at least two major alternatives to seeking unapproved drug treatments when facing a worst case scenario cancer death: seeking palliative care to control pain, or seeking drugs that can be used to end your life. This chapter continues the discussion (begun in Chapter 7) of the choices facing the terminally ill patient to include these options, and focuses on Supreme Court decisions involving the division of authority between the federal government and the states in regulating drugs used to control pain and produce death. In the first part of this chapter, I take up the question of whether the individual states have the authority to permit the use of marijuana for medical purposes in the face of a federal law outlawing such use. In the second part of the chapter, I examine the question of whether the US Attorney General can prohibit the states from permitting their physicians to write prescriptions for drugs with the intent that their terminally ill patients take them to commit suicide. Since both issues implicate highly volatile political questions, it seems reasonable to employ the great American writer, Mark Twain, to introduce the federalism issue at the heart of the marijuana question.

Mark Twain wasn't thinking about federalism or the structure of American government when he wrote "The Celebrated Jumping Frog of

Calaveras County."[1] Nonetheless, he would be amused to know that today, 150 years later, the Calaveras County Fair and Jumping Frog Jubilee not only has a jumping frog contest but also has its own Frog Welfare Policy. The policy includes a provision for the "Care of Sick or Injured Frogs" and a limitation entitled "Frogs Not Permitted to Participate," which stipulates that "under no circumstances will a frog listed on the endangered species list be permitted to participate in the Frog Jump."[2] This fair, like medical practice, is subject to both state and federal laws. Care of the sick and injured (both frogs and people) is primarily viewed as a matter of state law, whereas protection of endangered species is primarily regulated by Congress under its authority to regulate interstate commerce.

Not to carry the analogy too far, but it is worth recalling that Twain's famous frog, Dan'l Webster, lost his one and only jumping contest because his stomach had been filled with quail shot by a competitor. The loaded-down frog just couldn't jump. Until the California medical marijuana case, it seemed to many observers that the Supreme Court had succeeded in filling the Commerce Clause with quail shot—and had effectively prevented the federal government from regulating state activities. In the medical marijuana case, however, a new majority of justices took the lead out of the Commerce Clause so that the federal government could legitimately claim jurisdiction over just about any economic activity, including the practice of medicine.

Federalism, the Commerce Clause, and Medical Marijuana in California

The US Constitution specifies the areas over which the federal government has authority. All other areas remain, as they were before the adoption of the Constitution, under the authority of the individual states. Another way to say this is that the states retain all governmental authority they did not delegate to the federal government, including in areas such as criminal law and family law matters. These are part of the state's "police powers," usually defined as the state's sovereign authority to protect the health, safety, and welfare of its residents. Section 8 of Article I of the Constitution contains 18 clauses specifying delegated areas (including the military, currency, postal service, and patenting) over which "Congress shall have power," and these include the Commerce Clause—"to regulate commerce with foreign nations, and among the several states, and with the Indian tribes."

Until the Great Depression (and the disillusionment with unregulated markets), the Supreme Court took a narrow view of federal authority that could be derived from the Commerce Clause by ruling consistently that it gave Congress the authority only to regulate activities that directly involved the movement of commercial products (such as pharmaceuticals) from one state to another. Since then, and at least until 1995, the Court's interpretation seemed to be going in the opposite direction: Congress was consistently held to have authority in areas that had almost any relationship at all to commerce.

Under modern Commerce Clause doctrine, Congress has authority to regulate in three broad categories of activities: the use of the channels of interstate commerce (e.g., roads, air corridors, and waterways); the instrumentalities of interstate commerce (e.g., trains, trucks, and planes) and persons and things in interstate commerce; and "activities having a substantial relation to interstate commerce."[3] The first two categories are easy ones in that they involve activities that cross state lines. The third category, which does not involve crossing a state line, is the controversial one. The interpretation problem is the meaning and application of the concept of "substantially affecting" interstate commerce.

In a 1937 case that the Court characterized as a "watershed case" it concluded that the real question was one of the degree of effect. Intrastate activities that "have such a close and substantial relation to interstate commerce that their control is essential or appropriate to protect that commerce from burdens and obstructions" are within the power of Congress to regulate. Later, in what has become perhaps its best-known Commerce Clause case, the Court held that Congress could enforce a statute that prohibited a farmer from growing wheat on his own farm even if the wheat was never sold but was used only for the farmer's personal consumption. The Court concluded that although one farmer's personal use of homegrown wheat may be trivial (and have no effect on commerce), "taken together with that of many others similarly situated," its effect on interstate commerce (and the market price of wheat) "is far from trivial."[4]

The 1995 case that seemed to presage a states' rights revolution (often referred to as "devolution") was about the federal Gun-Free School Zones Act of 1990, which made it a federal crime "for any individual knowingly to possess a firearm at a place that the individual knows, or has reasonable cause to believe, is a school zone." In a 5-to-4 opinion, written by the late Chief Justice William Rehnquist, the Court held that the statute exceeded Congress's authority under the Commerce Clause and only the individual states had authority to criminalize the possession of guns in school.[5] The federal government had argued that the costs of violent crime are spread out over the entire population and that the presence of guns in schools threatens "national productivity" by undermining the learning environment, which in turn decreases learning and leads to a less productive citizenry and thus a less productive national economy. The majority of the Court rejected this argument primarily because they thought that accepting this line of reasoning would make it impossible to define "any limitations on federal power, even in areas such as criminal law enforcement or education where States historically have been sovereign."

In 2000, in another 5-to-4 opinion written by Rehnquist, using the same rationale, the Court struck down a federal statute, part of the Violence Against Women Act of 1994, that provided a federal civil remedy for victims of gender-motivated violence. In the Court's words: "Gender-motivated crimes of violence are not, in any sense of the phrase, economic activity." The Court continued, "Indeed, if Congress may regulate gender-motivated violence, it would be able to regulate murder or any other type of violence since gender-motivated violence, as a subset of all violent crime, is certain to have lesser economic impacts than the larger class of which it is a part."[6] The Court, specifically addressing the question of federalism, concluded that "the Constitution requires a distinction between what is truly national and what is truly local . . . we can think of no better example of the [state's] police power . . . than the suppression of violent crime and vindication of its victims."

The next Commerce Clause case is the one about medical marijuana, and whether California has the legal power to protect patients who used physician-recommended marijuana from federal criminal prosecution. In more technical terms, the question before the Court was, Does the Commerce Clause give Congress the authority to outlaw the local cultivation and use of marijuana for medicine if such cultivation and use complies with the provisions of California law?[7]

The California law, which is similar to laws in at least a dozen other states, creates an exemption from criminal prosecution for physicians, patients, and primary caregivers who possess or cultivate marijuana for medicinal purposes on the recommendation of a physician. Two patients for whom marijuana had been recommended brought suit to challenge enforcement of the federal Controlled Substances Act after federal Drug Enforcement Administration (DEA) agents seized and destroyed all six marijuana plants that one of them had been growing for her own medical use, in compliance with the California law. The Ninth Circuit Court of Appeals ruled in the plaintiffs' favor, finding that the California law applied to a separate and distinct category of activity, "the intrastate, noncommercial cultivation and possession of cannabis for personal medical purposes as recommended by a patient's physician pursuant to valid California state law," as opposed to what it saw as the federal law's purpose, which was to prevent "drug trafficking."[8] In a 6-to-3 opinion, written by Justice John Paul Stevens, with Justice Rehnquist dissenting, the Court reversed the appeals court's opinion and decided that Congress, under the Commerce Clause, did have authority to enforce its prohibition against marijuana—even state-approved, homegrown, noncommercial marijuana, used only for medicinal purposes on a physician's recommendation.

The majority of the Court decided that the Commerce Clause gave Congress the same power to regulate homegrown marijuana for personal use that it had to regulate homegrown wheat. The question was whether homegrown marijuana for personal medical consumption substantially affected interstate commerce (albeit illegal commerce) when all affected patients were taken together. The Court concluded that Congress "had a rational basis for concluding that leaving home-consumed marijuana out-side federal control" would affect "price and market conditions." The Court also distinguished the guns in school and gender violence cases on the basis that regulation of drugs is "quintessentially economic" when economics is defined as the "production, distribution, and consumption of commodities."

This left only one real question open: Is the fact that marijuana is to be used only for medicinal purposes on the advice of a physician, as the Ninth Circuit Court had decided, sufficient for an exception to be carved out of otherwise legitimate federal authority to control drugs? The Court decided it was not, for several reasons. The first was that Congress itself had determined that marijuana is a Schedule I drug, which includes only drugs that Congress believes have "no acceptable medical use." The Court acknowledged that Congress might be wrong in this determination, but the issue in this case was not whether marijuana had possible legitimate medical uses but whether Congress had the authority to make the judgment that it had none and to therefore ban all uses of the drug.

The dissenting justices argued that personal cultivation and use of marijuana should be beyond the authority of the Commerce Clause. The Court majority disagreed, stating that if it accepted the dissenting justices' argument, personal cultivation for recreational use would also be beyond congressional authority. This conclusion, the majority argued, could not be sustained, because it could start a worst case scenario in motion in which so many individuals would begin growing their own marijuana that it would have a substantial impact on both interstate commerce and legitimate federal drug enforcement.

The other primary limit to the effect of the California law on inter-state commerce is the requirement of a physician's recommendation on the basis of a medical determination that a patient has an "illness for which marijuana provides relief." The Court's discussion of this limit may be the most interesting, and disturbing, aspect of the case, at least to physicians. Instead of concluding that physicians should be free to use their best medical judgment and that it was up to state medical boards to decide whether specific physicians were failing to live up to reasonable medical standards—as the Court did, for example, in all but one of its cases related to restrictive abortion laws[9]—the Court took a much more cynical view of physicians and illegal drugs. The Court saw physicians as drug dealers, concluding that the broad language of the California medical marijuana law allows "even the most scrupulous doctor to conclude that some recreational uses would be therapeutic. And our cases have taught us that there are some unscrupulous physicians who overprescribe when it is sufficiently profitable to do so."

The California law defines the category of patients who are exempt from criminal prosecution as those suffering from cancer, anorexia, AIDS, chronic pain, spasticity, glaucoma, arthritis, migraine, and "any other chronic or persistent medical symptom that substantially limits the ability of a person to conduct one or more major life activities . . . or if not alleviated may cause serious harm to the patient's safety or physical or mental health." These strict limits are hardly an invitation for recreational use recommendations. Regarding "unscrupulous physicians," the Court cited two cases that involved criminal prosecutions of physicians for acting like drug dealers, one from 1919 and the other from 1975, implying that because a few physicians might have been criminally inclined in the past, it was reasonable for Congress (and the Court), on the basis of no actual evidence, to assume that many physicians may be so inclined today.

It was not only physicians that the Court found untrustworthy, but sick patients and their caregivers as well. The Court noted that the California exemption permitted patients to possess up to 8 ounces of dried marijuana and cultivate up to 6 mature or 12 immature plants, and simply assumed that the marijuana would not (and could not) be limited to medical use. In the Court's words, "The likelihood that all such production will promptly terminate when patients recover or will precisely match the patients' medical needs during their convalescence seems remote; whereas the danger that excesses will satisfy some of the admittedly enormous demand for recreational use seems obvious."

Justice Sandra Day O'Connor's dissent is especially relevant to bioethics, as she would leave the practice of medicine to state regulation. She argued that the Constitution requires the Court to protect "historic spheres of state sovereignty from excessive federal encroachment" and that one of the virtues of federalism is that it permits the individual states to serve as "laboratories," should they wish, to try "novel social and economic experiments without risk to the rest of the country." Specifically, she argued that the

Court's new definition of economic activity is "breathtaking" in its scope, creating exactly what the gun case rejected—a federal police power.

She also rejected reliance on the wheat case, noting that under the Agricultural Adjustment Act in question in that case, Congress had exempted the planting of less than 200 bushels (about six tons), and that when Roscoe Filburn, the farmer who challenged the federal statute, himself harvested his wheat, the statute exempted plantings of less than six acres. In O'Connor's words, the wheat case "did not extend Commerce Clause authority to something as modest as the home cook's herb garden." O'Connor was not saying that Congress cannot regulate small quantities of a product produced for personal use, only that the wheat case "did not hold or imply that small-scale production of commodities is always economic, and automatically within Congress' reach." As to potential "exploitation [of the act] by unscrupulous physicians" and patients, O'Connor found no factual support for this assertion and rejected the conclusion that simply by "piling assertion upon assertion" one can make a case for meeting the "substantiality test" of the guns in school and gender violence cases.

It is important to note that the Court was not taking a position on whether Congress was correct to place marijuana in Schedule I, or a position against California's law, any more than it was taking a position in favor of guns in schools or violence against women in the earlier cases. Instead, the Court was ruling only on the question of federal authority under the Commerce Clause. The Court noted, for example, that California and its supporters may one day prevail by pursuing the democratic process "in the halls of Congress." This seems extremely unlikely. More important to suffering patients are two unaddressed questions whether suffering patients have a substantive due process claim to access to drugs needed to prevent suffering or a valid medical necessity defense should they be prosecuted for using medical marijuana (or any other unapproved or illegal drug) on a physician's recommendation.[10] What is obvious from this case, however, is that Congress has the authority, under the Commerce Clause, to regulate both legal and illegal drugs whether or not the drugs in question actually cross state lines.

Whether the "states' rights" movement has any life left after the medical marijuana decision may ultimately be determined in the context of the Endangered Species Act. In this context, two US Circuit Courts of Appeals have upheld the application of the federal law to protect endangered species that, unlike the descendants of Mark Twain's jumping frog, have no commercial value. Even though the Supreme Court refused to hear appeals from both decisions, they help us understand the contemporary reach of congressional power under the Commerce Clause. One case involved the protection of six tiny creatures that live in caves (the "Cave Species")—three arthropods, a spider, and two beetles—from a commercial developer. The Fifth Circuit Court of Appeals noted that the Cave Species are not themselves an object of economics or commerce, saying: "There is no market for them; any future market is conjecture. If the speculative future medicinal benefits from the Cave Species makes their regulation commercial, then almost anything would be. . . . There is no historic trade in the Cave Species, nor do tourists come to Texas to view them." Nonetheless, the court concluded that Congress had the authority, under the Commerce Clause, to view life as an "interdependent web" of all species; that destruction of endangered species can be aggregated, like homegrown wheat; and that the destruction of multiple species has a substantial effect on interstate commerce.[11]

The other case, from the District of Columbia Court of Appeals, involved the arroyo southwestern toad, whose habitat was threatened by a real estate developer. In upholding the application of the Endangered Species Act to the case, the appeals court held that the commercial activity being regulated was the housing development itself, as well as the "taking" of the toad by the planned commercial development. The court noted that the "company would like us to consider its challenge to the ESA [Endangered Species Act] only as applied to the arroyo toad, which it says has no 'known commercial value'—unlike, for example, Mark Twain's celebrated jumping frogs [sic] of Calaveras County." Instead, the court concluded that application of the Endangered Species Act, far from eroding states' rights, is consistent with "the historic power of the federal government to preserve scarce resources in one locality for the future benefit of all Americans."[12]

Twain's short story has been termed "a living American fairy tale, acted out annually in Calaveras County."[13] An even more American "fairy tale" is that the government can effectively restrict the use of drugs by Americans through the criminal law. Like Twain's fairy tale, this one is retold over and over again, and most recently made its reappearance in the Supreme Court in the context of physician-assisted suicide by drug overdose.

Oregon's Physician-Assisted Suicide Law and Congress

The fact that Congress has authority over a particular subject, such as drug regulation, does not mean either that Congress will use it, or if it does, that its authority is unlimited. The Supreme Court also gets to determine the meaning of the laws Congress passes. This explains why it was not inconsistent for the Supreme Court to decide that California cannot permit patients of physicians who recommend marijuana, a Schedule I drug, to legally possess and use marijuana they may need to survive, but that Oregon can legally permit physicians to prescribe and patients to possess and use Schedule II drugs to end their lives.

The reason is that the California medical marijuana case was decided on the basis of determining the meaning of the Commerce Clause of the Constitution; the Oregon physician-assisted suicide case, on the other hand, was decided by determining the intent of Congress when it passed the Controlled Substances Act. In the California case, Congress had outlawed any use of marijuana by including it in Schedule I for drugs that have "no currently acceptable medical use." The legal question was whether Congress had the constitutional authority to do this under its Commerce Clause powers. In the Oregon case, the power of Congress to regulate the use of drugs in the practice of medicine was not at issue. Congress can set national drug prescribing rules. The question before the Court in the Oregon case was what, if anything, Congress had actually done when it enacted the Controlled Substances Act to limit the authority of states to set medical practice standards

As Justice Anthony Kennedy, the author of the 6-to-3 Oregon opinion, states it: "The question before us is whether the Controlled Substances Act (CSA) allows the United States Attorney General to prohibit doctors from prescribing regulated drugs for use in physician-assisted suicide, notwithstanding a state law permitting the procedure."[14] The opinion notes that in the 1997 physician-assisted suicide cases, the Court had unanimously concluded that there was no constitutional right to a physician's assistance in suicide. In that case, the Court had observed that "Americans are engaged in an earnest and profound debate about the morality, legality, and practicality of physician-assisted suicide."[15] Given this, the Court makes it clear that it is not determining whether Oregon's law is a good, bad, or neutral. Instead, its opinion is limited to interpreting the CSA to determine whether the Attorney General's action is authorized by the statute.

The Oregon statute, the first (in 2008 Washington's became the second) to grant immunity to physicians who write prescriptions for a lethal dose of drugs for their competent, terminally ill patients who ask for such a prescription at least twice, was adopted by ballot measure in 1994, and again in 1997.[16] In 1997, then Attorney General Janet Reno was asked by a group of senators to rule that prescribing drugs for suicide was not a "legitimate medical practice" (as required by the CSA), and that therefore writing such prescriptions could result in loss of DEA licensure and federal criminal prosecution. She refused because she believed that the CSA did not authorize her to "displace the states as the primary regulators of the medical profession, or to override a state's determination as to what constitutes legitimate medical practice."

John Ashcroft, who was one of the senators who had asked for Reno's intervention, was appointed Attorney General in 2001 after he had lost his bid for reelection to an opponent who died during the campaign. In November 2001, Ashcroft issued an Interpretive Rule that states:

> *Assisting suicide is not a "legitimate medical purpose"* within the meaning of 21 CFR 1306.04 (2001), and prescribing, dispensing, or administering federally controlled substances to assist suicide violates the Controlled Substances Act. Such conduct by a physician registered to dispense controlled substances may "render his registration . . . *inconsistent with the public interest*" and therefore subject to possible suspension or revocation . . . *regardless of whether state law authorizes or permits such conduct* by practitioners or others and regardless of the condition of the person whose suicide is assisted.[17] (emphasis added)

Every prescription filled under the Oregon law has been for Schedule II drugs; these drugs cannot be prescribed without a DEA registration, and dispensing controlled substances without a valid prescription is a federal crime. The Oregon law could simply not survive the Ashcroft rule. A lawsuit was filed in the US District Court of Oregon, which enjoined the enforcement of the rule.[18] The Court of Appeals for the Ninth Circuit affirmed, holding that the Ashcroft rule was invalid because, by making a medical procedure authorized under Oregon law a federal offense, it changed "the usual constitutional balance between the States and the Federal Government" without a clear Congressional statement authorizing this change.[19]

As a general rule, courts permit executive branch officials charged with administering statutes to interpret their meaning. Courts usually give their interpretations "substantial deference," at least when the statute is ambiguous and Congress has delegated authority to the executive agency to "make rules carrying the force of law, and that the agency interpretation claiming deference was promulgated in the exercise of that authority." Otherwise the interpretation is "entitled to respect" only to the extent it has the "power to persuade." Accordingly, the Court had to determine how much deference Attorney General Ashcroft's interpretation of the CSA deserved. The Court decided it didn't deserve much, for three basic reasons. First, the Court found the government's argument that the Attorney

General was really just interpreting one of his own regulations unpersuasive, since the regulation did "little more than restate the terms of the statute itself," like a parrot, and thus the Attorney General was actually interpreting the statute itself, not one of his own regulations. Second, the Court concluded that the CSA is not ambiguous: Congress did not delegate authority to the Attorney General to interpret it. Third, the Court concluded that what limited authority Congress had delegated to the Attorney General to register physicians is much more restricted than claimed. The Attorney General did have the power to revoke the registration of a physician who falsified an application or was convicted of a felony, but, the Court concluded, nothing in the CSA gives the Attorney General the power to "define the substantive standards of medical practice as part of his authority." Instead, the Court noted that it is the Secretary of Health and Human Services who has authority under the Controlled Substances Act to set medical standards, specifically those involving "the medical treatment of narcotic addiction."

To support this conclusion, the Court referred directly to an international treaty (something Justice Kennedy is more likely to do than the other justices), the Convention on Psychotropic Substances, which the United States had ratified. When passing a statute to enforce the Convention, Congress specifically stated that "nothing in the Convention will interfere with the ethical practice of medicine as determined by [the Secretary of Health and Human Services] on the basis of a consensus of the American medical and scientific community." The Court found that the structure of the CSA is the same as the structure of its law enforcing the Convention, and thus conveys an unwillingness on the part of Congress "to cede medical judgments to an Executive official who lacks medical expertise." Congress has the constitutional authority to delegate medical authority to the Attorney General. But the Court found that Congress did not do so because, among other reasons, the judgments the Attorney General claims legal authority to make are "quintessentially medical judgments . . . beyond his expertise and incongruous with the statutory purposes and design." Citing one of its prior cases, the Court concluded: "Congress, we have held, does not alter the fundamental details of a regulatory scheme in vague terms or ancillary provisions—it does not, one might say, hide elephants in mouseholes."

The final argument the Court considered is that the CSA itself prohibits physician-assisted suicide with controlled substances because this use of Schedule II drugs is not a "legitimate medical practice." In the California medical marijuana case, the Court concluded that in enacting the CSA, Congress sought to "conquer drug abuse and to control the legitimate and illegitimate traffic in controlled substances." The Court had not previously had occasion, however, to determine "the extent to which the CSA regulates medical practice beyond prohibiting a doctor from acting as a drug pusher instead of a physician." The Court had previously decided that the CSA prohibits "large-scale over prescribing of methadone" not consistent with accepted medical practice,[20] and in the California case, that Congress itself had expressly found that marijuana had no accepted medical use.

The Court ruled that the CSA cannot be reasonably read, based on its "text and design" as prohibiting physician-assisted suicide. This is because "the statute manifests no intent to regulate the practice of medical generally," and under basic principles of federalism, the states have "great latitude under their police powers to legislate as to the protection of the lives, limbs, health, comfort, and quiet of all persons." The Court not only concluded that the practice of medicine is a state-regulated activity and that Congress did not mean to make it federally regulated by the CSA, but also that the Oregon law itself is a good example of how states actually regulate the practice of medicine:

> Rather than simply decriminalizing assisted suicide, [the Oregon law] limits its exercise to the attending physicians of terminally ill patients, *physicians who must be licensed by Oregon's Board of Medical examiners . . . .* The statute gives attending physicians a central role, requiring them to provide prognoses and prescriptions, *give information about palliative alternatives and counseling, and ensure patients are competent and acting voluntarily.* Any eligible patient must also get a second opinion from another registered physician, and the statute's safeguards require physicians to keep and submit to inspection detailed records of their actions. (emphasis added)

Nonetheless, the Court found the Attorney General's contention that physician-assisted suicide is not a legitimate medical practice because it violates the position of prominent medical organizations, the federal government, and 49 states, "at least reasonable." Usually, a "reasonable" finding by the Court would lead it to defer to the Attorney General's interpretation of a statute. But the Court ruled it could not accept this "reasonable" conclusion because Congress did not authorize the Attorney General "to bar a use simply because it may be inconsistent with one reasonable understanding of medical practice." Instead, the Court concluded that the Attorney General's powers under the CSA are limited to drugs that have a potential for drug abuse, such as addiction or recreational use. The Court finished the opinion by characterizing its ruling as a "common sense" one in that "the background principles of our federal system . . . belie the notion that Congress would use such an obscure grant of authority to regulate areas traditionally supervised by the States' police powers."

The federalism background is simply the historical fact that states have traditionally licensed physicians and regulated the practice of medicine. Federal activity has been historically limited to regulating the manufacture and sale of drugs and devices, and controlling drug trafficking and recreational use. Once a drug is approved as "safe and effective" for a particular use, physicians are able to prescribe it for other uses consistent with the practice of medicine, as determined by state law and actual medical practice. Ultimately, the Court ruled, nothing Congress did in the CSA changed the respective roles of the states and the federal government.[21]

Justice Antonin Scalia would have deferred to the Attorney General's interpretation of the CSA, and he wrote a dissent. His most powerful argument, I think, is that Congress had set an objective federal standard of "legitimate medical practice" in the CSA. Under this federal standard it was (as the majority conceded) "at least reasonable" (a phrase Scalia describes as testing "the limits of understatement") for the Attorney General to conclude that, based on the laws of 49 states and the federal government, and on basic medical ethics standards, assisting in a patient's suicide is not a legitimate medical purpose for writing a drug prescription. Scalia argued that the majority has confused "the *normative* inquiry of what the boundaries of medical *should* be—which it is laudably hesitant to undertake—with the *objective* inquiry of what the accepted definition of medicine *is*." Justice Scalia continued, "The fact that many in Oregon believe that the boundaries of 'legitimate medicine' *should* be extended to include assisted suicide does not change the fact that the overwhelming weight of authority . . . confirms that they have not yet been so extended." (emphasis in original)

Justice Scalia also rejected the hiding "elephants in mouseholes" metaphor as an apt description of congressional intent, noting that the Attorney General had only attempted to regulate the uses of controlled substances outside addiction and recreational use in four areas: assisted suicide, aggressive pain management, anabolic steroid use, and cosmetic weight loss. In none of these four areas, Scalia argued, has the Attorney General's assertion of power done anything to undermine the statutory scheme. Scalia seemed intent on dismissing the mouseholes metaphor, possibly because it was he himself who first used it in a Supreme Court decision which he wrote for the majority.[22] The actual origin of the phrase is obscure, but may be related to, "fitting an elephant through a keyhole" which itself seems to have come from a phrase used by Samuel Richardson in *Clarissa*: "love will draw an elephant through a keyhole."[23] Of course, none of these actions is actually possible in the real world, and Scalia's attempt to construct a congressional intent to define a federal standard for the practice of medicine ultimately fails. Nonetheless, his argument is worth summarizing because it mostly concerns his views of medical ethics.

Scalia primarily argued that what is at stake in physician-assisted suicide has nothing to do with medical expertise, science, or medicine, but instead rests on a "naked value judgment" about the legitimacy of physician-assisted suicide, and that therefore the Attorney General is every bit as capable of making the judgment as the Secretary of Health and Human Services. In Scalia's words, the determination of whether physician-assisted suicide with drug overdoses is a legitimate medical procedure "no more depends upon a quintessentially medical judgment than does the legitimacy of polygamy or eugenic infanticide. And it requires no particular medical training to undertake the objective inquiry into how the continuing traditions of Western medicine have consistently treated this subject." Scalia knows better, as he seems to purposely conflate medical practice and medical judgment. The first involves a generic legal statement of what physicians can do; the second involves a normative ethical question of what physicians should do with individual patients. Justice Scalia closed his opinion by agreeing with the majority that Congress can outlaw physician-assisted suicide if it wants to:

> The federal commerce power to prevent assisted suicide is unquestionably permissible. The question before us is not whether Congress *can* do this, or even whether Congress *should* do this; but simply whether Congress *has* done this in the CSA. I think there is no doubt that it has. If the term "legitimate medical purpose" has any meaning, it surely excludes the prescription of drugs to produce death. (emphasis in original)

Like most judicial opinions devoted to interpreting a statute, this one about the CSA is not all that monumental, and Congress can rewrite the statute if it disagrees with the Court's interpretation. Although the vote was 6 to 3, the outcome of the case was difficult to predict in advance. I have never been all that enamored with the Oregon law, and I continue to believe that Oregon's approach to provide physicians with immunity for prescribing drugs for suicide is flawed both because it undercuts medical professionalism by making prescribing drugs for possibly suicidal terminally ill patients "much more bureaucratic and burdensome, and less private and accountable" and because it requires physicians to "specifically intend the deaths of their patients."[24]

Nonetheless, more than a decade after its enactment, in a contest between the seldom-used Oregon statute and a federal agency's assertion of power over all US physicians' scheduled drug prescriptions, it was not really possible to sympathize with the Attorney General. Moreover, the DEA had seemed much more menacing to physicians during the Bush administration.[25] End-of-life care specialists Timothy Quill and Diane Meier, for example, suggested that had the Court ruled the other way, "physicians may become hesitant to prescribe the best available medications to manage the pain, agitation, and shortness of breath that sometimes accompany the end stages of illness. As a result, they may, in essence, abandon patients and their families in their moment of greatest need."[26]

To the extent that their prophecy might have been correct, this opinion should be a major comfort to physicians, for two reasons. First, the majority found great significance in the fact that the Oregon statute sets procedures for physicians to follow and has explicit trust in physicians following them to exercise medical judgment. Thus, the Court's characterizations of some physicians as potential criminals in the California medical marijuana case now seems limited to physicians involved in drug trafficking of the type covered by the CSA. Second, the opinion strictly limits the jurisdiction of the DEA to physicians who are actually involved in traditional drug trafficking. Physicians treating terminally ill patients, or cancer patients at any stage of their illness, never had much to fear from the DEA; now they have nothing to fear from it at all. As Quill and Meier might put it, to the extent that "for better or worse, the DEA sets the tone and drives perceptions about legal risk associated with prescribing Schedule II drugs for seriously ill and dying patients," the tone should be nothing but supportive of palliative care designed to keep patients free from pain and discomfort.

Virtually anything that encourages what has been termed "a palliative ethic of care"[27] has strong public support, and is supported by the Court as well. This is probably why, although all nine justices agreed that Congress has the constitutional authority under the Commerce Clause to outlaw the prescription of controlled substances for physician-assisted suicide at any time, there has been no movement in Congress to do so. The lack of Congressional reaction to the opinion may also reflect the overwhelming condemnation by the public of Congress's bizarre and circus-like attempt to countermand the medical (and legal) judgments about the treatment of Terri Schiavo.

Now that there is no serious question that Congress has the authority to regulate the practice of medicine under the Commerce Clause, the issue of national medical licensure and national medical practice standards should receive more attention. The Court is certainly correct to note that, historically, Congress has been loath to legislate medical practice, preferring to see the areas in which it has legislated, like drug trafficking, recreational drug use, female genital mutilation, and even so-called partial-birth abortion, not as medical practice at all, but something outside the practice of medicine. Nonetheless, unsustainable tension exists between the historic role of the state in licensing physicians and setting medical practice standards, and arguments in favor of national practice standards. Any national healthcare access or financing reform will only increase this tension and move us closer to national licensing of physicians. Medical schools are all substantially identical in their training, and all their graduates must pass the same national examinations. State licensure seems a relic in a country where actual practice standards are national and where local variations from them are seen as both cost and quality problems. And Congress has acted to attempt to control medical practices that it has viewed as intolerable, most notably in the area of medical research standards to protect human subjects and emergency treatment standards in hospitals to protect patients experiencing a medical emergency from being turned away or transferred without medical assessment and stabilization.

The question is not whether national practice standards, for physicians and hospitals, could be a good thing—they could be. The question is who will have the authority to set the practice standards. It is one thing to decide that national standards will be set by the relevant specialty boards or other national medical organizations on the basis of evidence that supports their relevance to the health and welfare of patients. It is quite another thing to say they will be set by Congress or the Attorney General on the basis of the political winds of the day. This fear is currently driving much of the political concern with cost-effectiveness analysis in medicine, and is not entirely irrational. Chapters 10 and 11 deal with examples of politics overwhelming medicine and bioethics in the areas of partial-birth abortion and the removal of a feeding tube from Terri Schiavo. But before exploring these worst case bioethics scenarios, I address another case of Supreme Court–approved physician drug use: execution by lethal injection.

9

Toxic Tinkering

Michel Foucault opened his 1975 book *Discipline and Punish* with a gruesome account of a French execution in 1757 that included tearing the flesh away with hot pincers and applying boiling oil to what remained, followed by drawing and quartering of the body by four horses.[1] In the 18th century, the goals of torturing to death were retribution and deterrence by spectacle. Executions slowly moved away from worst case scenario, violent torture executions to methods that were seen as being more humane, such as hanging, shooting by a firing squad, electrocution, and lethal gassing. Executions also became much less public spectacle, usually with only a few members of the public permitted to witness the execution.

In the United States, a recurring question has been whether particular methods of execution are consistent with the Eighth Amendment to the Constitution, which states: "Excessive bail shall not be required, nor excessive fines imposed, nor cruel and unusual punishments inflicted." The most recent execution technique to raise this question is lethal injection. In 1977, Oklahoma became the first state to adopt lethal injection, and today it is used in 36 states and by the federal government. In this context, law professor Deborah Denno has argued persuasively that in adopting lethal injection execution, "The law turned to medicine to rescue the death penalty."[2]

After a number of statutes authorizing lethal injection were passed, but before the country's first execution by lethal injection in 1982, lawyer William Curran and physician Ward Casscells wrote an influential article arguing that physicians should not participate in executions by lethal injection. They suggested that lethal injection, unlike other methods, "presents the most serious and intimate challenge in modern American history to active medical participation in state-ordered killing of human beings... [since] this procedure requires the direct application of biomedical knowledge and skills in a corruption and exploitation of the healing profession's role in society."[3] The American Medical Association (AMA) and other medical societies quickly followed their advice, declaring the participation of physicians in executions by lethal injection unethical. Ethics, of course, is critical to the medical profession. But as bioethicist Robert Veatch noted at the time, no principle of medical ethics itself defines or sets legal limits to the physician's role in executions.[4] This helps explain why some physicians still participate in executions by lethal injection.[5]

Much of the Supreme Court's lethal injection decision, *Baze v. Rees*, reads like Foucault's *Discipline and Punish*. Foucault, for example, analyzed the manner of torture in executions as well as the movement to replace the vicious executioner with "a whole army of technicians . . . warders, doctors, chaplains, psychiatrists, [and] psychologists." Likewise, in *Baze*, the Supreme Court highlighted not only past uses of torture, but also issues of contemporary medical practice and medical ethics, including the drugs used, their method of delivery, and the qualifications of the persons involved. The Court also discussed the similarities and differences between veterinary euthanasia practices, as well as the Dutch protocols for euthanasia. The decision in *Baze*, which did not address the constitutionality of the death penalty itself, is fragmented and fractured, consisting of opinions written by seven different justices. Seven of the nine justices agreed that Kentucky's protocol for lethal injection, which was at issue in this case, is constitutional as is, but no more than three justices—Chief Justice John Roberts and two justices (Kennedy and Alito), who signed his plurality opinion—could agree on a specific standard that executions by lethal injection must meet.

In his plurality opinion, Roberts reviewed the previous use of hanging, electrocution, firing squad, and lethal gas in executions. He concluded that the motivation for adopting lethal injection as the exclusive or primary means of execution was "a desire to find a more humane alternative" to these brutal methods.[6] Thirty of the 36 states (including Kentucky) that have adopted lethal injection use a three-drug combination in their protocols:

The first drug, sodium thiopental is a fast-acting barbiturate sedative that induces a deep, comalike unconsciousness.... *The second drug, pancuronium bromide* is a paralytic agent that inhibits all muscular-skeletal movements and... stops respiration. *Potassium chloride, the third drug*, interferes with the electrical signals that stimulate the contractions of the heart, inducing cardiac arrest. The proper administration of the first drug ensures that the prisoner does not experience any pain associated with the paralysis and cardiac arrest caused by the second and third drugs. (emphasis added)

Kentucky's written protocol provides, among other things, that 3 grams of the first drug, 50 milligrams of the second drug, and 240 millimoles of the third drug be used. The intravenous catheters are placed by either a certified phlebotomist or an emergency medical technician with at least a year of experience. Other personnel mix the solutions and load them into syringes. The execution team administers the drugs from a control room, and the warden and deputy warden keep the prisoner under visual inspection. "A physician is present to assist in any effort to revive the prisoner in the event of a last-minute stay of execution" but by statute is prohibited from participating in the "conduct of an execution, except to certify the cause of death."

The petitioners, who were sentenced to death, sought to have the Kentucky protocol for lethal injection declared unconstitutional. A trial court concluded that the risk of improper administration of the drugs was minimal. The Kentucky Supreme Court agreed, holding that a method of execution violates the Eighth Amendment only if it "creates a substantial risk of wanton and unnecessary infliction of pain, torture or a lingering death."[7] This Kentucky opinion is the one that was appealed to the Supreme Court.

Chief Justice Roberts also reviewed previous Supreme Court execution opinions, noting an 1879 case in which the Court said simply, "it is safe to affirm that punishment of torture ... and all others in the same line of unnecessary cruelty, are forbidden by the Eighth Amendment." That opinion provided examples from England in which "terror, pain, or disgrace" were added to execution itself; these forms of punishment included being "emboweled alive, beheaded, and quartered" and sentenced to "public dissection... and burning alive." Roberts concluded that "What each of the forbidden punishments had in common was the deliberate infliction of pain for the sake of pain." In his words, the test of constitutionality must present more than a simple risk of needless suffering. To prevail, the condemned prisoner must "establish that the State's lethal injection protocol creates a demonstrated risk of severe pain ... that is substantial when compared to the known and available alternatives."

The condemned petitioners alleged that there was a risk that the dose of thiopental would be inadequate to render the prisoner unconscious, thus causing cruel suffering. Roberts, however, found that this risk was not substantial. He also concluded that the state had no constitutional obligation to adopt an alternative method, to adopt methods used to euthanize animals, or to assist in the suicide of terminally ill patients. The euthanasia of animals and assisted suicide both involve the use of a single overdose of a barbiturate.

Medical Ethics and Lethal Injection Executions

Justice Samuel Alito wrote a concurring opinion because he was concerned that the plurality opinion might be read as an invitation to litigants to suggest alternative methods of lethal injection that would "significantly reduce a substantial risk of severe pain." Alito noted that the majority of justices (including himself) proceed from two assumptions: the death penalty is constitutional, and lethal injection is a constitutional means of execution. Therefore, he argued, the use of lethal injection "must not be blocked by procedural requirements that cannot practicably be satisfied." The major practical constraint, he noted, is the ethics of the medical profession.

Physicians could, he wrote, make lethal injections even less risky, "But the ethics rules of medical professionals—for reasons that I certainly do not question here—prohibit their participation in executions." Justice Alito went on to cite the rulings of the AMA, as well as those of the American Nurses Association and the National Association of Emergency Medical Technicians, opposing participation in executions. He did this to make a point: Objections to current methods of lethal injection that can be remedied by medical participation cannot be regarded as being either "feasible" or "readily" available, and therefore cannot be constitutionally required. Moreover, he concluded, the Court should not get involved with micromanaging how executions by lethal injection are carried out, because this could "produce a de facto ban on capital punishment by adopting method-of-execution rules that lead to litigation gridlock."

Justice Clarence Thomas (in an opinion joined by Scalia) suggested his own constitutional standard. Thomas believes that the method of execution "violates the Eighth Amendment only if it is deliberately designed to inflict pain." He listed examples that would be unconstitutional under his standard: burning at the stake, gibbeting ("hanging the condemned in an iron cage so that his body would decompose in public view"), public dissection, emboweling alive, breaking on the wheel, flaying alive, crucifixion, "rendering asunder with horses," and mutilating and scourging to death.

The following penalty, pronounced on seven men convicted in England of high treason, would, Thomas wrote, be unconstitutional: "That you and each of you, be taken to the place . . . of execution, where you shall be hanged by the necks, not till you are dead; that you will be severally taken down, while yet alive, and your bowels be taken out and burnt before your faces—that your heads be then cut off, and your bodies cut in four quarters . . . ." Justice Thomas argued that the purpose of these "aggravated forms" of execution was to "terrorize the criminal," thereby deterring crime. He wrote that the "evil the Eighth Amendment targets is intentional infliction of gratuitous pain." Since lethal injection was adopted by the state legislatures and the federal government to make execution more humane, it could not be unconstitutional. The fact that the method might involve a risk of pain does not, in his view, raise a constitutional issue. If it did, Thomas expressed concern that the review of acceptable risks would require the Court "to resolve medical and scientific controversies that are largely beyond judicial ken."

Justice Stephen Breyer began his own opinion by adopting Justice Ruth Bader Ginsburg's test of constitutionality: Does the method create "an untoward, readily avoidable risk of inflicting severe and unnecessary suffering?" He believes that the key to making such a determination is found in the facts and evidence presented in the legal record of the case and in the medical literature. His reading of these sources did not persuade him that there was sufficient evidence to find that the Kentucky protocol poses a "significant and unnecessary risk of inflicting severe pain."

A 2005 article in the *Lancet* by Leonidas Koniaris and others has received wide attention in the courts in the United States, but it was not relied on by the litigants in this case.[8] Justice Breyer reviewed the study, which concluded that toxicologic testing at autopsy suggested that the amount of barbiturate used could leave the inmate conscious enough to suffer during the execution. He noted that others have criticized the study for relying on blood levels of thiopental taken hours to days after death (which may not indicate the level at the time of execution) and for a lack of scientific evidence of the person's actual awareness during the execution. Because of these criticisms, and because no one used the study in the case, Breyer concluded that "a judge, nonexpert in these matters, cannot give the *Lancet* study significant weight." Breyer also noted that the paralytic agent, pancuronium bromide, is used in the Netherlands for assisted suicide and euthanasia, which suggests that this method does not produce suffering. He concluded, nonetheless, that the call for better-trained executioners is not likely to be met by physicians who oppose participation in executions, so that even "finding better-trained personnel may be more difficult than might, at first blush, appear."

Justice Ruth Bader Ginsburg wrote the sole dissenting opinion, which Justice David Souter joined. She believes that the constitutionality of the Kentucky execution method turns exclusively "on whether inmates are adequately anesthetized by the first drug in the protocol, sodium thiopental . . . ." In her view, the Kentucky protocol fails to ensure unconsciousness because it "lacks basic safeguards used by other States to confirm that an inmate is unconscious before injection of the second and third drugs." She would have remanded the case for the trial court to determine whether the failure to use these safeguards "poses an untoward, readily avoidable risk of inflicting severe and unnecessary pain." In terms of simple safeguards adopted by other states, she noted that in Kentucky, "No one calls the inmate's name, shakes him, brushes his eyelashes to test for a reflex, or applies a noxious stimulus to gauge his response."

Of course it is death that is the elephant in the execution chamber, and it can certainly seem like it is being ignored by concentrating on the method of execution rather than on death itself. This helps explain why Justice John Paul Stevens used his concurring opinion to argue that the death penalty itself is unconstitutional, primarily for the reasons set forth in *Furman v. Georgia* (i.e., the risk of error, the risk of discrimination, and the excessiveness of the penalty).[9] But Stevens also added a new reason: In attempting to adopt a more humane method of execution, society has actually undermined its remaining primary purpose—retribution. In his words, by making execution less painful, "we necessarily [and appropriately] protect the inmate from enduring any punishment that is comparable to the suffering inflicted on his victim." Thus, the costs to society of the death penalty are not outweighed by any benefits. In addition, Stevens argued provocatively that Kentucky has outlawed the use of pancuronium bromide for animal euthanasia because of the risk of suffering and that, "It is unseemly—to say the least—that Kentucky may well kill petitioners using a drug that it would not permit to be used on their pets."

Justice Antonin Scalia wrote separately solely to refute what he characterized as Stevens' "astounding position that a criminal sanction expressly mentioned in the Constitution violates the Constitution." He argued that Stevens' position is based solely on "judicial fiat" and that it is not for individual justices but for state legislatures to decide whether the death penalty serves a public purpose such as retribution. Scalia opined, "I would think it difficult indeed to prove that a criminal sanction fails to serve a retributive purpose—a judgment that strikes me as inherently subjective and insusceptible of judicial review."

Fragmented as they are, the opinions speak pretty well for themselves. However, at least two points—the primary ones made by Justices Thomas and Alito—are dubious. Justice Thomas' insistence that it is only the "intentional" infliction of torture that is prohibited by the Eighth Amendment is almost the identical argument (although one made in the context of a statute, not the Constitution) that his former law clerk, John Yoo, made in the now infamous Department of Justice "torture memos" discussed in Chapter 4. In one of these memos, Yoo wrote that to constitute torture under federal law, "severe pain must be inflicted with specific intent . . . [and] knowledge alone that a particular result is certain to occur does not constitute specific intent."[10]

Justice Alito's point is similarly overstated. It is the role of the Court to determine what is and what is not constitutional. If the Court requires that procedures be followed to make the death penalty constitutional, and a state cannot follow them, then the state must stop executing convicted criminals. This is the teaching of the major death penalty case (*Furman*), in which all nine justices wrote separate opinions. In *Furman*, the justices held, among other things, that if procedures could not be put in place to minimize the risk of arbitrary and capricious death sentences, the death penalty simply could not be imposed. Thus, in the highly unlikely event that a future Court requires physician participation, and physicians refuse, the lethal injection method could not be used.

The Future of Physician Participation

Before *Baze* was decided, physician Atul Gawande had suggested that a fundamental question raised by the case was "whether physicians should take charge to make [lethal injection] deaths less painful."[11] Physician Robert Truog argued that if the inmate requests the involvement of a physician to prevent suffering, he could not think "of any principle of medical ethics that would say that this is an unethical thing for the physician to do."[12] Truog's position seems to rest on the proposition that the Hippocratic principle, "first, do no harm," is an insufficient guide, since it begs the question of whether it is proper to help in the prevention or alleviation of suffering in this context. He is not alone in this view.[13] But as bioethicist Arthur Caplan has persuasively noted, this argument rings hollow in the context of medical care in prison. On the one hand, in his words, "It seems a bit late for physicians to step forward in the context of an execution and say they are motivated by a duty of mercy given that many prisoners suffer miserably because of the poor state of prison-based medicine without eliciting any involvement from these same physicians."[14] On the other hand, one of the physicians interviewed by Gawande appeared to have provided continuous medical treatment to the death row prisoners before their execution, and in this admittedly rare circumstance a more principled argument for physician participation at the request of the condemned prisoner could be made.[15]

The more central principle at stake here, however, is that it is a violation of medical ethics for physicians to put their medical skills at the service of the state to facilitate the commission of crimes against humanity. Such crimes include murder and torture, as well as harmful experimentation without consent. Under the principles of the World Medical Association and the Geneva Conventions, these crimes also include cruel, inhuman, and degrading treatment, and the use of medical treatment as punishment.[16]

The majority of the Supreme Court does not believe that, as currently practiced, with or without the participation of physicians, executions by lethal injection are "cruel" as that term is used in the Eighth Amendment. Medical ethics is, of course, not synonymous with US constitutional law. Physicians may also reject this conclusion and refuse to participate on the grounds that even if it is not cruel or tortuous, execution by lethal injection is nonetheless inhuman and degrading to such an extent that it is unethical for physicians to participate by using their medical skills to kill in the service of the state. Nonetheless, at least some physicians would find it ethically acceptable to try to lessen the risk of suffering by improving on the existing protocols generally or even by changing them from a three-drug protocol to a one-drug protocol that produces death quickly and painlessly.[17]

The arguments for improving the methods of lethal injection are not entirely new. More than 20 years ago, for example, the Court heard a challenge to the three-drug protocol that argued that the Food and Drug Administration (FDA) should be required to certify these drugs as "safe and effective" for the purpose of execution.[18] The petition to the FDA noted that the FDA has certified drugs used to euthanize animals for the prevention of pain and discomfort, and it argued that humans should be treated at least as well as animals. This argument persists. The petition in *Baze* alleged that even a slight error in dosage could leave prisoners conscious but paralyzed while dying, a witness to their own slow, painful, and lingering asphyxiation. The FDA rejected the original petition, and the

Supreme Court later ruled unanimously that it was "solely in the FDA's discretion whether or not to exercise its enforcement authority over the use of drugs in interstate commerce."[19]

After *Baze*, it has also been suggested that states that have been trying to improve their methods of lethal injection are performing human experimentation involving prisoners, and are performing these experiments without either protocol review or informed consent, contrary to both medical ethics and federal and state regulations regarding human experimentation.[20] This is another way to recast the earlier argument that the FDA should have had to approve the drugs used for lethal injection as "safe and effective" for this purpose—by conducting research to demonstrate safety and efficacy. The FDA declined to do this, most likely because it did not want to get into the controversy regarding the death penalty and because it is difficult to see how any such study could be ethically conducted. This remains the case today when modifications of current protocols are proposed. Nonetheless, with or without physicians, courts and state legislatures may move to adopt single-drug protocols that have less risk of inflicting pain. An Ohio trial court did this, citing an Ohio law that requires that the drugs used "quickly and painlessly cause death."[21] Some states may also adopt Justice Ginsberg's suggestion. When Missouri, for example, carried out its first execution since *Baze* in May 2009 (of Dennis Skillicorn), curtains in the witness viewing area were closed for two minutes after the first drug was administered so the "medical staff" could make sure Skillicorn was unconscious and the catheters were functioning properly before the second and third drugs were administered.[22]

Curran and Casscells were correct in observing that lethal injection is not any part of "normal medical practice . . . but a corruption and exploitation of the health profession's role in society." Conducting medical research, even to achieve a more humane or less painful way of performing lethal injections, would be a similar perversion of the practice of medicine. Permitting a physician to administer the lethal injection at the prisoner's request to help reassure the prisoner that the process is likely to be painless would be another perversion. Consent cannot be voluntary in the execution chamber, and even if it could, consent cannot render an unethical act—such as torture, direct killing, or even physician-assisted suicide—ethical.

The Supreme Court did not and cannot solve this medical ethics problem for America's physicians. State legislatures continue to have the authority under the Constitution to determine whether or not to require executions by lethal injection, and physicians continue to have the legal freedom to determine whether placing their medical skills at the service of the state to execute condemned prisoners is consistent with medical ethics. In this regard, physicians could again come to the rescue of the law by helping corrections officials make executions by lethal injection less risky, less cruel, and more medicalized, routinized, and sanitized. This form of physician participation would follow Foucault's view of the "double process" of modern rituals of execution: "the disappearance of the spectacle and the elimination of pain."

None of the justices even suggested that physicians should be required to participate in or be present during executions by lethal injection. All the justices who mentioned medical ethics supported medicine's ethical stand against physician participation. The bottom line for physicians is clear: The law does not require physicians to be involved in administering the death penalty, and the future "involvement of physicians in executions will [continue to] be up to the medical profession."[23] To the extent that executions by lethal injection without physician participation could ultimately turn the public away from supporting capital punishment itself, this seems to be a much better outcome than medicalizing the death penalty in order to save it.

The relationship between capital punishment and more humane forms of execution is complicated. For example, like Gawande, one can be for the death penalty and yet be opposed to physician participation in it. Similarly, one can, like Human Rights Watch, be opposed to the death penalty but still insist that until it is abolished states must use the method that risks the "least possible pain and suffering of the inmate."[24]

Physicians should not lend their medical expertise to the state to make executions more palatable to the public, even by advising on drug protocols, doses, and routes of administration, any more than (as discussed in Chapter 4) they should lend their expertise to torturers even (or especially) with the goal of protecting the life and health of the person being tortured. Even physicians who support the death penalty should refuse to participate in executions, because the problem that the state seeks to solve by using physicians is one of the state's own making (by its refusal to abolish capital punishment and its insistence on execution by lethal injection).[25]

For physicians who oppose capital punishment, more than medical ethics is involved in refusing to participate in executions. Basic fairness in applying the death penalty is also at stake. By rejecting even the role of expert adviser in redesigning drug protocols, physicians will be joining Justice Harry Blackmun. After more than 20 years of attempting to fairly apply the death penalty, he abandoned his support for it, saying that it was wrong for the Court to substitute "mere aesthetics" for principles and that he would no longer "tinker with the machinery of death."[26]

Blackmun's concept of toxic tinkering is a powerful one, and can be used not just to describe ways in which to "improve" lethal injection techniques for condemned prisoners. In the next chapter, on abortion, I will explore why the Court adopts this strategy itself, when it instructs physicians how to kill near-term fetuses using the lethal injection technique to avoid potential criminal liability under the federal "partial-birth abortion" law.

10

....

Abortion

Abortion has been a central bioethics and biopolitics issue in America at least since the 1973 Supreme Court decision in *Roe v. Wade*. The political debate has been framed as pro-choice versus pro-life; protecting the rights of the pregnant woman against the life of the fetus. It has gotten us nowhere, and overall public attitudes toward abortion have not changed significantly in the past three decades. This makes the first two actions of the avowedly pro-choice President Obama regarding abortion especially noteworthy. In his first act, two days after becoming president and on the 36th anniversary of *Roe v. Wade*, he issued a short statement which encapsulated his views:

> On the 36th anniversary of *Roe v. Wade*, we are reminded that this decision not only protects women's health and reproductive freedom, but stands for a broader principle: that government should not intrude on our most private family matters. I remain committed to protecting a woman's right to choose.

The statement went on, however, to suggest common ground. "No matter what our views, we are united in our determination to prevent unintended pregnancies, reduce the need for abortion, and support women and families in the choices they make." To do this, President Obama wrote, "we must work to find common ground to expand access to affordable contraception, accurate health information, and preventative services ... [and] recommit ourselves more broadly to ensuring that our daughters have the same rights and opportunities as our sons ...." The following day President Obama rescinded the Mexico City Policy, first adopted by President Ronald Reagan in 1984, rescinded by President Bill Clinton in 1993, and re-adopted by President George W. Bush in 2001. That policy instructed the US Agency for International Development (USAID) to not only withhold aid to nongovernmental organizations (NGOs) that paid for abortions "as a method of family planning" or paid "to motivate or coerce any person to practice abortion" (a limitation on international aid funding placed by the Congress), but expanded this funding restriction to include NGOs that use non-USAID funds to engage in a wide range of activities, including providing advice, counseling, or information regarding abortion, or lobbying foreign governments to legalize or make abortion available. President Obama did this, he wrote, not only because the restrictions are "excessively broad" and "unwarranted," but also because "they have undermined efforts to promote safe and effective voluntary family planning programs in foreign nations."

In a statement the president issued to go with the policy change he said, "For too long, international family planning assistance has been used as a political wedge issue, the subject of a back and forth debate that has served only to divide us. I have no desire to continue this stale and fruitless debate." President Obama stated his objective of opening a "fresh conversation" on family planning with a goal to reduce unintended pregnancies but also to "promote safe motherhood, reduce maternal and infant mortality rates, and increase educational and economic opportunities for women and girls."

President Obama made it clear that he really does want to open a new American chapter in the abortion debate when he delivered the commencement address at Notre Dame University in May 2009. There he said, to an enthusiastic audience, that our abortion debate should be carried out with "open hearts, open minds, [and] fair-minded words." He told the graduates and their families, "Maybe we won't agree on abortion, but we can still agree that this heart-wrenching decision for any woman is not made casually. It has both moral and spiritual dimensions."

Few would disagree with the president's assessment of the abortion debate as "stale and fruitless," or with the president's call to reframe the debate in a more civil and potentially constructive direction. The continued power of this debate to divide the country, however, was underlined by the president himself in his healthcare address to a joint session of Congress in September 2009 when he said that there would be no funds in his health-care reform plan to pay for abortions. The real question is whether it is possible to move beyond the abortion debate by focusing on prevention of unintended pregnancies, making adoption more available, and guaranteeing good prenatal care for pregnant women. There is some hope, although a renewed discussion should include an appreciation of where we have been since *Roe v. Wade*, and an acknowledgment that the "partial-birth abortion" law, that has been at the center of political debate for more than a decade, has been a dangerous detour that has taken us to a dead end rather than a crossroads.

Partial Birth Abortion in the Supreme Court

The president concentrated his early remarks on abortion on women and girls, and did not mention the physicians who care for them until the murder of a prominent physician who performed abortions, George Tiller, shortly after his Notre Dame speech. Obama immediately denounced the killing, saying he was "shocked and outraged" by it and that differences over abortion "cannot be resolved by heinous acts of violence."

The Supreme Court would agree with the president on the murder, but a majority of the Court has also made it clear that they would also characterize at least some late-term abortions as heinous acts of violence. And it is because of this that the Court was, in its most recent abortion opinion, able to reverse itself and prohibit American physicians, for the first time in US history, from employing a legitimate medical procedure that the physician believes is medically indicated as the safest for the patient. The full implications of Court's 2007, 5-to-4 decision in *Gonzales v. Carhart*[1] will only be realized in the coming years. It is not too early to consider it a worst case bioethics scenario, made possible only by portraying "partial-birth abortion" as the most extreme and brutal medical procedure ever invented, and by accepting lethal injection killing of a near-term fetus as a reasonable alternative.

The opinion concerned a procedure that physicians, including the American College of Obstetricians and Gynecologists, term "intact dilation and extraction," (intact D & E) and that the anti-abortion community, the Congress, and a majority of states have labeled "partial-birth abortion." The partial-birth abortion label uses overtly inflammatory political language that ties abortion to childbirth to implicitly condemn this method of abortion as "infanticide." Like the Mexico City policy, presidential politics determined the fate of this legislation.

Previous bills to outlaw partial-birth abortions were twice passed by Congress, and twice vetoed by President Bill Clinton, who nonetheless said he would sign a ban if the Congress included an exception for the health of the woman.[2] In 2000, the Supreme Court ruled that substantially identical state statutes, which had been enacted in more than half of the states, were unconstitutional because the procedure they attempted to outlaw was too vaguely described, and because there was no exception for the health of the woman.[3] Nonetheless, political activism continued to seek prohibition. To improve its chances before the Supreme Court, Congress slightly modified the definition of the prohibited procedure, and in a preface declared that it was "never medically necessary." President George W. Bush signed the modified bill into law on November 5, 2003.[4]

By the time the Supreme Court reviewed the new law, it was a different Court than the one that had declared the substantially identical law unconstitutional in 2000. Most importantly, Justice Sandra Day O'Connor had been replaced by Justice Samuel Alito. Alito was nominated to the Court primarily because of the expectation that he would vote to reverse *Roe v. Wade*.[5] He did not disappoint, but joined with Chief Justice John Roberts and the Court's two most consistently anti-*Roe* members, Justices Antonin Scalia and Clarence Thomas, to give Justice Anthony Kennedy's opinion the five votes it needed to be the majority. In short, the political strategy to reframe the abortion debate in America to focus on a medical procedure—"partial-birth abortion"—rather than on either women or fetuses, succeeded in the Court.[6]

Justice Kennedy, who in 1992 had co-authored the joint opinion in *Casey*[7] that upheld the "core" of *Roe v. Wade*,[8] but who dissented in the 2000 *Stenberg* case (in which the Court found state laws prohibiting partial-birth abortions unconstitutional), was given the opportunity to turn his partial-birth-abortion dissent into the law of the land. Kennedy opens his opinion with descriptions of what "for discussion purposes" he termed "intact D&E," relying almost exclusively on first-hand accounts from one physician and one nurse who had described how the procedure was done in the early 1990s. The physician, Martin Haskell, described how after the fetus is partially delivered, the physician forces a "scissors into the base of the skull" and then "evacuates the skull contents" before removing the fetus "completely from the patient." In Kennedy's words, "This is an abortion doctor's clinical description."

The unnamed nurse described Haskell's procedure as beginning by grabbing the "baby's legs" with forceps, pulling the baby down the "birth canal" until "everything but the head is delivered.... The baby's little fingers were clasping and unclasping, and his little feet were kicking." She continued, "Then the doctor stuck the scissors in the back of his head, and the baby's arms jerked out . . . the doctor . . . sucked the baby's brains out . . . . He threw the baby in a pan, along with the placenta and the instruments he had just used." Kennedy concedes that the procedure "has evolved," and that other doctors do it differently. But these other methods, like squeezing the skull, crushing the skull, or even decapitating the fetus prior to removing it, do not seem much of an improvement.

Only after these descriptions does Kennedy quote the language of the 2003 federal law that was meant to respond to the constitutional defects in the Nebraska law that a majority of the Court had identified in *Stenberg:*

(a) Any physician who, in or affecting interstate or foreign commerce, knowingly performs a partial-birth abortion and thereby kills a human fetus shall be fined under this title or imprisoned not more than 2 years, or both. This subsection does not apply to a partial-birth abortion that is necessary to save the life of a mother whose life is endangered by a physical disorder, physical illness, or physical injury, including a life-endangering physical condition caused by or arising from the pregnancy itself . . . .

(b) (1) the term 'partial-birth abortion' means an abortion in which the person performing the abortion—

(A) deliberately and intentionally vaginally delivers a living fetus until, in the case of a head-first presentation, the entire fetal head is outside the body of the mother, or, in the case of breech presentation, any part of the fetal trunk past the navel is outside the body of the mother, for the purpose of performing an overt act that the person knows will kill the partially delivered living fetus; and

(B) performs the overt act, other than completion of delivery, that kills the partially delivered living fetus . . . .

It is worth noting in passing that, consistent with the California medical marijuana case and the Oregon physician-assisted suicide case discussed in Chapter 8, the Court does not even find it necessary to discuss whether the Commerce Clause gives the federal government authority to regulate abortions—it simply accepts this conclusion as a given (and I think properly so). Federal jurisdiction is not the constitutional problem here. All three US District courts and all three Courts of Appeal that had examined this federal law found it unconstitutional under the principles in *Casey* and *Stenberg*, primarily because of the vagueness of the procedure's definition, and the lack of a health exception for the pregnant woman. Most of Kennedy's opinion addresses these two central issues.

Regarding the vagueness argument, Kennedy thinks that the new federal law cures the defects of the Nebraska statute that had been found unconstitutional. The Nebraska law was held to create an "undue burden" on women because their physicians could not readily distinguish the prohibited procedure from the commonly performed D&E procedure, and thus might not perform even the legal D&E procedure for them. The Nebraska law, which carried a penalty of up to 20 years in prison, reads in relevant part:

> No partial-birth abortion shall be performed in this state, unless such a procedure is necessary to save the life of the mother whose life is endangered by a physical disorder, physical illness, or physical injury, including a life-endangering physical condition cause by or arising from the pregnancy itself.
> [a "partial-birth abortion" is] an abortion procedure in which the person performing the abortion partially delivers vaginally a living unborn child before killing the unborn child and completing the delivery....["partially delivers vaginally a living unborn child before killing the unborn child" means] deliberately and intentionally delivering into the vagina a living unborn child, or a substantial portion thereof, for the purpose of performing a procedure that the person performing such procedure knows will kill the unborn child and does kill the unborn child.

Kennedy believes that the new law is no longer vague because it "adopts the phrase 'delivers a living fetus' instead of 'delivering . . . a living unborn child, or a substantial portion thereof.'" He also finds that this new law makes the distinction between the prohibited procedure and standard D&E abortions clear. This is primarily because the federal law specifies fetal landmarks (e.g., the "navel") instead of the vague description used in the Nebraska law, "substantial portion" of the "unborn child."

Since the law applies to both previable and viable fetuses, Kennedy concedes that under *Casey* the law would be unconstitutional "if its purpose or effect is to place a substantial obstacle in the path of a woman seeking an abortion before the fetus attains viability." Kennedy, however, finds that Congress wanted to do two things: First, Congress wanted to "express respect for the dignity of human life" by outlawing "a method of abortion in which a fetus is killed just inches before completion of the birth process," because use of this procedure "will further coarsen society to the humanity

of not only newborns, but of all vulnerable and innocent human life . . . . ."
Second, Congress wanted to protect medical ethics, finding that this procedure "confuses the medical, legal and ethical duties of physicians to
preserve and promote life . . . . "

The key to Kennedy's legal analysis is his conclusion that these
reasons are constitutionally sufficient to justify the ban because under
Casey "the State, from the inception of pregnancy, maintains its own
regulatory interest in protecting the life of the fetus that may become a
child [and this interest] cannot be set at naught by interpreting *Casey*'s
requirement of a health exception so it becomes tantamount to allowing
the doctor to choose the abortion method he or she might prefer." His
conclusion follows:

> Where it [the State] has a rational basis to act, and it does not impose
> an undue burden, the State may use its regulatory power to bar
> certain procedures and substitute others, all in the furtherance of its
> legitimate interests in regulating the medical profession in order to
> promote respect for life, including the life of the unborn.

Kennedy then goes on to describe the majority's view of women. He
writes that "respect for human life finds an ultimate expression in the bond of
love the mother has for her child," and that "while no reliable data" exists on
the subject, "it seems unexceptionable to conclude some women come to
regret their choice to abort the infant life they once created and sustained . . . .
Severe depression and loss of esteem can follow." Such regret, Justice
Kennedy believes, can be caused or exacerbated if a woman later learns
the details of what the abortion procedure entailed. He suggests that physicians fail to describe the procedure to patients because they "may prefer not
to disclose precise details of the means [of abortion] that will be used . . . ."
From this he concludes that the new law, even though it cannot itself prevent
one abortion (only change the method used) is rationally based because it may
save some fetuses:

> It is a reasonable inference that a necessary effect of the regulation and
> the knowledge it conveys will be to encourage some women to carry
> the infant to full term, thus reducing the absolute number of late-term
> abortions. *The medical profession*, furthermore, *may find different and less
> shocking methods to abort* the fetus in the second trimester, thereby
> accommodating legislative demand. The *State's interest in respect for life*
> is advanced by the dialogue that better informs the political and legal
> systems, the medical profession, expectant mothers, and society as a

whole of the consequences that follow from a decision to elect a late-term abortion. (emphasis added)

The final, closely related issue is whether the prohibition would "ever impose significant health risks on women," and whether physicians or Congress should make this determination. Kennedy picks Congress: "The law need not give abortion doctors unfettered choice in the course of their medical practice, nor should it elevate their status above other physicians in the medical community. . . . Medical uncertainty does not foreclose the exercise of legislative power in the abortion context any more than it does in other contexts." Furthermore, Kennedy argues, the law does not impose an undue burden on women for another reason: Alternative ways of killing a fetus exist and have not been prohibited, and not only standard D&E. In his words, "If the intact D&E procedure is truly necessary in some circumstances, it appears likely *an injection that kills the fetus is an alternative under the Act that allows the doctor to perform the procedure.*" (emphasis added)

Writing for the four justices in the minority, Justice Ruth Bader Ginsburg opens her dissent by observing, "Today's decision is alarming. It refuses to take *Casey* and *Stenberg* seriously. It tolerates, indeed applauds, federal intervention to ban nationwide a procedure found necessary and proper in certain cases by the American College of Obstetricians and Gynecologists (ACOG)." She continues, " It blurs the line, firmly drawn in *Casey*, between previability and postviability abortions. And, for the first time since *Roe*, the Court blesses a prohibition with no exception safeguarding a woman's health."

Ginsburg argues (correctly in my view) that the majority of the Court have overruled *Stenberg*'s conclusion that a health exception is required as long as "substantial medical authority supports the proposition that banning a particular abortion procedure could endanger women's health [because a division in medical opinion] at most means uncertainty, a factor that signals the presence of risk, not its absence." This conclusion, bolstered by evidence presented by nine professional organizations, including ACOG, and conclusions by all three US District Courts that heard evidence concerning the Act and its effects, directly contradicts the Congressional declaration that "there is no credible medical evidence that partial-birth abortions are safe or are safer than other abortion procedures." Even the majority agreed that this Congressional finding was untenable, which is why the Court had to disregard the relevance of the pregnant woman's health altogether.

This leaves, Justice Ginsburg concludes, only "flimsy and transparent justifications" for upholding the ban. She rejects those justifications, arguing that the state's interest in "preserving and promoting fetal life" cannot be furthered by a ban that targets only a method of abortion and therefore cannot save "a single fetus from destruction" by its own terms. Nor, she believes, is the method condemned sufficiently different from methods approved to make the distinction rational. This is because the permitted alternative, lethal injection followed by delivering the dead fetus, also results in an intact fetus that resembles an infant.

Ultimately, she believes the decision rests entirely on the proposition, never before enshrined in a majority opinion, and explicitly repudiated in *Casey*, that "ethical and moral concerns" unrelated to the government's interest in preserving life can overcome fundamental rights of citizens. The majority seeks to bolster this reasoning by describing pregnant women as in a fragile emotional state that physicians may take advantage of by withholding information about abortion. The solution to this hypothetical problem, as Justice Ginsburg characterizes the majority opinion, is to "deprive women of the right to make an autonomous choice, even at the expense of their safety." The only woman on the Court continues, "This way of thinking [that men must protect women by restricting their choices] reflects ancient notions about women's place in the family and under the Constitution—ideas that have long since been discredited."

Justice Ginsburg also observes how at odds Kennedy's opinion is with existing precedents, especially *Roe* and *Casey*, which the majority insists they are only interpreting, not overruling. All previous cases, for example, had drawn the relevant line for outlawing abortion at fetal viability. But Kennedy's opinion (and the law he is interpreting) ignores this line, and instead approves of a law based on "where a fetus is anatomically located when a particular medical procedure is performed . . . . " She does not add, but could have, that application of the law prior to fetal viability makes its foundational concept, "partial-birth abortion," incoherent since if the fetus is not viable, the procedure becomes what can only be accurately described in the law's language as a "partial-abortion abortion."

Ginsberg notes further that the majority simply can't contain its contempt for the physicians who perform abortions:

> The Court's hostility to the right *Roe* and *Casey* secured is not concealed. Throughout, the opinion refers to obstetrician-gynecologists and surgeons who perform abortions not by the titles of their medical specialties, but by the pejorative label "abortion doctor." A fetus is described an "unborn child," and as a "baby"; second-trimester, previability abortions are referred to as "late-term," and the reasoned medical judgments of highly trained doctors are dismissed as "preferences" motivated by "mere convenience."

Ginsberg makes two final points. First, although the Court invites a lawsuit to challenge the Act "as applied," it gives "no clue" as to how such a lawsuit should be brought. Surely, she asks, "the Court cannot mean that no suit to challenge the ban [based on how it affects an actual woman or her physician] may be brought until a woman's health is immediately jeopardized." Second, she argues that the opinion threatens to undercut the rule of law and the principle of stare decisis, both of which the Court affirmed in *Casey*, concluding that, "A decision so at odds with our jurisprudence should not have staying power."

Abortion Bioethics

The major change in the law this opinion brings with it is the new willingness of the Court to disregard the health of pregnant women and the medical judgment of their physicians.[9] This was only possible by categorizing physicians as unprincipled "abortion doctors" and infantilizing pregnant women as incapable of making serious decisions about their lives and health. The majority opinion ignores longstanding principles of constitutional law, substituting the personal morality of Justice Kennedy and four of his colleagues. The rule of law, under intense pressure since the decision of *Bush v. Gore*, and reinforced in the aftermath of 9/11, has been all but replaced by the rule of personal opinion. The election of President Obama assures that *Roe* will not be overturned in the near future, although it is too early to tell how far the Court will ultimately go in "chipping away" at *Roe* and *Casey*.[10]

It is not, however, too early to tell what the majority of this Court thinks of physicians and of Congress' power to regulate physicians. The majority conclude that physicians, especially "abortion doctors" (Kennedy at least stopped calling physicians "abortionists" as he did in his *Stenberg* dissent), cannot be trusted either to tell their patients the truth or to act in their medical best interest. The majority asserts that giving Congress constitutional authority over medical practice is nothing new, but identifies no case in which Congress had ever outlawed a medical procedure. Its reliance on the more than 100-year-old *Jacobson v. Massachusetts* case in this regard is especially inapt. *Jacobson* was about mandatory smallpox vaccination during an epidemic. The statute had an exception for "children who present a certificate, signed by a registered physician, that they are unfit subjects for vaccination," and the Court implied that a similar medical exception would be constitutionally required for adults. It is not just abortion regulations that have had a health exception for physicians and their patients—all health regulations have.[11]

In *Roe v. Wade*, and even more centrally in its companion case, *Doe v. Bolton*, Justice Harry Blackmun, writing for a 7-to-2 majority in both opinions, had centered the privacy rights *Roe* articulated in the doctor–patient relationship generally, and on the doctor's right to practice medicine specifically.[12] In rejecting a Georgia statute that required a physician to obtain the concurrence of two other physicians before performing an abortion, Justice Blackmun wrote:

> If a physician is licensed by the State, he is *recognized by the State* as *capable of exercising acceptable medical clinical judgment*. If he fails this, professional censure and deprivation of his license are available remedies. Required acquiescence by co-practitioners has no rational connection with a patient's needs and unduly infringes on the *physician's right to practice*.[13] (emphasis added)

This new opinion is a wholesale vote of no confidence by the Court not only in the way physicians are licensed and regulated by state medical boards, but also in the ethics of physicians themselves. This is a stark change in the law, and what can reasonably be referred to as American biopolitics. I have, for example, told medical audiences that I did not believe the Supreme Court would *ever* prohibit a physician from acting in what he or she believed, on the basis of reasonable medical judgment and with informed consent, was in the patient's best medical interest. Even the suggestion that politicians understand more about the nexus between health risks and risks to life of specific patients than physicians do is irrational on its face. How can this radical change be accounted for, and what can or should be done about it?

One possible response is to pretend that this is an opinion only about abortion. And it will be tempting for physicians to believe that the legal change only applies to abortion, and even more narrowly, only to intact D&E. But this is a mistake. By its own words, the opinion applies to all physicians—in fact, the Court argues the case the other way around. Congress can, the Court holds, regulate abortion procedures and "abortion doctors" because it can regulate all other doctors—at least when there is medical uncertainty.

Another possible response is to believe that Congress and the Court think so little of medical ethics and the regulation of medical practice that they feel comfortable, in effect, practicing medicine without a license.[14] To do so both Congress and the Court had to find "medical uncertainty" regarding the necessity of a particular medical procedure under future unknowable specific circumstances. And they had to make this finding in the face of medical experts, including ACOG, who have consistently concluded that the procedure, although used extremely rarely, should remain available for the safety of their patients. On the other hand, the AMA actively supported the first partial-birth abortion law in Congress in 1996, not to protect patients, but in exchange for Congressional support for increases in Medicare reimbursement rates.[15] The AMA not only provided cover for Congress to vote for the ban, but also gave the Court some basis for finding medical uncertainty. Remarkably, in supporting the ban, the AMA explicitly conceded—long before the California medical marijuana case—that Congress has the authority under the Commerce Clause to regulate the practice of medicine throughout the United States.

Many physicians will surely be tempted to respond by ignoring the decision as an example of the political framing of abortion that was successful on its own terms, but is unlikely to have more than a marginal effect on medical practice. This is understandable, but misses the potential broader impact of the opinion on the practice of medicine generally. For physicians who are disturbed, dismayed, or even disgusted with this opinion—ACOG, for example, termed it "shameful and incomprehensible"[16]—there are concrete actions to consider.

The most direct and reasonable response to the opinion, I think, is to seek an amendment of the Act in Congress to protect women's health. This could be done, for example, by adding a specific exception when "in the reasonable medical judgment of the attending physician, an alternative procedure poses a significant risk to the health of the pregnant woman." While it would be better to simply repeal the law, this amendment could actually pass because it permits legislators to be against the unpopular, despised procedure, but at the same time to demonstrate concern about the health of women and to protect the doctor–patient relationship. This is also the position President Obama took when he was a senator in the Illinois legislature, and the same position President Bill Clinton took in twice vetoing a similar law—that he could only support banning the procedure if there was an exception to the ban to protect the health of the pregnant woman, as required by *Roe* and *Casey*.

The overwhelmingly negative reaction to Congressional intervention in the case of Terri Schiavo, the subject of the next chapter, will likely be sufficient to persuade the current Congress not to try to exercise its new regulatory power over the practice of medicine. President Obama is also likely to be able to lead a Democratic Congress to concentrate on voluntary family planning and education measures, and avoid further erosion of physician–patient autonomy. The president will not, however, be able to influence all of the state legislatures.

Many state legislatures have already used this decision to begin to enact new laws restricting abortion access. New proposals require physicians to present their patients with more and more information designed to discourage pregnant women from having abortions, such as offering to review ultrasound images of their fetuses with them. Some states will also likely attempt to outlaw other abortion procedures that the members of their legislatures find personally or religiously objectionable, including standard D&E.

In the past, it was easy for members of state legislatures to vote for an assortment of restrictions and bans, knowing that the courts would almost certainly find them unconstitutional. Now, however, the states have been given the green light to regulate medicine based on their own views of morals and ethics, detached from medicine and science. For the sake of their patients and the profession of medicine, physicians will have to pay much more attention to politics, in this case the new American biopolitics. This may itself seem like a worst case scenario, but the more life becomes the object of political action, the more necessary and appropriate political action by physicians, on behalf of themselves and their patients, becomes.

Justice Ginsburg was, I think, correct in seeing the partial-birth abortion act and its approval by the Court as reflective of a long discredited view of women and their capacity to make important decisions about their lives. Viewing competent women as incompetent is a brutal anachronism. But it is not only pregnant women for whom some men think they should be able to make medical decisions. As the next chapter illustrates, in an admittedly extreme and incredibly disturbing example of biopolitics, when a woman patient actually is incompetent to make her own decisions even the Congress and the president of the United States can see it as politically advantageous for them to try to make medical decisions for her under the spotlight of the national and international press.

As we will see, the goal for many in the strangely compelling morality play of Terri Schiavo was not to preserve her life or liberty, but to preserve their own political futures by avoiding imputed membership in the "culture of death."

11

Culture of Death

The case of Terri Schiavo is a worst case bioethics scenario in at least three senses: her case is one of the worst cases in American bioethics, it represents what can happen when opposing sides each take extreme positions, and the extreme positions taken are themselves a product of worst case scenario thinking.[1] The public's view of biopolitical intrusion into the medical care of Terri Schiavo, a young Florida woman in a permanent vegetative state, is well illustrated by two political cartoons. The first, by Tony Auth, published in the *Philadelphia Inquirer* shortly after Congress passed a law authorizing intervention by the federal courts, pictures a horde of members of congress charging mindlessly out of the Capitol, all dressed as physicians—one carrying a saw, another an IV pole—with the caption, "Coming Soon to a Sickbed Near You . . . The US Congress." The second, by Tom Toles, published in the *Washington Post* shortly after the results of the Schiavo autopsy were released, pictures an elephant being examined by two physicians. The elephant says, "I don't care what the autopsy says! I was right to intervene in the Terri Schiavo case and I'll do it again if I get the chance." In the corner of the cartoon one physician tells the other, "No hope for recovery."

Religious faith, by definition, does not depend on facts, but law and medicine should. Traditional advice to a young litigator is, "When the facts are against you, argue the law; when the law is against you, argue the facts; and when both are against you, scream like hell." The case of Terri Schiavo was never about the law—the law was unchallenged and left unchanged by seven years of litigation, a Florida statute, and a federal statute. Nor was her case really about the medical facts. Terri Schiavo was in a permanent vegetative state (PVS)—as demonstrated by consistent clinical and laboratory determinations during her life and the massive brain damage found on autopsy after her death. Although her parents and siblings disagreed with her husband, Michael, about her wishes for treatment, courts consistently concluded that if she was ever in such a hopeless condition, Terri Schiavo would not have wanted her life medically sustained and would have refused all treatment, including artificially delivered fluids and nutrition.

Few outside her friends and family ever knew Theresa Schiavo (or her husband, Michael). Nonetheless, almost everyone who has commented on her case, or tried to use it for personal or political gain, called her simply "Terri." This fake familiarity is the inevitable fate of those who become symbols in a political battle. Almost everyone with a cause seems to have believed that he or she was competent to speak on her behalf. That is why, outside the court system, the case of Terri Schiavo was never really about her and her medical condition and medical care, or even about her personal wishes. Her case instead was mostly about the fundamentalist religious right screaming into the ears of the governor of Florida; his brother, the president of the United States; the majority leader of the Senate; and the leaders of the House of Representatives.

What the name Terri Schiavo ultimately will stand for remains to be seen, although now Americans are more likely to say "I never want to be like Terri Schiavo" than they are to say "I never want to be like Karen Ann Quinlan" (or Nancy Cruzan). Whatever her legacy, during the last months of her life, Terri Schiavo became, at least to the politically active religious right, a symbol of an American judiciary out of control that was making antimajoritarian decisions on their core social issues, especially abortion, same-sex marriage, and the separation of church and state.

Her case even played a small role in the 2008 presidential campaign when Barack Obama was asked during a debate with Hillary Clinton in Cleveland on February 26, 2008, if there were any statements or votes he'd made that he'd like to take back. He didn't hesitate to identify his silence in the Senate's unanimous agreement to intervene in the Schiavo case. His answer was precise and eloquent:

> When I first arrived in the Senate that first year, we had a situation surrounding Terri Schiavo. And I remember how we adjourned with a unanimous agreement that eventually allowed Congress to interject

itself into that decisionmaking process of the families. It wasn't something I was comfortable with, but it was not something that I stood on the floor and stopped. And I think that was a mistake, and I think the American people understood that that was a mistake. And as a constitutional law professor, I knew better.

It was not only Obama who knew better—virtually everyone involved in this political theater knew better. Nonetheless, the fear of being branded as members of the "culture of death" should they oppose legislation aimed at keeping Terri Schiavo's feeding tube in place and in use was strong enough to silence most voices that should have supported her right to refuse treatment.

I have written about many right-to-refuse-treatment court cases since the 1976 Karen Ann Quinlan case. Nonetheless, I did not focus on the Terri Schiavo case until I was invited to participate in a Florida conference on her case in early 2005. That conference led me to write about it for the *New England Journal of Medicine*. My plan was to summarize existing law and to reassure my physician readers that no matter what they might have heard to the contrary, the Schiavo case did nothing to change existing law and they should not alter their medical practices because of it. Then, on Palm Sunday, to a chorus of religious platitudes about promoting the "culture of life," Congress passed a bill entitled "For the relief of the parents of Theresa Marie Schiavo."

The following day, as US District Court Judge James Whittemore was hearing arguments about the new law and deciding whether or not to grant a temporary restraining order, I rewrote my article to reflect the congressional action. And on the next day, March 22, the same day Judge Whittemore issued his precise and persuasive opinion, the *New England Journal of Medicine* released my article electronically.[2] With the Congressional action, the case of Terri Schiavo almost instantly went from one of only local interest, to one potentially affecting physicians and their patients around the country.[3] In this chapter, I concentrate on the worst case scenario worries of the religious right that in turn incited legislation at both the state and federal level, with a view toward learning something about the current state of American biopolitics, including the role physician-legislators in imagining worst case scenario visions that in turn produce meaningless symbolic legislation divorced from real life.

Culture of Life Politics

On Palm Sunday 2005, in a remarkable and unprecedented legislative event, the House of Representatives was recalled to Washington to convene in a special emergency session to pass legislation aimed at the medical care of one patient: Terri Schiavo. President George W. Bush encouraged the legislation, flying back to Washington, D.C. from his vacation in Crawford, Texas, to be on hand so he could sign it just after midnight, at about 1:30 A.M. Monday. In a statement three days earlier President Bush had said: "The case of Terri Schiavo raises complex issues . . . . Those who live at the mercy of others deserve our special care and concern. It should be our goal as a nation to build a culture of life, where all Americans are valued, welcomed, and protected—and that culture of life must extend to individuals with disabilities."[4] The imagined worst case scenario seemed to be a future determined by Terri Schiavo: If a feeding tube could be removed from Terri Schiavo, the lives of all Americans with disabilities were at serious risk.

The "culture of life" is a thinly coded label for the anti-abortion movement (sometimes called the "pro-life movement"), but also can include opposition to physician-assisted suicide and capital punishment, opposition to human embryonic stem cell research, and even opposition to war. In the United States, however, it has primarily come to mean a fundamentalist Christian position that is anti-abortion, anti-embryo research, and anti-same-sex marriage. Other than the Catholics in it, this movement has never taken issues like universal health insurance or access to medical care seriously and has had virtually nothing to say about cutting Medicaid benefits for millions. The rhetoric suggests that its opposite is a "culture of death" (a phrase popularized by Pope John Paul II). However, the legal and political mirror image is more properly seen as a "culture of liberty"—in which individuals are entitled to make their own deeply personal decisions free of government coercion, including decisions about pregnancy continuation, medical care, and marriage.

In President Bush's first term, the religious right seemed to be content with passing the "partial-birth abortion" ban (discussed in the previous chapter), limiting federal funding for human embryonic stem cell research to existing stem cell lines, and opposing state court decisions giving same-sex marriage constitutionally protected status. After President Bush's reelection, however, the religious right saw itself as significantly strengthened and, among other things, it moved to reopen a debate from the 1980s that had been decisively lost. The debate had been about whether artificially delivered fluids and nutrition should be classified as a medical treatment like any other, or should be seen as unique—and always obligatory—at least for incompetent patients. The courts had universally decided that feeding tubes were a form of medical treatment and so could be refused, like any other medical treatment. The Schiavo case seemed a good vehicle to reopen this debate.

Like the 2000 presidential election itself, the politicizing of the Terri Schiavo case began in Florida. Following the court-ordered removal of the feeding tube from Terri Schiavo in October 2003, and after intense lobbying by organized "right to life" groups, the Florida legislature passed a new law (2003-418), often referred to simply as "Terri's Law," which gave Governor Jeb Bush the authority to order the feeding tube reinserted, and he did so. The act applied only to a patient who met the following criteria on October 15, 2003; i.e., only to Terri Schiavo; a patient who

(a) ... has no written advance directive;

(b) [a] court has found that patient to be in a persistent vegetative state;

(c) ... has had nutrition and hydration withheld; and

(d) A member of that patient's family has challenged the withholding of nutrition and hydration.

The constitutionality of this law was immediately challenged. In the fall of 2004, the Florida Supreme Court ruled that it was unconstitutional because it violates the separation of powers, the division of the government into three branches, each with its own powers and responsibilities: the executive, the legislative, and the judicial. The doctrine states simply that no branch may encroach upon the powers of another branch, and no branch may delegate to another branch its constitutionally assigned power. The court held that for the legislature to pass a law that permits the executive to "interfere with the final judicial determination in a case" is "without question an invasion of the authority of the judicial branch." The court also found the law unconstitutional for an independent reason, because it "delegates legislative power to the governor" by giving the governor "unbridled discretion" to make a decision about a citizen's constitutional rights. In the court's words:

If the Legislature with the assent of the Governor can do what was attempted here, the judicial branch would be subordinated to the final directive of the other branches. Also subordinated would be the rights of individuals, including the well established privacy right to self determination.... Vested rights could be stripped away based on popular clamor.[5]

In January 2005, the US Supreme Court refused to hear an appeal brought by Florida's Governor Jeb Bush. Thereafter, the trial court judge ordered that Schiavo's feeding tube be removed in 30 days (at 1:00 P.M.,

Friday, March 18) unless a higher court again intervened. After this decision, the judge, George W. Greer of the Pinellas County Circuit Court, was picketed, threatened with death, and had to be accompanied by armed guards at all times. Schiavo's parents, again with the aid of a variety of religious fundamentalist and "right to life" organizations, sought review in the appeals courts, a new statute in the state legislature, and finally, congressional intervention. Both the trial judge and appeals courts—all of whom agreed that Terri Schiavo would not want her tube feeding continued—refused to reopen the case based on claims of new evidence (including the pope's 2004 statement on fluids and nutrition) and the failure to appoint an independent lawyer for Terri at the original hearing.

In Florida, the state legislature considered, and the House passed, new legislation aimed at restoring the feeding tube. The Florida Senate, recognizing, I think, that this new legislation, like the 2004 law, would be unconstitutional for the same reason, ultimately refused to go along. Searching for another way to proceed, Ken Connor, a prominent Florida trial attorney and Christian conservative who had represented Governor Bush on this issue, turned to his friend physician-Congressman Dave Weldon to try to devise a way for Congress to demand that the federal courts intervene. House majority leader Tom DeLay, who was under intense attack for alleged ethics violations, was only too happy to oblige. As he told a conference organized by the Family Research Council, a conservative Christian group in Washington, D.C. on Friday, March 19: "One thing that God has brought to us is Terri Schiavo to help elevate the visibility of what is going on in America . . . . This is exactly the issue that is going on in America, of attacks against the conservative movement, against me and against many others."[6]

"Right to life" advocates decided that a winning argument would be that Terri Schiavo deserves at least as much due process from the federal courts as a convicted murderer facing execution. Thereupon an event unique in American politics occurred: After only about a week of discussion, and after formally leaving Washington on their Easter recess without having taken action, Congress reconvened two days after the feeding tube was removed to consider emergency legislation written to apply only to Terri Schiavo.

Under rules that permitted a few senators to act if no senator objected (as President Obama now wishes he had), the US Senate adopted a bill entitled "For the relief of the parents of Theresa Marie Schiavo" on March 20, 2005, with only three senators present: Majority Leader Bill Frist, Senator John Warner of Virginia, and Senator Mel Martinez of Florida. In doing so, it took a private family dispute that the courts had resolved and transformed it into a worst case scenario medical science versus fundamentalist religion dispute. Three days earlier Senator Frist, a former heart transplant surgeon (who insisted on being called "Dr. Frist" even when he was the Senate Majority Leader), said:

> When I first heard about the situation facing Terri Schiavo I immediately wanted to know more about the case from a medical standpoint. I asked myself, just looking at the newspaper reports, *is Terri clearly in this diagnosis called a persistent vegetative state?* I was interested in it in part because it is a very difficult diagnosis to make and I've been in a situation such as this many, many times as a transplant surgeon .... *Persistent vegetative state, which is what the court has ruled—I question it. I question it based on a review of the video footage which I spent an hour or so looking at last night in my office here in the Capitol. And that footage, to me, depicts something very different from persistent vegetative state.* .... I mentioned that Terri's brother told me that Terri laughs, smiles, and tries to speak. Doesn't sound like a woman in a persistent vegetative state .... There just seems to be insufficient information to conclude that Terri Schiavo is persistent vegetative state. Securing the facts I believe is the first and proper step at this juncture.[7] (emphasis added)

Any senator could have stopped the madness with an objection—but none did. Apparently Republican senators were willing to go along with their leader—a physician whom they trusted on medical issues. Democrats were rudderless and afraid. They were afraid of being labeled the "party of death"—and more concretely of possibly hurting Florida Senator Bill Nelson's reelection chances. Nelson had refused to sign on as a sponsor of the bill. The contemporary view of the political implications of the bill was summarized in a memorandum written (it was later learned) by the legal counsel of Senator Mel Martinez (known by some in Florida as "Senator Bush" because of his "eagerness to please his political masters"). The memo, which Martinez helped circulate, characterized the Schiavo case as "a great political issue" for Republicans and "a tough issue for Democrats," especially Bill Nelson, who could be portrayed as Terri Schiavo's Democratic Angel of Death.[8] Because of the lack of courage or conviction in the Senate, the real legislative action was in the House of Representatives, where many physician members were eager to endorse Dr. Frist's virtual medical examination.

The House, a majority of whose members had to be physically present to vote under their rules, debated the same measure from 9:00 P.M. to midnight on Palm Sunday, and passed it by a 4-to-1 margin (203 to 58) shortly after midnight on Monday, March 21 (they were required to wait until Monday to vote under their rules). In substance the new law (S. 686), which was to set no precedent, provided that "the US District Court for the Middle District of Florida shall have jurisdiction" to hear a suit "for the alleged violation of any right of Theresa Marie Schiavo under the Constitution or laws of the United States relating to the withholding or withdrawal of food, fluids, or medical treatment necessary to sustain her life." The parents have standing to bring the lawsuit, and the court is instructed to "determine de novo any claim of a violation of any right of Theresa Marie Schiavo...notwithstanding any prior State court determination...."[9]

The brief debate on this bill in the House of Representatives (there were no hearings in either chamber, and, as noted, no debate at all in the US Senate) was notable primarily for its incredibly uninformed and frenzied rhetoric, and was covered live by C-SPAN. The primary sponsor of the measure, Majority Leader Thomas DeLay, for example, asserted, "She's not a vegetable, just handicapped like many millions of people walking around today. This has nothing to do with politics, and it's disgusting for people to say that it does."[10] Others echoed the sentiments of Senator Bill Frist, who had added earlier that day that immediate action by Congress was imperative because "Terri Schiavo is being denied life-saving fluids and nutrition as we speak."[11]

Almost all of the physician members of the House chimed in. Their statements are worth repeating because almost all of them turned their backs on the medical facts of the case and pandered instead to religiously inspired political passion. In the order in which they spoke, Congressman Phil Gingrey was first. His website features him as "Phil Gingrey, M.D." and on which he describes himself as "a pro-life OB-GYN" saying, "my 100% pro-life voting record reflects ... my commitment to support life at every stage." He said, "I am not playing doctor, for indeed I am one ... since Terri Schiavo's brain injury 15 years ago, she has been profoundly disabled. She is not, however, in a coma. *She responds to people around her; she smiles and she can feel. Terri is very much alive ... Terri's condition can improve.* Terri responds to verbal, auditory, and visual stimuli, normally breathes on her own and can move her limbs on command ... to uphold a culture of life and compassion it is important we act today to save Terri Schiavo's life and uphold the moral and legal obligation of our nation, indeed this poor woman's Constitutional right to life."[12] (emphasis added)

Congressman Dave Weldon, who brought the measure to Congress in the first place, remarked, "I practiced medicine for 15 years, internal medicine, before I came to the House of Representatives. I took care of a lot of these kinds of cases .... *Number one, by my medical definition she was not in a vegetative state based on my review of the videos, my talking to the family, and my discussing the case with one of the neurologists who examined her.* And, yes, I asked to get into the room and was unable to do so"[13] (emphasis added) Another physician-Congressman, Tom Price, said simply that he thought the law was reasonable because there was "no living will in place," and the family and experts disagreed.[14]

Physician-Congressman Jon Schwarz, a head and neck surgeon, said, "I shall not try to influence the opinion of anyone on this issue. I will simply share with you my opinion, the opinion of a physician of almost 41 years' duration ... Terri Schiavo has spontaneous respiratory activities and spontaneous cardiac activity. *She is not on life support* as we routinely define it. She is not intubated and she is not on a respirator ...*she does have some cognition and some cortical activity.*" He continued, "Removing her gastrostomy tube will ultimately cause her demise .... How many others in this country are now in long-term care facilities with feeding tubes, but breathe on their own, their hearts beating strongly? Should their feeding tubes be removed as well? I think not."[15] (emphasis added)

Finally, Congressman Charles Boustany's remarks were recorded, even though his flight to Washington was delayed, and he was not able to personally deliver them: "As a physician, I have been faced with many families in situations similar to that of Terri Schiavo's family .... But fortunately, *advances in medical technology have made recovery possible when before it was not possible.*" (emphasis added) Boustany continued, "I have seen people recover from illnesses to lead fulfilling lives when most thought all hope was lost. But Terri Schiavo's parents have not lost hope .... Her parents only ask that they be allowed to care for her. How can we deny her parents that possibility?"[16]

The only physician troubled by the public long-distance diagnosis of Schiavo by the Congress was psychiatrist-Congressman James McDermott, who chided his physician colleagues for making a diagnosis without examining the patient, noting that this was bad medical practice:

> And what troubles me, and I have heard my colleagues here, as a psychiatrist, I cannot make diagnoses of people I have not examined. That is contrary to my profession, and I can be disciplined for doing that. *The rest of you can be doctors.* You can come out here and tell us anything you want. *But a doctor cannot come out here and say anything really about somebody they have not examined.*[17] (emphasis added)

While deferring to the medical expertise of his congressional colleagues with medical degrees, Congressman Barney Frank, who vigorously led the floor fight for those opposed to the measure (most, but not all of whom were Democrats), recognizing that the chamber was not filled with physicians, quipped that the proper one-liner for the proceedings was, "We're not doctors, we just play them on C-SPAN."[18] The major slogans that recurred in the debate were that in a life-or-death decision we should "err on the side of life," that action should be taken to "prevent death by starvation" and ensure the "right to live," and that Congress should "protect the rights of disabled people," and give them at least the same rights to federal judicial review that convicted criminals have.

All of these have some abstract truth—but none have much to do with Terri Schiavo herself. No one was starving her. Like Nancy Cruzan, she was incapable of eating and a drug-like substance was being medically delivered to her body by a tube that had been surgically inserted, a continuing invasion of her body that she had a right to refuse. She was so far beyond "disabled" that the term could not accurately be used to describe her condition. She was permanently unconscious and unable to do anything; her upper brain was not "damaged" but absent. Finally, she was not a convicted criminal, and not in state custody. The medical decisions involving her care were all private, family, nongovernmental decisions.

After reviewing the new law, Judge Whittemore denied a request for a preliminary injunction to have the feeding tube reinserted, finding that her parents had failed to demonstrate "a substantial likelihood of success on the merits." In his well-reasoned opinion, subsequently upheld on appeal, he found that the claim that Schiavo had not been accorded due process was unpersuasive since the case had already been "exhaustively litigated"; that throughout all parties had been "represented by able counsel"; and that the First Amendment claim that Schiavo's right to practice her religion was being violated by the state was without merit since there was no state action involved.[19] Although the issue was never litigated, the statute itself would likely have been found unconstitutional for the same reasons the Florida Supreme Court found Terri's Law unconstitutional. Following Whittemore's opinion, unsuccessful appeals, demonstrations, and almost uninterrupted coverage by cable news stations, Terri Schiavo died on March 31. Her death, however, did not stop the screaming.

Feeding Tubes and Abortion

The challenge to Terri Schiavo's husband, Michael, was brought by her parents, Mary and Robert Schindler, and championed by a wide variety of "right to life" groups and fundamentalist religious organizations that politicians like Bill Frist found themselves unable to resist. Neither the public nor Congress could make a reasoned judgment about the case because of blatant misrepresentations of the facts. Most notable was the release of edited videotapes that seemed to show her interacting with visitors, and thus conscious and aware of her surroundings and able to suffer physically and mentally. The list of conservative lobbyists and special interest groups that sought to use Schiavo to further their agenda is long, but two examples illustrate their tactics.

The first is the conservative website RightMarch.com, whose publicity on the case featured a flyer (which could be printed from their website for distribution) with the headline "Tell Congress to Help Save Terri Schiavo from Starvation." The flyer included the following "facts" about her medical condition: "Terri laughs, Terri cries, she moves, and she makes childlike attempts at speech with her parents. Sometimes she will say 'Mom' or 'Dad' or 'yeah' when they ask her a question. When they kiss her hello or goodbye, she looks at them and 'puckers up' her lips." RightMarch was aided in its campaign by the Right Brothers, who agreed to let them use their anti-abortion song "I Want to Live." The chorus, which includes the refrain "Mama I want to live, Mama I want to breathe," was apparently seen as close enough for use in a tube-feeding campaign. And like a fetus, Terri Schiavo herself was silent. The assertions that she could communicate, and even say "I want to live," echoed the medically inaccurate arguments of the anti-abortion film *Silent Scream* (first shown in the mid-1980s) which features an ultrasound film of a 12-week fetus, who, again like Schiavo, is said to be in distress and struggling to survive.[20]

The second example involves more direct action demonstrations, and is illustrated by a photograph taken on March 18, the day the feeding tube was removed. Outside of the hospice, Rev. Bob Schenck and Rev. Ed Martin posed for photographers by crying in agony as if they had just learned that their only child had been killed (the color photo, by KRT, appeared on the front page of major newspapers on March 19, including the *Boston Globe*). Rev. Schenck works closely with Rev. Patrick Mahoney of Faith and Action, an umbrella religious organization that, among other things, was dedicated to abolishing the filibuster and replacing liberal judges with those who believe as they do that "every human being at every stage has dignity no matter what its dependency."[21]

Mahoney (now director of the Christian Defense Coalition), who has said about the fight for new judicial appointments, "let's make no mistake about it, this hinges on abortion," was originally a leader of the anti-abortion group Operation Rescue.[22] In 1990, he and his colleagues were trying to get media attention outside of Nancy Cruzan's nursing home after her tube feeding was discontinued by court order on the basis that it was her wish. He recalls how they had to beg the night clerk to use the fax machine. "That's how sophisticated we were. We were desperately trying to get the word out, desperately trying to get people out. There just wasn't much interest." Today, he says that by turning to the Internet, alternative media, and grass roots organizations, the "faith-and-values community" has "unleashed an avalanche of support for Schiavo's parents."[23]

Former Republican Senator and Episcopal minister John C. Danforth insightfully observed that in pushing the Schiavo legislation the Republican Party departed from its principles, especially those involving government intrusion into private decisions and federal courts overruling state courts, and "can rightfully be interpreted as yielding to the pressure of religious power blocs." Danforth went further, concluding that the Republican Party's "current fixation on a religious agenda has turned us in the wrong direction."[24]

To the extent that medical facts mattered, the autopsy report on Schiavo settled them. It was released on June 13, 2005. Although the clinical diagnosis of persistent or permanent vegetative state cannot be determined on autopsy, the physical findings were consistent with a PVS. With specific reference to her brain the report concluded:

> Mrs. Schiavo's brain showed marked global anoxic-ischemic encephalopathy resulting in massive cerebral atrophy. Her brain weight was approximately half of the expected weight. Of particular importance was the hypoxic damage and neuronal loss in her occipital lobes, which indicates cortical blindness. Her remaining brain regions also show severe hypoxic injury and neuronal atrophy/loss.[25]

This confirms that the only functioning part of her brain was her brain stem. She had no upper brain activity and therefore no ability to interact with her environment, and certainly no ability to speak. Although she could open her eyes, she was incapable of sight. The injuries to her brain were irreversible and no potentially beneficial therapy was possible. The ultimate cause of her "severe anoxic brain injury" could not be determined with reasonable medical certainty, and the medical examiner left the case open, as is the policy of his office "that no case is ever closed and that all determinations are to be reconsidered upon receipt of credible, new information."

A week before the autopsy report was released, I had the privilege of participating in a program sponsored by the District of Columbia Bar Association on the Schiavo case with two of the post–Congressional action appellate litigators, one from each side: Professor Robert Destrow (for the parents) and Attorney Thomas J. Perrelli (for the husband). I gave the first presentation, essentially summarizing the law, and as an aside on the facts, said that if the autopsy report was inconsistent with permanent vegetative state I would be the first to say I was wrong to rely on the judge's evaluation of the medical testimony. Professor Destrow, on the other hand, made it clear that whatever the autopsy report concluded, it would not affect the opinions of many of those who, like him, sided with the parents. In his words, "The autopsy is interesting. But we wanted to know what her living brain could do, not what her dead brain can do."[26]

Destrow was attempting to preemptively deny the relevance of whatever medical facts would be found at autopsy. Similarly, the parents and brother of Terri Schiavo, understandably, could not accept the autopsy results. But more politically motivated people tried to use the autopsy report for their own purposes. Governor Jeb Bush, for example, used it to make it appear that he was right to question Michael Schiavo's competence to speak for his wife, by maliciously and without any evidence asking a prosecutor to investigate Michael to determine if he delayed calling 911 on the night of Terri's heart attack.[27] As prosecutor Bernie McCabe told a columnist for the *New York Times*, he had no basis for the investigation (which turned up no evidence against Michael) and agreed to do it only because Governor Bush asked him to.[28]

William Hammesfahr, one of the two primary medical witnesses for Terri's parents at trial, and whose testimony at trial that he could treat Terri was discounted by Judge Greer as not credible, also refused to accept the medical facts. In a June 19 statement released by the Christian Communication Network he wrote,

> Dr. Maxfield [a radiologist who was the other expert witness for the parents] and myself both emphasized that she was a woman trapped in her body, similar to a child with cerebral palsy, and that was borne out by the autopsy, showing greater injury in the motor and visual centers of the brain. *Obviously, the pathologists' comments that she could not see were not borne out in reality*, and thus his assessment must represent sampling error . . . . *That she could not swallow was obviously not borne out by the reality that she was swallowing her saliva* . . . . Thus there appears to be some limitations to the clinical accuracy of an autopsy in evaluating function . . . . Ultimately, *based on the clinical evidence and the autopsy results, an aware woman was killed.*[29] (emphasis added)

President Bush was also unmoved by the autopsy findings. His spokes-person, Scott McClellan, said at a June 15 press briefing, "It [the autopsy] doesn't change the position that the president took. The president took the position he did for a reason. *The president believes we should stand on the side of defending and protecting life.* That's why he stood with those who supported efforts to defend her life. This is a sad case. Our thoughts and prayers continue to be with her family and friends."[30] (emphasis added)

Senator Frist, on the other hand, tried almost desperately, but ultimately without success, to distance himself from his original comments made as a physician-senator, saying, "I never made a diagnosis.... I wouldn't ever attempt to make a diagnosis based on a videotape." But, of course, Frist's comments questioning the diagnosis were recorded by C-SPAN, and among others, Jon Stewart replayed them on *The Daily Show*. Stewart observed, "Not only do I believe that Senator Bill Frist may be a terrible doctor, I think he doesn't realize C-SPAN has cameras."[31] Republican political strategist Tony Fabrizio noted, "It is never good when you say you didn't do something when you are on camera doing it.... [Frist's adversaries] will use it time and time again."[32] Columnist David Brooks, who is very sympathetic to Frist, nonetheless accurately and succinctly summed it up: "It's not quite fair to say that Frist diagnosed Schiavo from a TV screen, but he did put himself on the wrong side of the autopsy .... He did betray his medical training, which is the core of his being, to please a key constituency group."[33] Political cartoonist Mike Luckovich was less kind, picturing Frist at the new King Tut exhibit saying of Tut, "This young man's the picture of health." It does not seem to be an exaggeration to say that Frist's leadership in making the Schiavo case one of national concern was the major factor disqualifying him to run for the Republican nomination for president in 2008.

The autopsy report, of course, also vindicated the primary expert medical witness for Michael Schiavo, neurologist Ronald Cranford, perhaps the country's leading expert on vegetative states, and certainly the country's most experienced examining physician in courtroom controversies featuring this diagnosis. Over the years of his involvement in this case, Cranford lost all respect for the opinions of Maxfield and Hammesfahr, whom he came to see simply as quacks. As he has put it:

> The following is a sample of the completely fallacious opinions rendered about Terri's medical condition by Drs. Maxfield and Hammesfahr. Twelve years after an hypoxic-ischemic insult, and serial CT scans showing extremely severe atrophy of the cerebral hemispheres, both doctors said their was a "chance of recovery," with the potential for response to treatment. Dr. Maxfield, the radiologist, testified that "abnormal brain dissolves," so what's left

[as seen in the CT scans] is "normal, functioning brain." He further stated that the most recent CT scan shows "improvement." They gave no published data to support their opinions on their proposed treatments of HBO [hyperbaric oxygen] or vasodilator therapies as effective treatment for patients with chronic brain damage. The articles on the Internet on vasodilator therapy, including those by Dr. Hammesfahr, are extremely poorly written, and only a cursory examination of these articles would tell any medical professional that they could not have possibly been peer-reviewed.[34]

After the feeding tube had been removed and Congress had tried to intervene, another neurologist-"bioethicist," William Cheshire, saw Terri Schiavo and told Governor Bush, "Although Terri did not demonstrate during our 90-minute visit compelling evidence of verbalization, conscious awareness, or volitional behavior, [there is] a distinct presence of a living being who seems at some level to be aware of some things around her." Asked to comment on this new finding, Cranford gave the opinion of his fellow neurologist all the respect he believed it deserved, saying simply, "I have no idea who this Dr. Cheshire is. He has to be bogus, a pro-life fanatic."[35]

Post-Schiavo Biopolitics and Bioethics

The fact that Cheshire, whom no one in mainstream American bioethics had ever heard of, could simply call himself a bioethicist and be accepted by many in the media as one disclosed something about the politicization of bioethics itself. Whether dated from the early 1970s, as many do, or from the Nuremberg Doctors' Trial, as I do, American bioethics has welcomed religious thinkers into its ranks, but has remained secular and pragmatic.[36] Under President George W. Bush, however, government-sponsored bioethics turned overtly political when he charged his President's Council on Bioethics with the primary mission of justifying his ban on federal funding of human embryonic stem cell research, and chose the neoconservative thinker Leon Kass to chair it. The Council quickly developed an embryo-centric, anti-abortion and anti-regulation agenda which it never effectively transcended.[37] This narrow agenda helps explains why, even though the president was personally involved in the Schiavo case, and even though it was at heart a bioethics dispute that involved issues that have been at the core of the work of national bioethics panels for more than two decades, President Bush never sought the advice of his own highly political bioethics council on this premier biopolitical dispute.

But there is more to it than this. American bioethicists have largely stayed away from the politics of abortion. When they have engaged in it, mainstream bioethicists have found that the compromise and pragmatism that has characterized American bioethics was totally unacceptable to the "right to life" organizations—who have themselves begun to call some of their own anti-abortion spokespersons "bioethicists." It was probably inevitable that bioethics and bioethicists get more involved in politics. But must bioethics accept rigid fundamentalist believers as colleagues in the bioethics field just because they self-identify as bioethicists? The fact that religious views are relevant to bioethics should not mean that bioethics can be equated with religious beliefs. The question of whether it is good or bad for bioethics to be embroiled in American politics is no longer relevant; the only question is whether bioethicists can retain credibility in a political world much more interested in opinion and controversy than in facts and principles.

The reason the Schiavo case did not turn out to be a watershed event on the bioethics/religion front can be attributed primarily, I think, to the influence of America's two best known bioethicists—Leon Kass and Art Caplan. As the president's bioethicist, Kass would have been expected to play a prominent role, and I believe he did. His public silence was deafening, and can be explained by the fact that Kass has consistently and eloquently attacked vitalism and has argued against prolonging life at all costs, as well as against seeing immortality as a reasonable medical goal. After *Quinlan*, but before *Cruzan*, he wrote, "even people in the so-called persistent vegetative state must have healthy vegetative functions .... But few of us would accept the preservation of such a reduced level of function as a proper goal for medicine...."[38] Although Kass might or might not support discontinuation of fluids and nutrition in any particular case, he does not accept death as always evil or the continuation of life by medical means as always good. In his words, "I think one can walk between the extremes of vitalism and 'quality control' and uphold in so doing the respect that life itself commands for itself."[39] And although he became a political animal under President Bush, he could not have been comfortable with the sloganeering in the Terri Schiavo case, having written perceptively that questions of life prolongation

> Will not yield to simple formulae such as "death with dignity" or "life is sacred" or "dispense with extraordinary means." Such terms as "incurable," "dying," "terminal," and "hopeless" are notoriously vague, not to speak of "dignity" .... Measures that can be said to be life-preserving span a continuum from respirators and dialysis

machines, through antibiotics, insulin, to intravenous glucose and water, even to food and drink.[40]

Kass' silence on Schiavo was at least somewhat reassuring; politics had not totally hijacked bioethics, even in the intensely biopolitical Bush administration. But bioethicists also have an obligation to speak up when power politics and religious fundamentalists threaten to reverse the good that bioethics has done. And many bioethicists did. Of them, the most articulate was the bioethicist who has become the public face of bioethics in America, Arthur Caplan. Caplan came out early and strongly against Congressional intervention, writing a powerful editorial for MSNBC entitled "The Time Has Come to let Terri Schiavo Die" on March 18, 2005. He argued that both bioethics and law supported Michael Schiavo as the decision maker, and that should be the end of it. He also noted, both in the editorial and later in other venues, including many CNN and network appearances, that honoring the right to refuse any medical treatments also serves to protect religious practices, at least of adults, including Christian Scientists and Jehovah's Witnesses. And in calling for more people to designate a health care proxy to make decisions for them when they cannot make decisions themselves, he joined a veritable chorus of bioethicists urging Americans to take actions that might help avoid getting them and their families into similar circumstances.[41] Caplan did not "save" American bioethics in the Schiavo controversy, but he should get credit for postponing a decisive, but seemingly inevitable, confrontation between secular bioethics and religious anti-abortion bioethics.

The major heroes in the Terri Schiavo case are Judges George Greer and James D. Whittemore, both of whom resisted intense political pressure to render opinions based on the law and the facts in the highest tradition of American law. The primary villains are Senator Bill Frist and Representative Tom DeLay, both of whom attempted to use the plight of Terri Schiavo and her family for their personal political gain and neither of whom should be forgiven. Jeb and George Bush were, I think, more pawns than players in this saga—and neither ever claimed to be anything but a fundamentalist Christian politician. That they succumbed to intense pressure from the religious right came as no surprise to anyone.

In terms of winners and losers, conclusions must be tentative, and like the medical examiner's autopsy report, subject to revision upon receipt of additional credible information. Nonetheless, it seems fair to conclude that the big loser in the Schiavo debate was Congress and the big winner was the judiciary. This is because the primary message of the radical religious right turned out to be widely mistaken—both in their medical diagnosis of Terri

Schiavo, and more importantly in their diagnosis of the wishes of the American people. Overwhelming majorities of Americans in every major poll taken after Congress passed the Theresa Schiavo Act found that Americans do not want Congress involved in life-and-death medical decisions, but believe these should be made by families who know the individuals involved and can best articulate their wishes.[42]

As important, the public agreed with the determination of the judges in the Schiavo case itself.[43] In short, as Professor Jeffrey Rosen has astutely observed in a broader context, including not only Schiavo, but also the judicial filibuster debate and even *Roe v. Wade*, "the conservative interest groups have it exactly backward. Their standard charge is that unelected judges are thwarting the will of the people by overturning laws passed by elected representatives. But in our new topsy-turvy world, it's the elected representatives who are thwarting the will of the people, which is being channeled instead by unelected judges."[44]

The Schiavo case may have changed politics and bioethics by making the public more cynical about both, but it did not change the law. It is probably too much to hope that the case will help demonstrate the shallowness and vapidity of the slogan "err on the side of life" in this context, which has about as much depth as slogans like "look before you leap" and "he who hesitates is lost." Life-or-death decisions are easy. But when a person's brain is irreversibly destroyed, life has no side—it's only a question of how the dying process will proceed. To deny this is to not only to deny the medical facts, it is to revert to mindless vitalism—a concept no religion that believes in an afterlife can support. We all "want to live," but most Americans recognize that ultimately we will all die, and that dying in America remains more fearsome than death—and immortality is not an option.[45]

Terri Schiavo was abused by the political system and used as a voiceless vessel for anyone with a cause to claim to speak on her behalf. Although she and her husband ultimately prevailed in court, it was a bitter legal victory, and no person's private life should be subjected to such intense and vicious public scrutiny for trying to do what a family member would have wanted.

There is no escaping the fact that when we are unable to make medical decisions for ourselves, someone else will have to make them for us. It will be farier to all our friends and family if we each designate the person we want to make decisions for us ourself. The "health care proxy" is the name for both the document and the person you designate to make decisions for you when you are no longer able to make them yourself. It is, I believe, everyone's personal responsibility to name a proxy; and the fact that almost no attention was paid to health care proxies during the temporary political insanity of the "death panel" debate in August 2009 reflects both our desire to keep end of life decisions out of politics, and our desire to simultaneously deny that decisions at the end of life will ever have to be made. Making decisions at the end of life will never be easy and should never be formulaic, and families that were dysfunctional when everyone was healthy are not usually healed when a family member becomes incapacitated. But we should nonetheless maintain the presumption that close family members are the best people to make decisions and insist that decisions regarding medical care at the end-of-life stay within the family and out of the hands of politicians. Courts must remain available, but used only in cases, like the case of Terri Schiavo, where family conflicts are irreconcilable.

Terri's tombstone accurately summarizes her life and her husband's efforts to fulfill her wishes: "Schiavo, Theresa Marie, Beloved Wife, Born December 3, 1963, Departed this Earth February 26, 1990, At Peace March 31, 2005, I Kept My Promise." Terri Schiavo is beyond being further abused by the political system, but fundamentalist religious fanatics remain capable of inflicting further harm on society and only an informed citizenry that insists on keeping highly personal decisions out of the hands of government, insists on separation of church and state, and insists that the courts, not Congress, interpret the Constitution can save us all from a "salvation" we neither seek nor can live with on this earth.

We Americans like stories and can relate to the plight of individuals and their families, which enables us to obsess over one life. But when the numbers become large, and the individuals are not identified, we quickly lose interest and turn to another subject. This is not only true in extremes like war, famine, and even genocide; it is also true in medical care, and helps explain why, as I address in the next chapter, Americans have not been able to confront the issue of patient safety in our hospitals, even though we know that more than a million Americans have died needlessly in our hospitals as a result of preventable medical errors in the past decade. When it comes to saving lives, it is primarily those with a politically useful story to tell make the cut.

12

Patient Safety

B eing killed in a hospital where you went for care, or by a drug you took for cure, can reasonably be termed a worst case scenario. I will deal with both of these hazards in this chapter, exploring the very tentative steps the law has taken to date to try to improve patient safety and thus help save the lives of patients, rather than being indifferent to their deaths.[1] In most areas of life and politics, saving lives, especially by improving safety and security, are very powerful motivators. But not, it seems, in healthcare itself, where cost savings continue to be more compelling than quality improvements. I examine safety in the hospital first—an issue that has not made it to the Supreme Court—and then examine drug safety, an issue the Court has considered.

Hospital Safety

Consumers Union reported in mid-2009 that after more than a decade of trying, "we have failed to make the systematic changes in health care needed to end preventable medical harm" that has taken more than a million lives since the Institute of Medicine's (IOM) 1999 report on patient safety, *To Err is Human*.[2] New training programs, new organizations, and new journals are devoted to patient safety. We have made "a little progress," but major changes in practice that might actually help protect the lives and health of hospital patients have been rare.[3] What can explain this overall failure to take patient safety seriously and what, if anything, can be done about it?

The IOM made its point dramatically by equating the approximately 100,000 hospital deaths annually caused by medical errors to a jumbo jet crashing every day. This makes death from medical error in hospitals one of the leading causes of death in the United States, representing, for example, more than double the number of Americans killed in automobile accidents. The airlines would take immediate action; why don't hospitals? Since the IOM report, much has been written on lessons that hospitals can learn from the airline industry about safety, including the use of checklists in the operating room. But the airline analogy appears to have simply created another problem, rather than serving as part of the solution. This is because providing safe, quality medical care in a modern hospital has virtually nothing to do with flying passengers from one city to another.

In an airplane, all passengers can be treated identically (with the possible exception of what they want to eat—and this can be taken care of by discontinuing food service on airlines), and they all want exactly the same thing: to get from New York to San Francisco, for example, safely and efficiently. Moreover, passengers are given no say in when, whether, or how their plane actually flies. Their only choice is to take the flight or not. Every patient in a hospital, of course, is unique; each has his or her own problems, values, and expectations; and each patient is seen by dozens of people who make decisions about their care. There are few standard measurements of quality, and outcomes will vary.

Keeping a plane in good working order, and making sure the pilots are competent to fly it is a comparatively easy task—and standard for all airlines, even low-cost, no-frills airlines. Machines are basically all the same and are repaired in standard ways. Hospital-based medical care is many things, but it's not rocket science—it's much more difficult. Using the airline analogy doesn't help because it is too far removed from medical care. Instead, the airlines analogy returns us to the early days of managed care, when all hospital problems were going to be solved by treating hospitals just like "ball bearing factories," and arguably, treating patients just like ball bearings.[4]

Patient safety experts are fond of saying that we have learned two major lessons about safety: "It's a systems problem," and "We need to create a culture of safety."[5] In arriving at these conclusions, the experts rely heavily on the work of psychologist James Reason. In his classic text, *Human Error*, Reason makes many useful distinctions, including one between active errors (whose effects are felt immediately) and latent errors (whose adverse consequences lie dormant within the system for a long time and only become evident when combined with other factors). Reason concludes that in complex systems (he studied Three Mile Island, Bhopal, Chernobyl, and the *Challenger* disaster, among others—all worst case scenarios in their respective industries) "latent errors pose the greatest threat to safety."[6] Perhaps the most important latent error in the complex hospital system is that patient safety is still seen as an optional activity, or a low-priority one, instead of as a primary organizational obligation. We really do need to promote a culture of safety, but how?

The IOM report noted that to be successful, "safety must be an explicit organizational goal that is demonstrated by clear organizational leadership ... this process begins when boards of directors demonstrate their commitment to this objective by regular, close oversight of the safety of the institutions they shepherd." Medical safety experts Lucien Leape and Don Berwick agree, noting that safety cannot become a priority "without more sustained and powerful pressure on hospital boards and leaders—pressure that must come from outside the health industry."[7] In hospital care, the challenge is to reform corporate governance to make hospital boards take their responsibilities to patients in their hospitals at least as seriously as they take the hospital's financial condition.

Most physician patient safety experts continue to believe that the threat of liability is the primary barrier to the development of effective and comprehensive patient safety programs in hospitals. I suggest, on the contrary, that judicial recognition of an explicit "right to safety" for hospital patients, with a correlative duty of hospitals to implement patient safety measures, can become the primary motivator for the development of systems to improve patient safety. Hospitals that do not take specific actions to improve safety are negligent and should be subject to malpractice lawsuits when a violation of the right to safety results in patient injury or death. We take rights seriously in this country, and a rights frame could do more to both encourage patients to insist on a safe hospital environment, and to work with physicians and other healthcare providers to insist that hospitals, and especially the members of hospital boards, take seriously their obligation to maintain an environment in which patient safety is the number one priority.

Patients have rights, even when they are in the hospital. As I noted in Chapter 1, except in emergencies, Americans do not have the right *to* healthcare, but we do have rights *in* healthcare, and we do not check our rights at the hospital door. Patient rights, most centrally, include the right to information, often called informed consent or informed choice; the right to refuse any treatment; the right to privacy and confidentiality; the right to emergency treatment; and the right to be treated with dignity.[8] A new patient "right to safety" could be derived, as most patient rights are, from the fiduciary nature of the doctor–patient relationship. But since physicians do not and cannot control all possible risks of injury in the hospital setting, it is more appropriate to define the scope of this right as a reflection of corporate responsibility: the obligation of a hospital to maintain a safe environment for patients and their healthcare providers.

Hospitals are corporations (artificial persons created by law), and their obligations are imposed on them by civil and criminal law, their own by-laws, their mission statements, and their internal rules. Hospitals are responsible for their own negligence under the doctrine of corporate responsibility, which a number of courts have already applied directly to hospitals. The law usually lets industries, like the hospital industry, set their own standards of practice and permits juries to find a hospital negligent only if the hospital fails to live up to the standard of care adopted by the industry itself.

Thus, theoretically at least, if no hospitals take patient safety seriously—and all of them, for example, refuse to adopt computerized medical records generally, or a computerized physician ordering system specifically—a court could conclude that they have not violated the industry's standard of care and so are not negligent. If a court followed this standard, a patient who has been given the wrong drug and has died as a result, for example, might not be able to successfully sue the hospital on the basis that the death would have been avoided had a computerized physician ordering system been in place.

In real life, however, the law does not permit industries to create preventable risks by adopting unreasonably low standard for themselves. Courts have consistently ruled that the real standard of care is not deter-mined by "custom" (another word for what hospitals actually do), but by "reasonable prudence" (another term for what the hospitals should do to prevent harm). Courts have found that entire industries or professions can be negligent by failing to adopt new technologies, especially those that are inexpensive and effective.

The famous 1932 *T. J. Hooper* case, for example, involved the question of whether it was negligent for a tugboat not to have a wireless radio on board to get weather reports. The tugboat sank with the plaintiff's cargo during a storm that had been predicted, a storm that the tugboat could easily have avoided had the captain listened to the weather forecasts. The practice in the tugboat industry was not to adopt wireless radios. Commenting on this "nobody else does it" defense the court observed:

In most cases reasonable prudence is in fact common prudence; but strictly it is never its measure; a whole calling may have unduly lagged in the adoption of new and available devices. It never may set its own tests, however persuasive be its usages [custom]. Courts must in the end say what is required; *there are precautions so imperative that even their universal disregard will not excuse their omission.*[9] (emphasis added)

Hospitals have been successfully sued for endangering patient safety by, for example, having inadequate nurse staffing and having inadequate facilities. Since providing a safe environment for patient care is a corporate responsibility, understaffing is corporate negligence. The best-known case of this kind is the *Darling* case, in which the Supreme Court of Illinois determined that a jury could find that a hospital was negligent for not having a sufficient number of qualified nurses to properly monitor a patient. The 18-year-old patient in this case lost his leg because the fact that his cast had been put on too tightly and had cut off his circulation was not dealt with effectively by the nursing staff.[10]

In a similar case, the Supreme Court of Mississippi held that it was for the jury to decide if a hospital was negligent for failing to keep an operating room available should a high-risk patient undergoing elective cardiac catheterization require surgery to survive (about a 1% risk). The patient, a judge, died because all of the hospital's operating rooms were in use when he needed emergency surgery to repair an injury he suffered during his cardiac catheterization. Even though other hospitals followed this same practice, the court ruled: "In assessing reasonable conduct there is a vast difference between taking a chance when unavoidable and when avoidable. Taking a 1% chance when necessary might be exemplary, but taking the same chance when unnecessary might be negligence."[11] Common sense, and almost any attention at all to the patient's safety, would have dictated postponing his elective procedure until emergency backup was available.

Although courts have not explicitly adopted a right to safety, courts have been discussing the specific content of such a right in the context of corporate responsibility for almost two decades. In 1991, for example, the Pennsylvania Supreme Court stated simply, "Corporate negligence is a doctrine under which the hospital is liable if it fails to uphold the proper standard of care owed the patient, which is to *ensure the patient's safety* and well-being while at the hospital."[12] (emphasis added) The court also listed four specific examples that previous courts had identified as hospital safety obligations: the maintenance of safe and adequate facilities and equipment;

selection and retention of competent physicians; oversight of medical practice within the hospital; and adoption and enforcement of adequate rules
and policies to ensure quality of care for patients.

Specific hospital obligations would flow from the recognition of a
patient's right to safety. For example, courts could determine that a hospital's failure to adopt new technology to prevent patient injury, such as a
computerized physician ordering system, could subject the hospital to
liability for injury in cases in which it could be demonstrated that adoption
of the technology would not have been prohibitively expensive and would
probably have prevented the injury. Nosocomial infections resulting from a
hospital's failure to adopt or enforce hand-washing policies would be even
easier to demonstrate as a breach of a hospital's duty to keep patients safe.[13]
The 100,000 Lives Campaign of the Institute for Healthcare Improvement
has actively promoted six evidence-based patient safety interventions:
deployment of rapid-response teams, reliable care for acute myocardial
infarction, medication reconciliation, and prevention of central line infections, surgical site infections, and ventilator associated pneumonia.[14] A
majority of US hospitals have already joined this campaign, which helps
make these six safety interventions the standard of care for all hospitals.
Potential liability for not adopting these safety measures (and others backed
by similar evidence of effectiveness) should give hospitals an added incentive
either to adopt such measures, or to explain to the public why particular
evidence-based safety interventions will not improve safety in their hospital.
The National Patient Safety Goals of the Joint Commission can also be
reasonably viewed as setting national standards of care for patient safety,
although these are pretty rudimentary.

In the absence of a comprehensive national patient protection system,
the patient's right to safety can be enforced only by a legal claim against the
hospital. The hospital, not the physician, satisfies or breaches the duty to
ensure patient safety. And more liability suits against hospitals may be
necessary to motivate hospital boards to take patient safety more seriously.
The question of whether to take the additional step of moving to enterprise
liability—in which all medical malpractice suits (including those alleging
negligence by physicians working in hospitals) are brought against hospitals—also deserves more serious consideration than it has had to date. It
should be emphasized that the goal is not to encourage more litigation for its
own sake. The goal is prevention of injury ("saving lives"), and litigation
provides a strong incentive for hospital boards of directors to insist that their
administrators make their institutions safer.

Patient safety experts almost uniformly insist that hospitals track
errors and near misses, whether required by federal or state law, or by

accreditation requirements. Patients should also be informed when their injuries are caused by medical errors. Most experts also believe that reporting by physicians cannot be achieved without drastically limiting or eliminating legal liability. The view that physicians fail to report errors (to both patients and hospitals) because they are afraid of being sued is plausible and has intuitive appeal. But the intuitive view is not supported by empirical evidence. As David Hyman and Charles Silver found, no empirical study has shown a negative correlation between "the intensity of malpractice risk and the frequency of error reporting, or has shown that liability correlates inversely with health care quality."[15] A 2005 survey of patients also found that only one-quarter of US physicians disclosed errors to their patients; but the result was not that much different in New Zealand, a country that has had no-fault medical malpractice for more than three decades, and where fewer than 40% of physicians report errors to their patients.[16]

Thus, to the extent that the patient safety movement seeks to be "evidence-based," the confidentiality/immunity model may produce little or no change in actual error reporting by physicians. Nor should this be surprising. There are many reasons why physicians don't report errors, including a general reluctance to communicate with patients and fear of disciplinary action or loss of privileges.[17] If this analysis is correct, the passage of the Patient Safety and Quality Improvement Act, which establishes federal confidentiality protections for a new system of reporting medical errors, will have little or no effect on error reporting by physicians, and even less on patient safety.[18]

Physicians have historically complained that most malpractice suits are frivolous and that there are few legitimate patient-victims. Now that the facts of widespread error-related injury are well-documented and accepted, nothing has changed. The evidence has not altered the desire for tort reform. As physician-lawyer and malpractice expert William Sage has pointed out, "Tort reform is not an intuitive solution to rampant medical error. Why should the medical profession, which historically criticized lawyers for inventing medical errors where none existed, receive even greater protection from lawyers now that we know errors to be widespread?"[19]

Nonetheless, if we believe the real problem is defective systems, not defective physicians and nurses, doesn't holding individual physicians and nurses responsible for their negligence make patient safety reforms, such as mandatory error and near miss reporting that the airlines use, less likely? The answer is that it is not all or nothing. Bad systems are the major problem, but negligent physicians and nurses are part of the problem as well, and there is no evidence that protecting negligent healthcare providers from accountability for actions that cause death and injury results in more reporting and makes patients safer—the opposite seems to be true. As patient safety expert Robert Wachter has noted, not only does the current system lack accountability for bad nurses and doctors, but also, as hospitals try to implement new patient safety systems, "a new problem has emerged: what to do with providers who willfully violate reasonable safety rules. Nothing undercuts an institution's effort to fully comply with safety regulations more than having an individual provider (particularly a prominent physician) regularly ignore the regulations."[20]

Even those who espouse an exclusively systems approach to patient safety would probably agree that the most important case driving the patient safety movement was the death of *Boston Globe* medical reporter Betsy Lehman from a series of chemotherapy overdoses, a case highlighted in the IOM report. Lehman's widely publicized death did result in the hospital, Boston's Dana-Farber Cancer Institute, adopting state-of-the-art drug ordering software and initiating a system-wide patient safety program. But accountability was also crucial. The hospital itself early on settled a medical malpractice suit, four physicians were sued (two successfully), and 18 nurses were disciplined by the state licensing board. It is also not irrelevant that the Lehman case occurred in Massachusetts, or that the Massachusetts Board of Registration in Medicine has moved forward more aggressively on patient safety as a result of it.

One myth, for example, is that medical malpractice litigation is unrelated to medical quality of care and thus the fact that a physician has been sued multiple times tells us nothing about the physician's competence. The data paint a different picture. In a survey of medical malpractice in the Commonwealth of Massachusetts, the Board identified 98 physicians (4% of the 2,307 who made a malpractice payment in the period 1994–2003) who had made three or more malpractice payments. An examination of these 98, who were collectively responsible for 13.5% of all claims paid, found that approximately half (48) were removed by the Board from practice, retired, allowed their licenses to relapse, or are inactive or deceased; nine of the remaining 50 have been disciplined by the Board.[21] In short, a high correlation exists between multiple malpractice payouts and competence, and the Board's "three strikes and you are reviewed" policy seems just right (versus a "three strikes and you're out" rule, which seems overly harsh).

The most important point is that continuing our 30-year-plus battle to make marginal changes in state medical malpractice laws does nothing to improve patient safety. As Peter Budetti noted in a *JAMA* editorial on two studies of the effects of medical malpractice litigation on physician practice and the patient safety movement, positions "cannot be reconciled as long as the patient safety movement and tort reform initiatives proceed along separate tracks. What is needed is to link new approaches of legal accountability with mandatory active participation in advanced, systematic measure to ensure high-quality care ... rather than a continuance of actions reflecting the visceral antipathy of many physicians and lawyers to one another."[22] Having the courts (or legislatures, or even regulatory agencies, like boards of medicine) establish a basic patient right to safety could do more to encourage hospitals, through their boards of directors, to adopt a culture of safety than any other patient safety reform so far suggested.

With respect to patient safety, lawyers and physicians should see each other as natural allies rather than as predator and prey. The patient safety problem is complicated, and no single change in the tort system (including the recognition of a right to safety) will solve it, any more than the elimination of legal liability for vaccine manufacturers will solve our chronic vaccine shortages.[23]

A right to safety will have to be implemented by hospitals. Nonetheless, physicians will be central to its success. The most appropriate model for physicians to emulate is not the airline industry, but the anesthesiologists. Because of the successful 25-year program to make anesthesia safer for patients, the risk of death from anesthesia has dropped from 1 in 5,000 to about 1 in 250,000; and as a consequence their malpractice insurance rate, once the highest in medicine, is now among the lowest.[24] As their experience illustrates, high malpractice premiums can themselves be a motivator to develop safer practices that can ultimately end in a win-win situation for both patients and physicians. The Massachusetts Board of Registration in Medicine likewise based its "Medical Malpractice Analysis" on its philosophy that its job was to improve patient safety by preventing medical malpractice in the first place, and not to worry about flaws in the legal system. In the Board's words: "The Board's primary responsibility is patient safety, and so this Report focuses on proposals whose effects will be felt *before* malpractice even happens."[25]

Less helpful is a Joint Commission patient safety initiative that encourages physicians to wear a button that reads, "Ask me if I have washed my hands." This is an example of putting responsibility for patient safety in the hands of patients themselves. The fact that the Joint Commission sees patient self-defense as a major safety strategy is a symptom of the problem, not a solution. Patients should, of course, be encouraged to participate actively in their care, but they should not be responsible for their own safety in an environment over which they have little, if any, control.

How misguided this strategy is can be illustrated by a story one of the country's leading patient safety advocates, physician Don Berwick, tells about himself. A friend had asked him to come with her when she had a cardiac catheterization (the procedure that killed the judge in the earlier mentioned Mississippi case), telling him, "I would feel so much better if you were there with me in the cath lab." Berwick says he immediately agreed. When they came together for the procedure, however, the nurse informed them, "It's not possible. We have a policy against that." And when the cardiologist arrived, he backed up the nurse, telling the patient, "I am just not comfortable with that. We don't do that here. It doesn't work." Berwick continues, "Moments later, my friend was wheeled away, shaking in fear and sobbing." He asks, "What's wrong with this picture?," and concludes that it is a system that exerts "its power over reason, respect, and even logic in order to serve its own needs, not the patient's . . . [an] exercise of a form of violence and a tolerance for untruth, and needless harm."[26]

Berwick's story speaks volumes about why there is no right to safety, as well as why it is misguided to expect patients to protect themselves. His story could have been told literally decades ago, during the early 1970s, when obstetricians were becoming accustomed to having fathers in the delivery room, and hospitals were becoming accustomed to having parents stay with their sick children. But for anyone to have to tell this story in the 21st century is, I agree with him, outrageous. Patients have legal rights, and one of them is to have a friend, who can be called a patient advocate or not, with them at all times. There is literally no excuse for the self-serving and anti-patient behavior of the cardiologist or the nurse. Berwick should also have known better—he wasn't sick, and as a physician he should know that almost every time a doctor, nurse, or hospital official says that something you want to do is "against [hospital] policy" it's a lie. The response should be, "OK, can I see a copy of the policy so I can see if it applies to us?" Most likely there is no such policy, and if there is, there are always exceptions that can be made. Ultimately, patients have a right to refuse any treatment, and patients and their friends and family can use this leverage to obtain the quality of care they want—by refusing to be treated in such a grossly rude and medically risky manner.

Hospitals can decide on their own to take the patient's right to safety seriously. But the continued extraordinarily high rate of death and injury from medical errors in hospitals indicates that most hospitals have not. Effective pressure for a change in the safety culture seems most likely to come from an increased risk of liability, which is signaled by an increase in patient safety lawsuits, one incentive to which hospitals (at least those not still covered by the old doctrine of charitable immunity) seem to respond. Legal actions that are focused on patient safety systems in hospitals, rather than on the actions of individual physicians, could help encourage more serious consideration of other reforms as well.[27]

One such reform is making medical products (rather than places) safer. It involves the FDA, and the way we approve and market prescription drugs in the United States. Most studies, for example, show even more patients are killed and injured by adverse drug reactions than are killed and injured by preventable medical errors in our hospitals. A recent opinion of the Supreme Court helps frame the issue of drug safety and the role of legal liability in encouraging greater safety measures.

Drug Safety

The *New York Times* editorialized "A Win for Injured Patients,"[28] while the *Wall Street Journal* opined that the Supreme Court was "Pre-empting Drug Innovation."[29] To the *Times*, the Court's decision in *Wyeth v. Levine* was "wise and surprising"; to the *Journal* it was a "defeat for drug innovation and public health." There was surprise because the Court had earlier ruled that Congress had preempted (forbidden) state civil lawsuits for medical device misbranding (incomplete drug labelling), and many thought that the Court had turned relentlessly pro-business and would therefore also rule that civil lawsuits for drug misbranding were also preempted.[30] Medical commentators had also been very concerned with the outcome in *Wyeth v. Levine*.[31] Some argued, for example, that should Wyeth prevail, the result would "undermine the confidence that doctors and patients have in the safety of drugs . . . ."[32]

The case drew wide attention both because of its facts and its ideological policy underpinnings. The facts led dissenting Justice Samuel Alito to proclaim, "This case illustrates that tragic facts make bad law," a paraphrase of Oliver Wendell Holmes famous 1904 saying, "Great cases, like hard cases, make bad law."[33] Put another way, Holmes could have said simply, "Don't make law or policy based on worst case scenarios." The ideological policy question was whether FDA approval of a drug should immunize its manufacturer from liability suits by injured patients. The pharmaceutical industry had long argued that FDA approval should immunize it from lawsuits, and although its position had been consistently rejected by the FDA itself, under the Bush administration the FDA changed its mind and joined hands with industry to argue for such immunity from lawsuits.

The heated debate about the *Wyeth* case specifically, and preemption generally, has focused on three components, and understanding which component one is addressing is critical to understanding the case itself. In short, one can argue the facts of the case, the law of preemption, and public policy regarding the role of the FDA in drug regulation. Most scientific and medical commentary prior to the decision dealt with the public policy component: How can the FDA be strengthened to better protect the pubic from the dangers of drugs that are discovered only after the drugs have been approved (and are in wide use) for marketing?[34] As an IOM panel put it, an understanding of the risks and benefits of a drug changes "over the drug's lifecycle, and the attention paid to safety and efficacy before approval must therefore be sustained as a drug enters and diffuses through the market and is used by a growing number of patients ... preapproval clinical trials do not obviate continuing formal evaluations after approval."[35] These policy questions are critical, but the policy component is primarily for Congress and the FDA. In *Wyeth*, the Court dealt mainly with preemption and the facts of the case.

As summarized by the Court, the facts in *Wyeth* were not really in dispute. The plaintiff, Diana Levine of Vermont, was a professional musician who suffered from migraines for which she was treated at a local clinic. She had previously been given an intramuscular injection of Demerol for her headache, and a Wyeth drug, Phenergan, for her nausea. On April 7, 2000, she got this same treatment. This time it turned out to be ineffective. So she returned to the clinic later in the day and received a second injection of both drugs. At this second visit, the physician assistant administered the drugs by the intravenous (IV)-push method. Because the drug was not administered correctly, Phenergan came into contact with her arterial blood, which caused her to develop gangrene. This eventually resulted in the amputation of her right hand, and later in the amputation of her entire forearm.

Levine settled her malpractice claim against the health center. She then sued Wyeth for failure to properly warn healthcare providers of the dangers of administering the drug by IV-push. Wyeth argued that this claim was preempted by federal law because it would be impossible for Wyeth to both follow the FDA's labeling requirements for the drug as well as following additional warnings required by individual states. The trial judge instructed the jury that it could consider evidence that Wyeth complied with FDA requirements, but that FDA compliance alone did not prove that the warnings were adequate. The jury awarded Levine $7,400,000, which the judge reduced by the amount of her earlier malpractice settlement with the clinic. The Vermont Supreme Court affirmed the jury verdict, finding, among other things, that the verdict did not conflict with FDA labeling requirements because those requirements "create a floor, not a ceiling, for state regulation."[36] The Supreme Court's opinion, written by Justice John Paul Stevens, is premised on the jury's finding that Levine's injury would not have occurred if Phenergan's label had included an adequate warning about the risks of the IV-push method of administering the drug.

Preemption means that when Congress legislates in an area in which it has authority, the Supremacy Clause of the Constitution provides that federal law is the "supreme law of the land" and displaces any state law in that area, if that is what Congress intends or if the federal and state laws are in conflict.[37] The preemption issue in *Wyeth* is not one of conflicting state and federal laws. Instead, the question is whether Congress has forbidden state legislatures and courts from imposing more stringent labeling standards than those imposed by the FDA. The Court states the question before it as "whether federal law preempts Levine's claim that Phenergan's label did not contain an adequate warning about using the IV-push method of administration." In addressing this question, the Court declares that it must be "guided by two cornerstones of our preemption jurisprudence": (1) the purpose of Congress is the "ultimate touchstone" and (2) Congress is not to be understood as exercising its Supremacy powers in areas affecting the "historic police powers of the States" unless this is the "clear and manifest purpose of Congress."

Since Congress did not explicitly preempt the area of drug labeling, as the Court had previously held it did in the area of device labeling,[38] the only question is whether preemption should be implied in this case. Wyeth made two arguments for implied preemption: that it is impossible for Wyeth to comply with both federal and state rules, and that the potential operation of state law in the area of labeling would obstruct the effective operation of federal drug laws. The Court discussed both arguments in some detail, but ultimately rejected each of them. As to impossibility, FDA premarket approval of a new drug application includes with it the approval of the text of the proposed label. Also, as a general rule, a drug company may only alter the label with the approval of the FDA. Nonetheless, there is an exception in FDA regulations: The manufacturer need not wait for FDA approval for new language on a drug label to change the label to "add or strengthen a contraindication, warning, precaution, or adverse reaction" or to "add or strengthen an instruction about dosage and administration that is intended to increase the safe use of the product." Wyeth argued that this exception only applied if the change was made in response to new information; that is, information that the FDA had not previously considered. The Court disagreed, noting that FDA regulations also permitted "new analyses of previously submitted data." The record also indicated that in at least 20 incidents prior to Levine's injury, Phenergan injection had resulted in amputation.

Wyeth's most sweeping claim, however, was that the FDA, not the drug manufacturer, has the primary responsibility for the content of the drug label. Again, the Court disagreed, noting that "it has remained a central premise of drug regulation that the manufacturer bears responsibility for the content of its label at all times." The FDA does, of course, have the authority to reject changes to a drug's label, but in this case the Court found no clear evidence that such a change would have been rejected, and "absent clear evidence that the FDA would not have approved a change to Phenergan's label, we will not conclude that it was impossible for Wyeth to comply with both federal and state requirements."

Wyeth's second argument was that requiring it to comply with both federal and state law would "obstruct the purposes and objectives of federal drug labeling regulation." The basic argument is that Congress placed the responsibility for making drug labeling decisions in the hands of an expert agency, the FDA, and that to permit juries of untrained lay people to second-guess the FDA in this regard would undermine the FDA's role and authority. The Court again disagreed, concluding that if Congress thought that state lawsuits were an obstacle to achieving federal objectives, "it surely would have enacted an express preemption provision at some point during the FDCA's [Food, Drug and Cosmetic Act's] 70-year history."

Nor was the Court persuaded by the policy change adopted by the Bush administration's FDA. In the preamble to its 2006 regulations governing prescription drug labels, the FDA proclaimed that its rules establish "both a 'floor' and a 'ceiling,'"[39] so that "FDA approval of labeling ... preempts conflicting or contrary state law." Recognizing that an agency regulation could result in a finding of preemption if the regulations were well-reasoned and persuasive, the Court nonetheless found the FDA's newly discovered 2006 position a "mere assertion" that "is entitled to no weight." Instead, the Court concluded that FDA and Congressional history, as well as good public policy, support the continued use of state lawsuits to protect the public from dangerous drugs. As the Court noted, "The FDA has limited resources to monitor the 11,000 drugs on the market, and manufacturers have superior access to information about their drugs, especially in the post-marketing phase as new risks emerge. State tort suits uncover unknown drug hazards and provide incentives for drug manufacturers to disclose safety risks promptly."

Justices Stephen Breyer and Clarence Thomas each wrote concurring opinions. Justice Breyer wanted to make clear that, even though he agreed with the judgment, he thought that there might be times when the FDA could adopt a drug labeling regulation that would have a preemptive effect. Justice Thomas wrote about federalism, essentially arguing that, to be constitutional and preserve the federalist system, the Supremacy Clause should be read so as to require explicit language in legislation that Congress intends to preempt state law, at least in cases where no direct conflict exists between the federal and state law.

Justice Samuel Alito wrote a dissenting opinion in which Chief Justice Roberts and Justice Antonin Scalia joined. Alito seems convinced that the jury made a bad decision, and that to avoid such bad decisions the Court should have concluded that only the FDA should make determinations regarding the adequacy of drug warnings. His first sentence is instructive: "This case illustrates that tragic facts make bad law." This is followed up in the next paragraph with an assertion that even a stronger warning would not have helped Levine, and the case should have been tried solely as a malpractice case: "The physician's assistant who treated her disregarded at least six separate warnings that are already on Phenergan's labeling, so [Levine] would be hard pressed to prove that a seventh would have made a difference." This is at least curious, since this is just what she had proven to the jury. Alito then restated his view of the case, which is different from the majority's, and seems fanciful since no other judge at any level in this case had challenged the FDA's authority to find Phenergan "safe": "the real issue is whether a state tort jury can countermand the FDA's considered judgment that Phenergan's FDA-mandated warning label renders its intravenous (IV) use 'safe.' "

Justice Alito continued by arguing that the FDA, "whether wisely or not" had consistently concluded during its long history with Phenergan that it was safe and effective when used following the labeling, and that nothing in the FDA's history suggested that juries may "second-guess" the FDA on a labeling determination. If it could, Alito argued, it would run afoul of the Court's conflict preemption cases. Specifically, Alito argued that this case should be decided just like a previous case involving airbags (a case which the majority found easy to distinguish). That case involved a woman who was seriously injured when she drove her 1987 Honda automobile into a tree. She was wearing a seat belt, but she sued in state court alleging that her Honda was negligently and defectively designed because it lacked a driver's side airbag.[40] Congress had empowered the Secretary of Transportation to set "minimum standards" for vehicle safety, and in the statute had specifically said that "compliance with any Federal motor vehicle safety standard issued under this subchapter does not exempt any person from any liability under common law." Nonetheless, Alito noted, the

Court found the state claim of the injured woman preempted because the Department of Transportation's regulations permitted manufacturers to install "alternative protection systems" (rather than any specific one) in their vehicles, and the Secretary had determined that using a menu of safety devices was "safe." Alito concluded that this case should be seen as controlling because the FDA had found Phenergan "safe and effective," and Levine was trying to get a state court to reverse this finding. In Alito's words: "Federal law does not prohibit Wyeth from contraindicating IV-push, just as federal law did not prohibit Honda from installing airbags in all its cars. But just as we held that States may not compel the latter, so, too, are States precluded from compelling the former."

Finally Alito argued that, as a factual matter, the FDA had made a decision based on "ample evidence" that the warning label, which said among other things (in bold lettering): "Inadvertent intra-arterial injection can result in gangrene of the affected extremity," was adequate, and that the FDA decision should control. This is true, in Alito's view, primarily because "juries are ill-equipped to perform the FDA's cost–benefit-balancing function . . . " because they only see patients who have "suffered a tragic accident" whereas the FDA "has the benefit of the long view," including those who would suffer without access to the product.

To emphasize this point, Alito used the example of "vesicant" drugs used for chemotherapy, drugs he characterized as "much more dangerous than drugs like Phenergan," but drugs that, nonetheless, do not disallow IV-push administration. Alito uses the example of mechlorethamine, which is "highly toxic" and he believes much more dangerous than Phenergan. His conclusion: "Regardless of the FDA's reasons for not contraindicating IV-push for these drugs, it is odd (to say the least) that a jury in Vermont can now order for Phenergan what the FDA has chosen not to order for mustard gas [i.e., no IV-push administration]." Alito then set forth an appendix to his opinion that lists 23 specific dangerous drugs, 21 of which either IV-push is not specifically prohibited or is specifically allowed. While Alito's argument is interesting, it is ultimately beside the point: The question was not about the safety of Phenergan, or even about approved routes of administration, but about the content of its label.

The Court's earlier decision in the medical device case of *Riegel v. Medtronic* had led many commentators to predict that the Court could rule the same way in this case, based on an anti-regulation market ideology. It should thus be comforting to see the Court rule based on a reasonable interpretation of the drug law. In the devices case, there was specific Congressional language on preemption, which eight of the nine justices found decided the case in favor of preemption. In this drug case, on the other hand, there was an absence of any statutory preemption language, so the Court had to decide the case based on whether preemption was implied by either an impossibility of complying with both federal and state rules, or whether the state rule would "obstruct the purposes and objectives" of federal drug labeling regulation. Six of the nine justices had no real problem finding that the federal and state rules could coexist, as they have since the FDA was created.

Even the dissenting justices seemed to argue only half-heartedly about legal principles of preemption. Instead, Justice Alito really disagreed with the jury's finding of facts. He wanted the injured plaintiff to be content to sue the physician assistant who administered the drug that caused her injury, and barring this, he wanted the jury (or trial judge) to find as a fact that the drug's label could not be considered the cause of her injury. And, because the jury did not come to the conclusion he believed the jury should have reached, Alito decided that juries should never be permitted to make such decisions— the FDA's determination should be unchallengeable.

Justice Thomas' opinion was based entirely on the law of preemption and was unaffected by the specific facts of this case. Justice Thomas makes a federalist argument, that the states and their inherent powers are vital to our federalist system, so vital that if Congress wants to use the Commerce Clause to take over and preempt an area of law historically regulated by the states (like health and safety regulations), it should only be permitted to do so by adopting explicit statutory language. Thomas would therefore entirely do away with the doctrine of implied preemption. Unlike all the other justices, he would never permit a federal agency to preempt an area through agency regulation. All the other justices allow for the possibility of agency preemption, but the majority at least would require very compelling reasons for agency preemption and a determination that it was consistent with (if not specifically authorized by) Congressional delegation of authority.

In the wake of *Levine*, it has been suggested that the current state of the law, in which failure-to-warn lawsuits are preempted for medical devices but not for drugs, is a "perplexing state of affairs [that] defies all logic."[41] This statement is true if one believes (and many, if not most, physicians probably do) that there is little difference between an inadequately labeled drug and an inadequately labeled medical device in terms of patient safety. But, as these cases illustrate, preemption is a legal doctrine, and its application is primarily determined by interpreting statutory language. Under the Supremacy Clause, federal law is the supreme law of the land. But federal law is exclusive in a particular area only if Congress deems it to be, or if it is impossible for both federal and state laws to coexist.

The Court's conclusion that Congress intended to preempt state level device litigation, but not state level drug litigation, is persuasive as a matter of law given the differing language of each statute. The result may well be described as a "perplexing" state of affairs from a medical or even consumer point of view, but it is perfectly permissible from a legal point of view. The different preemptive language in the drug and device laws is the result of the political process (including intense industry lobbying) when these two different statutes were adopted, not of the legal process of interpreting these statutes. As a result, a very effective way exists to make both device and drugs laws the same: Congress can either simply delete the preemptive language from the device amendments or add the preemptive language of the device law to the drug law. This is a policy decision.

Because the safety of patients cannot be assured by the FDA or by prescribing physicians, and because we learn more and more about both risks and benefits of drugs and devices the longer they are used, the most reasonable public policy position for Congress to take is to continue the American tradition of permitting state level lawsuits for failure to adequately warn of drug dangers and to amend the device law to be consistent with the drug law. Like patient safety in hospitals, patient safety in the context of prescription drugs will be improved by litigation, even though both pharmaceutical companies and hospitals will likely continue to view litigation as a worst case scenario.

The Obama administration has also taken the position that preemption should not be decreed by executive department agencies unless Congress has explicitly acted, or where preemption would be justified under "legal principles governing preemption"; that is, the principles outlined by the Court in *Wyeth*. The president has instructed all departments and agencies to review all regulations issued within the past 10 years that have language meant to support preemption of state law and amend them if the language is not legally supportable by Congressional language or impossibility of coexistence. The rationale for the president's May 2009 memorandum is to uphold the traditional role the states have played to protect the health and safety of Americans: "Throughout our history, state and local governments have frequently protected health, safety, and the environment more aggressively than has the national government."[42]

It may seem strange for a federal government that is entirely dominated by one party to encourage states to actively engage in health and safety regulation. It is an understandable Congressional tradition that the party in power usually seeks to use preemption to impose its policy views on the entire country, while the minority party seeks to retain at least some power in the hands of the states. But, I think, the Obama memo persuasively quotes the explanation given by Justice Louis Brandeis more than 70 years ago as its justification: "It is one of the happy incidents of the federal system that a single courageous state may, if its citizens choose, serve as a laboratory and try novel social and economic experiments without risk to the rest of the country." At least in the area of drugs (and devices, should Congress change the law), the states can also serve to supplement federal regulators when the safety of the public cannot be adequately protected by the federal government.

Because patient safety is a quintessential public health issue, this chapter also serves as a reasonable bridge to the third and final section of the book, Disaster and Public Health. In it, I will deal with major public health challenges faced by populations in which prevention of disaster rather than simply preparing to respond to worst case scenarios is the goal. In attempting to avoid global disasters I will argue that human rights is a much more powerful framework for action than bioethics (or even social justice). Moreover, as illustrated in the opening chapter of Disaster and Public Health, it will often be the case that physicians are critical to public health effectiveness, and bioethics and human rights are each more powerful as allies than strangers. I will make the case that the future of an integrated health law, bioethics, and human rights agenda is a global. Nonetheless, as most of the worst case scenarios I have examined so far illustrate, medical decisions will continue to be made on the local, doctor-patient level, and the way physicians, hospitals and health systems perform locally will continue to be the major determinant of the quality of care people obtain.

III

....

DISASTER AND PUBLIC HEALTH

13

Global Health

After 9/11 it became fashionable to ask, at least in the arena of global health, if human rights had any special relevance anymore. This question is still being asked as the second year of the Obama administration approaches. The president picked Joseph O'Neill's post-9/11 novel *Netherland* to read shortly after taking office. The novel's narrator, Hans van den Broek, simply refuses to consider many of the questions that I have concentrated on in *Worst Case Bioethics*. In his words:

> I found myself unable to contribute to conversations about the value of international law or the feasibility of producing a dirty bomb or the constitutional rights of imprisoned enemies or the efficacy of duct tape as a window sealant or the merits of vaccinating the American masses against smallpox or the complexity of weaponizing deadly bacteria or the menace of the neoconservative cabal in the Bush administration, or indeed any of the debates, each apparantly vital, that raged everywhere—raged, because the debaters grew heated and angry and contemptuous . . . I had little interest. I didn't really care. In short, I was a political-ethical idiot.

Hans is, of course, not the only one who has lost interest in these topics. *Netherland* has deservedly been blessed with gushing reviews and a presidential endorsement. Nonetheless, my own choice for pursuing a conversation about "the value of international law" in the context of global health is *Falling Man*. The conflicting perceptions of the value of international human rights are echoed in the decidedly mixed reviews Don DeLillo's *Falling Man,* garnered. The novel (like human rights?) has been described by reviewers as "frustratingly disjointed," "masterly polyphonic fizzling," "a terrible disappointment," "setting the standard," and "a display of cumulative brilliance." My own view is that the post-World War II human rights movement in general, and its much more recent health and human rights application to global health, sets the "standard" and even represents "a display of cumulative brilliance."

DeLillo's last great novel, *Underworld,* published in 1997, portrays the Cold War and its fallout as well as anything in fiction or nonfiction. Its cover, surely not meant to be purposely prophetic, pictures the twin towers on both the front and back (one a photo positive, the other a negative) with a church steeple and cross in front of them, and a bird of prey flying in their direction. The cover of *Falling Man* is self-consciously derivative. The front cover is illustrated by a blue sky as seen from above cloud cover; the back cover contains the same cloudscape with the twin towers breaking through. Both books are about our fear and confusion, followed by our death and decay, which we cover up—with more or less success—with consumption and by building massive monuments to ourselves. But *Falling Man* has more bite than *Underworld,* no doubt because of the fall of the towers. It is filled, as we are, with loss and self-destruction. Memory loss is its central obsession, but it is also filled with assorted ways and reasons to commit suicide in the midst of plenty. The main character of *Falling Man,* a survivor from the first tower, is almost universally described by reviewers as a shallow, middle-aged businessman (the typical American?). DeLillo describes his plight at the end of the novel (which ends where it begins, with the main character escaping from the tower, and observing what is happening): "He could not find himself in the things he saw and heard."

Human rights advocates usually don't have a hard time finding them-selves, and their general quest is to change the things they see and hear. But they may see more blue sky than threatening clouds on the horizon, and may or may not have faded memories of the horrors of World War II that gave birth to modern human rights. Nonetheless, 9/11 changed the inter-national human rights movement as well. Former Yale Law School Dean Harold Koh, for example, the leading human rights expert in the Obama administration, has perceptively identified four eras of human rights: (1) the

Era of Universalism (1941–56), beginning with Roosevelt's Four Freedoms speech (freedom of speech and religion, freedom from want and fear), and containing the founding of the United Nations and the adoption of the UDHR; (2) the *Era of Institutionalization* (1965–76) when the treaties were adopted and the institutional structures of human rights were formed, mostly at the UN; (3) the *Era of Operationalization* (1976–89), with the formation of national and regional human rights regimes, constitutional law applications, special reporters, and specialized nongovernmental organizations (NGOs); and finally (4) the *Era of Globalization* (1989–present). Koh divides the globalization of human rights into two periods: (1989–2001) the Age of Optimism, from the fall of the Berlin Wall to 9/11; and the Age of Pessimism from 9/11 to today.[1] He delineated these eras before the election of Barack Obama, and there is at least the hope that the Obama presidency could mark a turning point in the Age of Pessimism concerning human rights. Nonetheless, reasons for continued pessimism abound.

The United States used 9/11 as a rationale to abandon not only our rhetorical role of global leader in human rights (always contested by some), but also to abandon human rights itself as a professed guide to our own actions, adopting methods we had consistently condemned since World War II, including preemptive war, torture, cruel and humiliating treatment, indefinite detention, disappearances, and grave breaches of the Geneva Conventions. As described in some detail in Chapter 4, we became a human rights outlaw in promoting the use of torture, and our country is no longer credible as a moral, or even rhetorical, leader in this arena.[2]

This is disheartening. But does it mean that it is also time to abandon the nascent health and human rights movement as a potential fundamental underpinning for global health? I think not. In spite of our recent disgraceful and illegal behavior in the human rights arena labeled "civil and political rights," in the health portion of "economic, social, and cultural rights," as Solly Benatar and Renee Fox have argued, "the United States is the country with the most *potential* for favorably influencing global health trends."[3] (emphasis in original)

Health and Human Rights

Jonathan Mann is rightly identified as the father of the (public) health and human rights movement. As he first noted, it is neither health nor human rights alone that provide the prospect of motivating a global public health movement, but the combination of health and human rights. Not only do negatives in one area exacerbate negatives in the other, positives in both amplify each other.[4]

World War II, arguably the first truly global war, led to a global acknowledgment of the universality of human rights and the responsibility of individuals and governments to promote them. Jonathan Mann also perceptively identified the HIV/AIDS epidemic as the first global epidemic because it is taking place at a time when the world is unified electronically and by swift transportation. Like World War II, this worldwide epidemic requires us to think in new ways and to develop effective methods to treat and prevent disease on a global level. Globalization is a mercantile and ecological fact; it is also a public health reality. The challenge facing medicine and public health, both before and after 9/11, is to develop a global language and a global strategy that can help to improve the health of all of the world's citizens.

To address the HIV/AIDS epidemic it has been necessary to deal directly with a wide range of human rights issues, including discrimination, the rights of women, privacy, and informed consent, as well as education and access to healthcare. Although it is easy to recognize that population-based prevention is required to effectively address the HIV/AIDS epidemic on a global level (as well as, for example, tuberculosis, malaria, and tobacco-related illness), it has been much harder to articulate a global public health ethic, and public health itself has had an extraordinarily difficult time developing its own ethical language. Because of its universality and its emphasis on equality and human dignity, the language of human rights is well suited for public health.

Similarly, Paul Farmer has asked, "What can a focus on health bring to the struggle for human rights?" and answered, "A 'health angle' can promote a broader human rights agenda in unique ways." Using the example of TB in Russian prisons, he noted that he and his colleagues would not have been invited in if they were seen as human rights workers— but as physicians with expertise in TB treatment, they were welcomed in the spirit of "pragmatic solidarity" which, Farmer noted, "may in the end lead to penal reform as well."[5]

Health and human rights experts Sofia Gruskin and Daniel Tarantola have made it crystal clear that the health and human rights movement is based on the human rights movement itself, including the corpus of human rights law articulated in international human rights treaties. As such, primary obligations to respect, protect, and fulfill human rights, including the right to health, fall on the governments of those countries that have signed these treaties and have adopted their own domestic laws to oper- ationalize them. Most fundamentally, human rights law is itself founded on the principle of nondiscrimination: All people everywhere should be treated equally.[6] Women and children also merit special protection under the right to health, and their rights are also reinforced by specific treaties, the Convention on the Elimination of Discrimination Against Women (CEDAW), and the Convention on the Rights of the Child (CRC). Gruskin insists that human rights obligations are legal obligations that bind countries, and it is the legal dimension of the health and human rights field that distinguishes it from the more aspirational field of social justice.[7]

Gruskin is, I believe, quite correct. Nonetheless, as a public health advocate, she would likely agree that spending time mining for differences between the human rights and the social justice approaches, rather than seeking commonalities that can lead to public health action, is counterproductive. Human rights is action- and advocacy-oriented, characteristics that also commend it for global public health.

More than ten years ago I was asked to review a conference-generated book entitled *Ethics, Equity, and Health for All.* The 1997 conference was intended to develop an action plan to promote equity in health and was based on four principles for action: (1) take an inclusive approach to the governance of ethics and human rights in health; (2) give priority to the involvement of countries and groups that are underrepresented in ethics and human rights deliberations; (3) combine shorter- and longer-term efforts to incorporate ethical practice and respect for human rights in the applications of science and technology to health policy and practice; and (4) give priority to the development of human and institutional capacity to ensure sustainability of effort. These principles are reasonable, but the ultimate action plan suggested by the participants, perhaps unsurprisingly, was not. It called primarily for more work to "prepare working definitions of such key terms as ethics, equity, solidarity, [and] human rights, to take account of international . . . and cultural diversity."

Writing this chapter on global health reminded me of the conference, as well as of my initial thoughts about it. Just as books often end by suggesting other books, so conferences have a tendency to end by suggesting more conferences. I wrote at the time:

> The conference wound up calling for more conferences. *Academic conferences have an important place in health and human rights work, but do we really need more conferences to define "equity, ethics, and human rights" in our world?* Aren't the inequalities gross enough and obvious enough to warrant direct attention to actions to deal with the problem itself, rather than to refine the "ethics" of approaching it? Moreover, strong

theoretical works already exist that provide astute analyses of
the relationships between equity (and ethics) and development.
Of special note are two books by Amartya Sen, *On Ethics and
Economics*, and *Inequality Reexamined*.[8](emphasis added)

Today it is worth asking again, Do we really need more conferences
(or books?) to define equity, ethics, and human rights before engaging in
advocacy and direct health action? I remain skeptical. I think we can
conference and write ourselves and the would-be beneficiaries of direct
public health action to death. On the other hand, it must be recognized,
as Sudhir Anand, Fabienne Peter, and Amartya Sen have suggested in
their *Public Health, Ethics, and Equity*, that "the commitment of public
health to social justice and to health equity raises a series of ethical
issues which, until recently, have received insufficient attention."[9] Their
book however, has not satisfied everyone. Bioethicists Madison Powers
and Ruth Faden, for example, suggest that we do need more conferences
and books, when they argue that "the foundational moral justification for
the social institution of public health is social justice," and that "commentary on ethics and public health is, at best, thin."[10] Nor is their view
idiosyncratic.

Jennifer Ruger has argued that although "global health inequalities
are wide and growing ... [and] pose ethical challenges for the global
health community ... we lack a moral framework for dealing with them,"
and suggests pursuing equality from a theory of justice.[11] Elsewhere,
Ruger has suggested that on the specific question of the human right to
health, "One would be hard pressed to find a more controversial or
nebulous human right than the 'right to health'" (although she has also
suggested that a philosophical justification for this right can be provided).[12] Others, including physician-anthropologist and activist Jim
Kim, president of Dartmouth College, has argued that the human rights
approach to health disparities and inequality is more rhetoric than reality,
akin to singing "Kumbaya."[13]

It is easy to be cynical about or disenchanted with human rights. Law
professor David Kennedy has catalogued the major critiques of human
rights, noting that human rights can be legitimately critiqued for driving out
other emancipatory possibilities, for framing problems and solutions too
narrowly, for overgeneralizing and being unduly abstract, and for expressing a Western liberalism. Kennedy's list continues: human rights promises
more than it can deliver, the human rights bureaucracy is itself part of the
problem—it can strengthen bad government, and it can be bad politics in

particular contexts. In his words, "The generation that built the human rights movement focused its attention on the ways in which evil people in evil societies could be identified and restrained. More acute now is how good people, well-intentioned people in good societies, can go wrong, can entrench and support the very things they have learned to denounce. Answering this question requires a pragmatic reassessment of our most sacred humanitarian commitments, tactics and tools."[14]

There is a measure of truth in all these observations, and effective action does require defined goals and specific actions to reach them. But as Joseph Kunz observed almost 60 years ago in regard the Universal Declaration of Human Rights, "In the field of human rights ... it is necessary to avoid the Scylla of a pessimistic cynicism and the Charybdis of mere wishful thinking and superficial optimism."[15] No other language than rights language seems as suitable for global health advocacy. All people have (inherent) human rights by definition, and people with rights can demand change, not just beg for it. And rights matter—and will matter even more as judicial structures to enforce them, like the International Criminal Court, continue to be established and nourished. Values of course underlie rights, but it would be incomprehensible to adopt a "Bill of Values" rather than a "Bill of Rights" to protect people.

In the language of contemporary human rights, governments don't simply have an obligation to act or not to act. Governments have obligations to *respect* the rights of the people themselves, to *protect* people in the exercise of their rights, and to *promote* and *fulfill* the rights of people. Of course, not all governments can immediately fulfill economic rights, like the right to health, because of financial constraints. International human rights law therefore provides that a government's obligation can be defined as working toward the "progressive realization" of these rights within their resource constraints. Some countries are so limited in their resources that they require assistance from the world community. The novel but potentially powerful right to development speaks to the obligations of the world community to provide that assistance, as do the goals of the UN's Millennium Declaration.

In public health, of course, it is well-recognized that many countries require the support of the world community to deal effectively with epidemic diseases, like SARS and the H1N1 flu, and that such support is in everyone's collective interests. (Epidemics are dealt with in the next two chapters.) Another development, the globalization of clinical research trials, provides a good example of the conflicting agendas and conflicts of interest that both call for and seek to avoid universal human rights norms.

The Globalization of Clinical Trials

The globalization of clinical research trials calls for more effective ethical and legal rules to protect research subjects, as well as to guard the scientific integrity of the research.[16] Nonetheless, as the former editor of the *New England Journal of Medicine*, Marcia Angell, observed more than a decade ago in this context, "there appears to be a general retreat from the clear principles enunciated in the Nuremberg Code and the Declaration of Helsinki as applied to research in the Third World."[17] The situation has not improved.

In the last chapter, on patient safety, I examined how the Supreme Court dealt with a Bush administration change in Food and Drug Administration (FDA) policy in which the FDA sought to immunize pharmaceutical manufacturers from state lawsuits asserting that FDA-approved drug labels inadequately warned healthcare providers of their risks. This was not the only step the Bush administration's FDA took to aid the pharmaceutical industry by undermining protections for the public. Another involved research trials. Near the end of the Bush administration, the FDA decided that research studies submitted to it for review need no longer follow the Declaration of Helsinki, but instead could follow the less-exacting, industry-sponsored, International Conference on Harmonization's Guidelines for Good Clinical Practice.[18]

There is another choice—the human rights choice as articulated in the Nuremberg Code. The Declaration of Helsinki is a statement of research ethics by physicians. But what is the legal status of the Nuremberg Code? Does it, like Helsinki and the Harmonization Guidelines, also represent a collection of bioethics rules that researchers can ignore with impunity? Or has the Nuremberg Code, and especially its uncompromising informed consent requirement, arrived at the status of international human rights norm that must be followed? Just as controversy over the US-sponsored 076 maternal-to-child HIV transmission interruption trials in Africa in the mid-1990s gave rise to a continuing debate about standard of care and benefit obligations, so another mid-1990s research trial in Africa has brought international research rules and the doctrine of informed consent back to center stage.

Four years after it occurred, the *Washington Post* broke the story of a 1996 medical experiment conducted by Pfizer researchers in Kano, Nigeria, during a meningitis epidemic. The story created a sensation, especially its lead, which described the slow death of a 10-year-old little girl known only as subject 6587-0069. The researchers monitored her dying without modifying her treatment, but simply followed the research protocol designed to test their potential breakthrough antibiotic, Trovan, on children. The *Post* noted that the story was hardly unique, their investigation having discovered corporation-sponsored experiments in Africa, Asia, Eastern Europe, and Latin America that were "poorly regulated," "dominated by private interests," and that "far too often betray" their promises to research subjects and consumers.[19]

Following the expose, the families of the children-subjects in the Kano experiment brought suit against Pfizer in Nigeria, and later in the United States as well, charging Pfizer with conducting medical experiments without informed consent. The lawsuits initially met dogmatic and sometimes zealous resistance by judges in both the United States and Nigeria. Pfizer had successfully argued both that there was no international norm that required the company physicians to obtain informed consent to experimental drugs, and that in any event, any lawsuit against them by the subjects and their families should be tried in Nigerian, not US courts. Pfizer abandoned this latter claim in 2006 when a copy of an internal report by the Nigerian Ministry of Health on the experiment was made public. The report concluded, among other things, that the study violated Nigerian law, the Declaration of Helsinki, and the Convention on the Rights of the Child (CRC). Following the release of the report, the Nigerian government filed both a criminal and a civil suit against Pfizer in Nigeria. Pfizer settled the Nigerian cases in mid-2009 for $75 million.

More important in human rights terms than the Nigeria litigation, is the litigation in the United States, especially the 2009 opinion of the Second Circuit Court of Appeals, which reversed a lower court dismissal of the lawsuit and sent it back for trial.[20] In the area of human rights, the Second Circuit is best known for its 1980 opinion that a physician from Paraguay could sue the inspector general of police of Asuncion, Paraguay, in the United States for the murder and torture of his son in Paraguay under the Alien Tort Statute. The reason, according to the court, was because torture is universally condemned as a violation of international human rights law, and "The torturer has become—like the pirate and the slave holder before him—*hostis humani generis*, an enemy of all mankind."[21] To oversimplify (but not much), at issue in the Pfizer case before the Second Circuit was whether the researcher who experiments on humans without their informed consent violates a substantially similar international human rights law norm.

It is worth underlining that there has never been a trial in this case, and that the facts alleged by the Nigerian families may not be able to be proven in court. Nonetheless, for the purposes of deciding whether they should have their day in an American court, the Second Circuit had to assume the facts as alleged in the complaint are true. These allegations are primarily that, in the midst of a meningitis epidemic in Nigeria, Pfizer dispatched physicians to go to the Kano Infectious Disease Hospital to do a study on

200 sick children to compare the efficacy of their new drug, Trovan, with the FDA-approved antibiotic Rocephin. Trovan had never before been tested on children in its oral form. The experiment was conducted over a two-week period, then the Pfizer team precipitously left. In the court's words, "According to the appellants, the tests caused the deaths of eleven children, five of whom had taken Trovan and six of whom had taken the lowered dose of ceftriaxone, and left many others blind, deaf, paralyzed, or brain-damaged." The central allegation is that "Pfizer, working in partnership with the Nigerian government, failed to secure the informed consent of either the children or their guardians and specifically failed to disclose or explain the experimental nature of the study or the serious risks involved," or the immediate availability of alternative treatment by Mèdecins sans Frontières (MSF) at the same facility.

The Supreme Court has cautioned lower courts to be conservative in determining whether a particular category of actions contravene "the law of nations" accepted by the "civilized world" as a norm of customary international law.[22] For the Second Circuit to permit this case to proceed it had to conclude that the requirement of informed consent to medical experiments on humans has become a norm of customary international law. The court so concluded because it found the informed consent requirement is sufficiently "(i) universal and obligatory, (ii) specific and definable, and (iii) of mutual concern," to be a customary international law norm that can support a claim under the Alien Tort Statute.

Perhaps of most interest from the global health perspective is that the court found the war crimes trials at Nuremberg, especially the Doctors' Trial, to provide the legal foundation for its conclusion. The major war crimes trial, the International Military Tribunal (IMT), was the only multinational trial at Nuremberg. Nonetheless, the court found that the US military trials that followed the IMT, including the Doctors' Trial, "effectively operated as extensions of the IMT." The Doctors' Trial, of course, produced the 1947 Nuremberg Code in the judgment, the first precept of which is the requirement for voluntary, competent, informed, and understanding consent of the research subject. In the court's words, "The American tribunal's conclusion that action that contravened the Code's first principle constituted a crime against humanity is a lucid indication of the international legal significance of the prohibition on nonconsensual medical experimentation." As important, the Nuremberg consent principle has been widely adopted in international treaties, including the International Covenant on Civil and Political Rights (ICCPR); the Geneva Conventions; and domestic law, as well as in nonbinding international ethics codes like the Declaration of Helsinki.

The court found that in addition to being universal, the Nuremberg norm is specific in its requirement (so researchers could understand it), and is of mutual concern among nations. To make this last point the court concluded that promoting global use of essential medicines can help reduce the spread of contagious disease, "which is a significant threat to international peace and stability." Contrariwise, conducting drug trials in other countries without informed consent "fosters distrust and resistance . . . to critical public health initiatives in which pharmaceutical companies play a key role." The example the court cited is the impact of local distrust of international pharmaceutical companies that caused the Kano boycott of the 2004 effort to stem a polio outbreak there that later spread across Africa, making global eradication of polio all the more difficult.[23]

Post-World War II ethical standards of clinical research have not effectively protected subjects or ensured scientific integrity. The Second Circuit's persuasive opinion that the doctrine of informed consent has attained the status of an international human rights norm that can be enforced in the world's courts should help persuade international corporations and researchers alike to take informed consent, and perhaps the other principles of the Nuremberg Code, much more seriously. If so, it will provide a powerful example of the beneficial impact of human rights on the health and welfare of subjects in clinical trials. But could social justice do the job just as well or better? As I have already suggested, I don't think arguing for one approach or the other is terribly fruitful, and that working together is much more likely to promote the publics' health than working separately. In Senator Edward Kennedy's last letter to President Obama on healthcare (which, as described in Chapter 1, the president read from in his September 2009 speech on the subject to a joint session of Congress), for example, Kennedy referenced both "fundamental principles of social justice" and making healthcare "a right and not a privilege" as complimentary rationales for universal access. It is, nonetheless, worth noting that even commentators who seem to believe in social justice alone is the preferable frame for public health action can't help coming back to the health and human rights movement.

Social Justice and Human Rights

In their discussion of social justice and public health, Powers and Faden describe what they characterize as "one of the most compelling recent examples of work in public health on behalf of an oppressed group. . . ." The example is the documentation of the rights of women by Physicians for Human Rights (PHR) during pre-9/11 Taliban rule. The authors write,

"Research conducted by the group Physicians for Human Rights provides powerful evidence that the denial of basic rights to women resulted not only in horrible injustices with regard to respect, affiliation, and personal security, but also with regard to health."[24] Of course, this research project by PHR can be characterized as public health research and as documenting a major injustice to women. But neither characterization accurately describes what PHR itself thought it was doing.

PHR's name could not be more descriptive of their membership and their goals: Physicians for Human Rights. Nor could the subtitle of its' Taliban report be any more explicit: *The Taliban's War on Women: A Health and Human Rights Crisis in Afghanistan.* The first sentence of their report says it again: "This report documents the results of a three-month study of women's health and human rights concerns and conditions in Afghanistan by Physicians for Human Rights." The report continues: "Taliban policies of systematic discrimination against women seriously undermine the health and well-being of Afghan women. Such discrimination and the suffering it causes constitute an affront to the dignity and worth of Afghan women, and humanity as a whole."

PHR's report is extremely powerful and merits the praise it has received. Nonetheless, it is a report by a physician group, not a public health group, and it is a group dedicated to doing health and human rights work, here especially founded on the ICCPR and CEDAW, not engaged in social justice. Although primarily focused on health, the report also noted that "The Taliban's edicts restricting women's rights have had a disastrous impact on Afghan women and girls' access to education, as well as health care. One of the first edicts issued by the regime when it rose to power was to prohibit girls and women from attending school."[25]

Since the beginning of the ongoing post-9/11 war in Afghanistan, conditions for women have marginally improved, but much remains to be done. Leadership in human rights has been since its creation in the hands of a physician, Sima Samar, chair of the Afghan Independent Human Rights Commission. This is the first human rights commission in Afghanistan's history and it has a wide-ranging mandate, including the promotion of health and human rights, especially the health and human rights of women. When this Commission speaks of justice, it means bringing the perpetrators of war crimes in Afghanistan to justice. And when it speaks of health, it does so in the language of human rights, for example in its 2006 report on "Economic and Social Rights in Afghanistan." Of special note is the Commission's recommendation regarding women and children's health: "The Government should prioritize reproductive (prenatal and postnatal) and child healthcare, according to their obligations under international treaties to which Afghanistan is a party. Afghan women should have universal access to reproductive health care."[26]

It is easy for Americans to criticize the marginalization of human rights and health of women in other countries. But when the health of women in the United States is directly undermined by our government, silence seems the preferred response. Thus, as noted in Chapter 10 on abortion, when our Supreme Court ruled that it is constitutionally acceptable for Congress to make it a crime for a physician to use a specific medical procedure that the physician believes is the best one to protect his female patient's health, most commentary focused on abortion politics, rather than the health of women. Few noted that American physicians have never before been prohibited from using a recognized medical procedure, or that prohibiting its use only affected the health of women. The Taliban must have been smiling. As human rights expert Rebecca Cook noted in the broader context of abortion availability globally, "Whether it is discriminatory and socially unconscionable to criminalize a medical procedure that only women need is a question that usually goes not simply unanswered but unasked."[27]

Globalization and Human Rights

American bioethics has had a major positive impact on the way medicine is currently practiced in the United States, especially in the areas of care of dying patients, including advance directives and palliative care, and medical research, including federal regulations to protect research subjects and institutional review boards. It is noteworthy that these accomplishments all came by enacting specific laws related to health. American bioethics has not exhausted what it can usefully accomplish in these spheres, but has of late seen most of its efforts and energy devoted to the interrelated fields of abortion, embryo research, and cloning.

Given the decade-long embryo-centric US activity (although as noted in Chapter 1, Obama's national healthcare plan did produce renewed political interest in discussing "death panels"), I think it is fair to conclude that bioethics is likely to have a stunted future in the real world without a significant reorientation of its focus and direction. I suggest that the most useful reformulation involves recognition and engagement with two interrelated forces reshaping the world and simultaneously providing new frameworks for ethical analysis and action: globalization and public health.

In *American Bioethics*, I argued that the boundaries between bioethics, health law, and human rights are permeable, and border crossings are common. That these disciplines have often viewed each other with suspicion or simple ignorance tells us only about the past. They are most constructively viewed as integral, symbiotic parts of an organic whole, with a common birthplace: Nuremberg.[28]

Globalization, of course, does not depend upon physicians, ethicists, or lawyers, anymore than it depends upon health law, bioethics, or human rights. It does not even depend primarily upon the actions of governments. Rather, two relatively new players dominate globalization: the transnational corporation, and to a lesser extent, the NGO. Both, I think, can be usefully viewed as new life forms on our planet that are increasingly evolving and changing our environment. A notable health-related example of an NGO is Medecins sans Frontiers (MSF), a humanitarian-human rights organization founded on the belief that human rights transcend national borders and thus human rights workers cannot be constrained by borders, but should cross them when necessary. MSF expands medical ethics to include physician action to protect human rights, blending these two fields and treating the law that protects government territorial boundaries as subordinate to the requirements of protecting human rights. Other human rights and health NGOs, like Physicians for Human Rights, view their primary mission as advocating for human rights.[29]

Transnational corporations deserve our attention because of their incredible potential to both help and harm the planet and its people. Corporations have historically seen at least part of their social responsibility as providing charity to the communities in which they have a large presence. They have, however, been quick to argue that this is purely voluntary and that the responsibility to provide direct services to people, including drugs and medical treatment, rests with the government. A nascent movement to articulate the human rights obligations of transnational corporations is now underway, both in the UN and among corporations themselves. It is too soon to tell whether the global recession, which required governments to rescue both large corporations and banks, will lead to a new recognition of the interdependence of governments and corporations, and thus of their complementary obligations to the people of the world.

Prior to the global financial meltdown, John Ruggie, the Special Representative of the Secretary-General on the issue of human rights and transnational corporations released his report on "Business and Human Rights." The report identifies five avenues to introduce human rights law into corporate behavior (in order, from the strongest to the weakest): (1) the state's duty to protect its citizens against non–state actor human rights abuses; (2) corporate responsibility and accountability for international crimes (including the use of slave labor, child soldiers, and the use of torture) under complicity theories; (3) corporate responsibility for other human rights violations under international law (e.g., under the Universal Declaration of Human Rights, although this is currently "not necessarily legal in nature"); (4) "soft law" mechanisms, such as voluntary international agreements, like the Kimberley process, which seeks to prohibit international trade in "conflict diamonds"; and (5) self-regulation, in which at least some of the 77,000 transnational corporations and their 770,000 subsidiaries voluntarily adopt and follow human rights standards in their businesses.

Approximately 3,000 transnational corporations, including some major pharmaceutical companies, have joined the UN's Global Compact and committed themselves to its principles, the first two of which are that corporations should support and respect the protection of internationally proclaimed human rights, and that corporations should make sure that they are not complicit in human rights abuses. In the conclusion to his report, Ruggie makes three points that have special importance to global health: (1) "human rights and the sustainability of globalization are inextricably linked"; (2) corporations can be tried in "courts of public opinion" for human rights violations; and (3) "no single silver bullet can resolve the business and human rights challenge."[30]

In our current climate, where transnational corporations like Pfizer seem intent on fostering protection of intellectual property more than the protection of people, is there any room for optimism? I think there is. This is because it is becoming critical for transnational corporations to respect human rights for their own sakes. As already discussed, for example, transnational corporations are becoming involved in human rights and bioethics because of their desire to do clinical trials around the world. Corporations may want to set their own rules. But most corporations recognize that they must follow generally accepted international norms of informed consent to conduct their clinical trials if they expect to use the results to have their products certified by government regulators. In short, in at least some cases, transnational corporations must adopt and follow human rights norms to accomplish their business goals. In addition, the human rights and bioethics issues that confront corporations continue to expand, and now include patenting, pricing, and access to their products by people who need them to survive or thrive, but who (either individually or through their governments) simply cannot afford them. These are basic human rights issues that have not been addressed by bioethics.

DeLillo would likely think that human rights and transnational corporations make too unlikely a combination to take seriously. In *Underground*, he saw the transnationals simply taking over from the exhausted Cold War governments. He pictured, for example, waste disposal done in secret by private corporations using underground nuclear explosions. One Kazakhstan company, named Tchaika (meaning seagull, a "nicer name" than rat or pig), is looking for an American broker to recruit US customers:

> They want us to supply the most dangerous waste we can find and they will destroy it for us. Depending on the degree of danger, they will charge their customers—the corporation or government or municipality— between three hundred dollars and twelve hundred dollars per kilo. Tchaika is connected to the commonwealth arms complex, to bomb-design laboratories and the shipping industry. They will pick up waste anywhere in the world, ship it to Kazakhstan, put it in the ground and vaporize it. We will get a broker's fee.[31]

DeLillo may be right. But little progress is likely to be made in global health without the active engagement of the transnational corporations. This could be done either through private–public agreements, or by holding transnationals themselves accountable for not only respecting human rights themselves, but also for protecting and fulfilling them in their spheres of business. In real life, Tchaika, for example, should be legally responsible for all the radiation-caused health consequences of its activities, and should therefore seek to prevent them. The currently contested question, of course, is whether transnationals should have obligations to help fulfill human rights as well, including the right to access to the potentially life-saving drugs whose supply and price they control.[32]

The hero of *Netherland*, Chuck Ramkisoon, tells Hans that his dream is to bring peace to the planet (or at least New York City) through cricket: "I'm saying that people, all people, Americans, whoever, are at their most civilized when they're playing cricket. What's the first thing that happens when Pakistan and India make peace? They play a cricket match."[33] Chuck is a dreamer, but has an abiding belief in the cornerstone of human rights: all human are fundamentally the same, and will recognize this fact when they get to know each other.

On a grander scale, Tony Blair entitled his thoughts on 9/11 in *Foreign Affairs*, "A Battle for Global Values." Much in his essay, especially about the continuing wars in Iraq and Afghanistan, is easy to disagree with. But his basic message is sound: We are not in a war that can be won by force of arms. "This is a battle of values [and] we have to show that our values are not Western, still less American or Anglo-Saxon, but values in the common ownership of humanity, universal values that should be the right of the global citizen." A name exists for those universal values that are the "right of the global citizen," and that name is human rights. Blair goes further, noting,

> The challenge now is to ensure that the agenda is not limited to security alone. There is a danger of a division of global politics into "hard" and "soft," with the "hard" efforts going after the terrorists, whereas the "soft" campaign focuses on poverty and injustice. That divide is dangerous because interdependence makes all these issues just that: interdependent. The answer to terrorism is the universal application of global values, and the answer to poverty and injustice is the same. That is why the struggle for global values has to be applied not selectively but to the whole global agenda.[34]

In the sphere of global health, another way to make Blair's point is, as Jonathan Mann put it, health and human rights are inextricably linked. In the next two chapters, Statue of Security and Pandemic Fear, I explore the link between health and human rights in the post-9/11 attempt to remodel public health as a national security activity, and the attempt of public health itself to regain the public's trust in the context of pandemic flu preparedness and response.

14

....

Statue of Security

Immediately after the 9/11 attacks, the United States government closed the Statue of Liberty to the public.[1] It took almost three years to reopen Liberty Island, just in time for the 2004 Republican National Convention. The public could again visit the island, but little was the same. Visitors had to submit to airport-like screening, bag checks, and bomb-sniffing dogs, at the dock to take the ferry. On the boat trip, the National Park Service had a new recorded welcome, asserting that although historically the Statue of Liberty symbolized freedom, it is now "a symbol of America's freedom, safety, and security." It was not until the 4th of July 2009, during the first year of the Obama administration, that the crown of the Statue of Liberty was reopened.

Intrusive screening is also required to see the Liberty Bell in Philadelphia. We have not yet renamed the Statue of Liberty the "Statue of Security" or the Liberty Bell the "Safety Bell," but since 9/11 safety and security have been consistently promoted as at least as important as liberty, and often more important. Even though President Obama has vowed to change the balance toward liberty, national security remains a potent rationale for just about every government action. Nor is the Obama administration above using the Statue of Liberty for its own purposes.

The announcement of the reopening of the crown, for example, seems to have been timed to help distract attention from the incredibly stupid decision to have Air Force One buzz the Statue of Liberty so that publicity photographs could be taken. The photos themselves were briefly suppressed, perhaps because the juxtaposition of Air Force One onto the Statue of Liberty suggested 9/11 more than America's new president.

The next stop after Liberty Island is Ellis Island, the site of intake screening for more than two million immigrants to America in the early 20th century. The most rigorous part of immigrant screening involved uniformed federal public health service physicians, whose main duty was to prevent immigrants with contagious diseases from entering the country. Few federal public health officials wear military uniforms any longer, and most public health activities now take place under state or local jurisdiction. 9/11, however, drastically affected public health, as public health officials were called upon to prepare the nation for a bioterrorist attack utilizing lethal disease agents, such as smallpox or anthrax.

Many public health officials hoped that public health would gain increased recognition from this new role. They also hoped to take advantage of the new funding available for terrorism preparedness not only to do their part in national security, but also to make "dual use" of the funding to help public health fulfill its core missions. Others argued that the traditional role of public health should be abandoned, and that it should be merged into the national security apparatus (at least in the area of biological threats) under the rubric of "biosecurity." Adding a "bio" to a noun has, of course, been common at least since Foucault's vision of biopolitics and biopower, and Van Rensselaer Potter's vision of bioethics. Biosecurity, biowarfare, bioterrorism, bioengineering, and biotechnology are just a few more examples (others include bioart, discussed in Chapter 2, and bioidentifiers, which will be discussed in Chapter 16).

In this chapter I focus primarily on public health responses to bioterrorist threats; in the next chapter, Pandemic Fear, I take up public health responses to pandemics. 9/11 was an event, not an epidemic, but the United States reacted to it as if it portended an epidemic of terrorist attacks. As former vice president Dick Cheney continues to say, this is a September 12th world, and we should be doing whatever it takes to prevent "another 9/11." 9/11 has, perhaps understandably, been viewed by many in the public health community as a signal of a coming pandemic, akin to the rise of severe acute respiratory syndrome (SARS) in China, a novel form of bird flu in Asia, or even swine flu in Mexico. Moreover, public health has been asked to prepare for both natural and terrorist-induced epidemics simultaneously, under the muddled "all-hazards" preparedness model.

Does 9/11 mean we must make fundamental changes in public health practices regarding epidemic control and revert to 19th-century, Ellis Island-type quarantine and forced treatment? Must we trade human rights and civil liberties for increased safety and security? These are important and complex questions. In this chapter I argue that the answer to both of these questions is "no," and that the movement in public health toward the adoption of a health and human rights should continue.

Osama bin Laden and his homicidal al Qaeda followers present a real danger to Americans, and the United States should bring them to justice for their crimes. The United States is more vulnerable to terrorist attacks than previously believed, and we do need to be on guard to prevent future attacks. However, we should not undermine our lives and our values by overreacting to the threat of terrorism encapsulated in the phrase "a second 9/11." Preserving and promoting human rights both protects core American values and makes it more likely that we will prevail in the long run. Ignoring or marginalizing human and constitutional rights, and treating Americans themselves as suspects or actual enemies, is counterproductive and dangerous itself—a conclusion I will support with specific post-9/11 examples, such as public health preparedness plans for mass smallpox vaccination, and the enactment of extreme state public health mandatory treatment and quarantine laws. Public health professionals are the "good guys" and rightly want to protect the public's health. However, the world has changed since the early 19th century, and reliance on coercion and police rather than education and consent is no longer either legally justifiable or likely to be effective. In this regard, what might be labeled "public health fundamentalism" is as dangerous to the health and safety of Americans as religious fundamentalism.

The language of human rights also has the great advantage of being universal and thus global. Neither the fight against terrorists nor the fight against epidemics can be successfully waged on a local, state, or even national level alone; both easily cross national boundaries and both can only be effectively confronted by a global, cooperative strategy. "Safety first" is a good thought, as is the Hippocratic injunction, "first, do no harm," but neither safety nor inaction are ends in themselves, only means to promote health and human rights.

In the previous chapter on global health, I gave a brief introduction to the human rights framework. In this chapter, I expand on that introduction. The modern human rights movement, like American bioethics, was born from the devastation of World War II. The multinational trial of the major Nazi war criminals at Nuremberg was held on the premise that there is a higher law of humanity, derived from natural law or rules based on an understanding of the essential nature of humans (sometimes termed our moral intuition of inherent rights), and that individuals may be properly tried for violating that law. Universal criminal law includes war crimes and crimes against humanity, such as murder, genocide, torture, and slavery. Obeying the orders of superiors is no defense; the state cannot shield its agents from prosecution for war crimes or crimes against humanity. Perhaps because we do not contemplate these horrible crimes in the abstract, it is only when we are forced to confront them on a large scale that we recognize them as gross violations of basic human rights—and thereby are able to articulate human rights themselves.

Unlike ethical precepts that primarily govern individual conduct, human rights are primarily rights individuals have against governments (although we all have them and are all expected to respect them). As to governments, human rights require governments to respect humans by refraining from doing certain things, such as torturing them or limiting their freedom of religion. Governments are also required to protect human rights by preventing their violation by private actors, and to work to fulfill human rights, such as by providing education and nutrition programs. The United Nations adopted the Universal Declaration of Human Rights (UDHR) in 1948 as a statement of inherent human rights. The legal obligations of governments were to derive from formal treaties that member nations would individually sign and then incorporate into their domestic law.

Because of the Cold War, with its conflicting governmental ideologies, it took almost 20 years to get agreement on the texts of the two major human rights treaties. The International Covenant on Civil and Political Rights (ICCPR) and the International Covenant on Economic, Social, and Cultural Rights (ICESCR) were both adopted by the UN General Assembly and opened for signature and ratification in 1966. The United States ratified the ICCPR in 1992, but not surprisingly, given our capitalist economic system with its emphasis on private property, has yet to act on the ICESCR. We have, nonetheless, signed other treaties that have special significance in the war on terror, including the Geneva Conventions, the Genocide Convention, and the Convention Against Torture.

The rights spelled out in the ICCPR include equality, liberty, security, and freedom of movement, religion, expression, and association. The ICESCR focuses on human well-being, including the right to work for fair wages, to a decent living, to safe and healthy working conditions, to be free from hunger, to education, and "the right of everyone to the enjoyment of the highest attainable standard of physical and mental health." The UDHR and the two subsequent treaties (together referred to as the International Bill of Rights) form a global human rights framework for action and have a special relevance for global health. The World Health Organization (WHO) has, for example, adopted the health and human rights framework as its own. By broadening our perspective, human rights language highlights not only human freedoms, such as self-determination, but also basic human needs, such as education, nutrition, and sanitation, the improvement of which will have a major impact on improving human health.[2]

Like World War II, pandemics (including HIV/AIDS) require us to think in new ways and to develop effective methods to treat and prevent disease on a global level. The challenge facing medicine and healthcare, both before and after 9/11, is to develop a global language and a global strategy that can help improve the health of all of the world's citizens. Clinical medicine is practiced one patient at a time, and the language of medical ethics is the language of self-determination and beneficence: doing what is in the best interests of the patient with the patient's informed consent. This is powerful, but has little direct application in countries where physicians are scarce and medical resources extremely limited.

Public health deals with populations and prevention—the necessary frame of reference in the global context. In a one-to-one physician–patient relationship, for example, a combination of antiretroviral drugs for AIDS treatment makes sense. In the worldwide pandemic, however, such treatment may be available to fewer than a quarter of the world's people with AIDS. The availability of a vaccine against a pandemic flu will also be severely limited. This is not just a matter of money, but also a matter of healthcare infrastructure and a lack of basic knowledge regarding how to deliver drugs effectively. In dealing with the AIDS pandemic, it has become necessary to deal directly with issues of discrimination, immigration status, the rights of women, privacy, and informed consent, as well as with education and access to healthcare.

As suggested in the previous chapter, because of its universality and its emphasis on equality and human dignity, the language of human rights is well suited for public health. On the occasion of the 50th anniversary of the UDHR, I suggested that the UDHR itself set forth the ethics of public health, since its goal is to provide the conditions under which humans can flourish. This is also the goal of public health. The unification of public health and human rights workers around the globe would be a powerful force to improve the lives of everyone.

Cynicism is understandable, but not only are democracy and human rights being taken more seriously by governments, they are also increasingly a major driving force in NGOs. Of course, there are different kinds of rights and more or less effective ways to enforce them. The new International Criminal Court can, for example, help to deter and punish those who engage in torture and genocide, but can do nothing to governments who fail to provide basic healthcare to their citizens. Moreover, to conclude that human rights is a more powerful language for good than bioethics is not to conclude that bioethics is irrelevant. On the contrary, bioethics not only is necessary to make basic human rights a reality (e.g., as has been previously discussed, by prohibiting physician involvement in torture and executions), but it also can advance an antipaternalistic public health agenda that supports public education and democracy in public health practice. Thus, it seems more fruitful to explore the ways in which bioethics and human rights can work together synergistically in preparing for and coping with bioterrorism and epidemics than to ignore either of them.

Bioterrorism and Public Health

In the immediate aftermath of 9/11, it was easy for human rights advocates and civil libertarians to despair. Congress almost immediately passed the Orwellian-named USA Patriot Act and authorized an international (and 1984-like perpetual) global war on terror. The Bush administration also announced that it would disregard not only the UN but also fundamental international human rights and humanitarian law as expressed in the Geneva Conventions. Even before the election of President Obama, however, the tide seemed to be changing, and at least some governmental actions were met with considerable skepticism and even active resistance. The color-coded terrorist warning system was all but abandoned as too vague to do anything more than scare the public. Duct tape and plastic sheeting remain punch lines in jokes about personal protection from che-mical and biological agents, although airline passengers are still required to remove their shoes because a mentally-challenged would-be terrorist once bumblingly attempted to explode a bomb in his shoe.

We continue to be bombarded with worst case bioterrorism doomsday scenarios, although the major terrorist threats are not from biological agents. Rather they are from conventional weapons (e.g., firearms and bombs—including "dirty bombs"—conventional explosives containing radioactive material), delivered either in trucks or by individual suicide bombers, as evidenced by terrorist activities in Israel for decades, by insurgent attacks in Iraq and Afghanistan, and by terrorists worldwide, including the attacks in London, Madrid, and Mumbai. These create panic, but the most dangerous weapons are not chemical or even biological, but nuclear. Although there were many inconsistent rationales given for going to war with Iraq, no one suggested it was because the country possessed chemical or biological weapons; we had known about these weapons for more than two decades, and Iraq had used its chemical weapons on both civilian and military targets. It was the prospect of Iraq possessing nuclear weapons that ultimately moved the country to accept the war.

Nonetheless, as underlined in Chapter 2 on bioterror and bioart, bioterrorism is hyped beyond all scientific or historic reality, not only in the biosecurity industry, but also in the public health community, which should know better. A leading public health lawyer, for example, asserted, "a single gram of crystalline botulinum toxin, evenly dispersed and inhaled, could kill more than one million people."[3] However, when he examined the actual data, the same lawyer admits that when Aum Shinrikyo, the Japanese terrorist cult, actually "attempted to disperse aerosolized botulinum toxin in Tokyo and at several US military installations in Japan," the result was not millions dead or even thousands or hundreds, rather all of these attacks "failed to kill anyone." Likewise, it has been asserted that the "release of 100 kilograms of aerosolized anthrax over Washington, D.C." could kill up to three million people. The real anthrax attacks, launched through the US mail, were highly effective in sowing terror in the population, but resulted in only five deaths, the number killed in American hospitals by negligence every 30 minutes or on our nation's highways every hour.

The scariest scenario involves smallpox because, unlike botulinum or anthrax, smallpox can be transmitted from person to person. This is why the Bush administration used the threat of a smallpox attack from Iraq as one reason for us to fear Iraq, and as the almost sole justification for its massive, national, three-phase smallpox vaccination program. That soon-abandoned program was a public policy and public relations disaster, reaching only about 40,000 of the initially proposed 500,000 healthcare workers the government planned to have vaccinated during phase one (phase two would have encompassed up to 10 million first responders and public safety personnel, and phase three would have included all willing civilians). Why?

The major reason for this policy disaster is that the administration failed to persuade physicians and nurses that the known risks of serious side effects of the smallpox vaccine were justified, given the fact that no evidence existed that Iraq (or anyone else) had both smallpox virus and the wish to use it in a terrorist attack. The information provided on this issue to the physicians and nurses was in the same spirit as the Iraq nuclear threat information, except that it contained no facts at all, not even misleading or phony ones. Julie Gerberding, the Director of the Centers for Disease Control and Prevention (CDC) and the person in charge of the smallpox vaccination program, for example, told a US Senate Appropriations Subcommittee on January 29 2003, about a month after the smallpox vaccination campaign began,

> I can't discuss all of the details because some of the information is, of course, classified. However, I think our reading of the intelligence that we share with the intelligence community is that there is a real possibility of a smallpox attack either from nations that are likely to be harboring the virus or from individual entities, such as terrorist cells that could have access to the virus. Therefore, *we know it is not zero. And, I think that's really what we can say with absolute certainty that there is not a zero risk of a smallpox attack.*[4] (emphasis added)

This is wonderful doubletalk that proves nothing except that the CDC's director did not seem to know much about the risk of a smallpox attack. No human activity is "zero risk." Most importantly, if the US government knows that an individual, group, or nation has smallpox and is planning to use it as a weapon, this information should be made public. It is the terrorists who want to keep their methods and intentions secret. The best defense of a potential target is to make this information public. Since most Americans probably know this, the failure of the administration to offer any evidence at all of any person or country possessing weaponized smallpox meant it was highly probable that the administration had no such evidence. Thus, the real risks of the vaccine could not be offset by any measurable benefit.

Few people were surprised, then, when after the commencement of the Iraq war, in August 2003, an Institute of Medicine panel recommended that smallpox vaccination for civilians be abandoned. By the summer of 2004, the entire effort was abandoned. The bottom line is that the potential for biological terrorism is real (i.e., greater than zero) but very low, and in almost any foreseeable attack the number of deaths is likely to be low (as evidenced in the only real biological attacks to date, in which between no one and five people died). Planning is reasonable, but overreaction by focusing on worst case scenarios has unintended negative consequences and creates more problems (including predictable adverse reactions to the vaccinations themselves) than it solves.

But what about a real epidemic, such as a new, worldwide pandemic? A repeat of the 1918 flu epidemic could prove devastating, but the possibility is remote and the world has changed so greatly since 1918 that possible repetition seems to be invoked primarily as a scare tactic rather than a planning tactic. We would no more fight a 2018—or 2009—recurrence of the 1918 flu epidemic with the ineffective remedies available at the turn of the last century than we would fight an expanded war in Afghanistan today with the trench warfare strategy used in World War I. Nor will we act as if cell phones, the Internet, and 24/7 cable news networks don't exist.

Of course, flu epidemics are real, and they can arrive in an unpredictable manner. We can and should produce vaccines against the flu, and we should continue research to develop a universal flu vaccine, effective against all variants. Our new emphasis on bioterrorism, however, has actually drained public health resources away from traditional public health, including flu vaccine preparation. As the WHO warned in late 2004, and again in 2009, we need much better planning and international cooperation to prepare for an influenza pandemic. Instead, we are diverting funds away from this traditional public health concern: Influenza causes tens of thousands of deaths a year in the United States alone, and it will cause a predictable worldwide pandemic at some point. Nonetheless, the government is diverting limited public health resources to try to protect us against an extremely unlikely bioterrorist attack. In addition, it is here that we can determine whether "dual use" is a reality or just a marketing slogan.

I agree with those who argue that public health infrastructure generally must be improved. However, where I disagree is with the assertion that bioterrorism preparation will improve or modernize public health infrastructure. I wrongly and naively expected the federal government to provide increased funding for public health in the wake of 9/11. There has been some additional funding for bioterrorism, but mostly state public health departments have been left to struggle with more unfunded federal mandates and suggestions, and have had to divert funds from public health programs we know work to save lives and improve health, to bioterrorism preparation that has little or no public health payoff.

Massachusetts, for example, always a national leader in public health, made major cuts in tobacco control, domestic violence prevention, and immunizations against pneumonia and hepatitis A and B. Public health spending decreased 30% in one two-year period, during which time Massachusetts received $21 million for bioterrorism-related activities, some of which could be categorized as dual-use. Public health expert David Ozonoff of the Boston University School of Public Health accurately described what happened: "The whole bioterrorism initiative and what it's doing to public health is a cancer, and it's hollowing out public health from within . . . . This is a catastrophe for American public health."[5] This reality was dramatically illustrated nationally in the fall of 2004 when the United States experienced a shortage of flu vaccine and was initially forced to ration it to Americans most at risk of death and hospitalization from the flu. Cartoonist Matt Davies caught the irony in his cartoon picturing a citizen coming to the door of the "Homeland Security Bio-Terror Readiness Unit" only to be greeted by a note pinned to the door reading, "Out with the Flu."[6]

Other public health experts have put the weakening of public health in even more disturbing biosecurity terms, noting, "Worse, in response to bioterrorism preparedness, public health institutions and procedures are being reorganized along a military or police model that subverts the relationships between public health providers and the communities they serve."[7] To the extent that these experts are correct, an exaggerated fear of bioterrorism is resulting in already counterproductive overreaction that is harming both public health's effectiveness and its relationship with the communities that public health serves.

Exaggerated risks produce extreme responses that are based more on fear than facts, so it is not surprising that they have unintended consequences. Public health planning should be based on science, not on free-floating anxiety and fear of worst case scenarios. Instead of using the tools of public health, especially epidemiology, to gather data, and to perform risk-assessments to identify most likely risks and work on them, our post-9/11 federal government adopted the bizarre preparedness doctrine that all threats are equal and that all states and localities should equally prepare for all of them ("a threat anywhere is a threat everywhere"). This philosophy has produced two interrelated epidemics in the United States: an epidemic of fear and an epidemic of security screening.

It cannot be emphasized enough that the primary goal and purpose of public health is prevention of disease in the first place. In the case of bioterrorism, this means prevention of an attack is much more important to public heath than responding to it after the fact. In addition, contemporary public health prevention of epidemics and bioterrorism is not primarily a local or state issue, but is fundamentally a global security issue that must be dealt with by the community of nations working together. National laws and treaties, with realistic inspection and sanctions devoted to preventing the development and production of biological weapons, are the most important tool in the prevention of bioterrorism. As the swine flu pandemic of 2009 illustrated, we are right to want to modernize the WHO's International Health Regulations. However, as the WHO recognizes, to be effective, revised regulations must be founded on respecting and protecting human rights, not trampling them.

All healthcare is delivered locally, one patient at a time. But this is not true of public health, and state and local laws, no matter what the CDC and its consultants say, simply cannot prevent or control bioterrorism. By seeming to grant unconstitutional power over citizens' lives and liberty, bad state public health emergency laws undermine public trust and, thus, are a danger to public health itself. This is because the key to any effective response to a public health emergency is an informed public that trusts its government.

State Public Health Emergency Laws

In the immediate aftermath of 9/11 the CDC encouraged individual states to enact laws that gave public health officials broad, unaccountable powers over their citizens in the event of a public health emergency. Florida's crude summary of the CDC-sponsored "model act," which seeks to trade off human rights for safety and security, provides the country's starkest example. As I have already discussed in Chapter 11, Culture of Death, Florida can act in uniquely strange ways. Nonetheless, Florida's public health emergency statute helps illustrate why honoring rather than destroying human rights is the most effective public health strategy for the 21st century.

A post- 9/11 epidemic of state laws to expand public health powers in the event of a bioterrorist attack continued into the 2009 swine flu outbreak. Florida's response, nonetheless, remains the most extreme. Perhaps because it was the site of the first anthrax letter attack, Florida proved to be fertile ground for all sorts of so-called antiterrorist legislation. Within a year of 9/11, the Florida legislature passed, and Governor Jeb Bush signed, eleven bills related to terrorism. One of these eleven bills (2002-269) was based at least in part on the CDC-sponsored model, adopting the scheme of declaring a public health emergency to trigger additional government powers and vesting this power in the state's health officer. The state officer's emergency powers are in four categories: (1) the shipment of drugs in the state, (2) the provision of bulk drugs by pharmacists, (3) the temporary licensing of certain healthcare practitioners, and (4) power over individuals.[8]

There are major problems with all of the provisions (especially the extraordinarily broad definition of public health emergency which, for example, would include the annual flu epidemics and HIV/AIDS). But Section 4, on the power over individuals, is so extreme and out of step with anything else in the country, and so inconsistent with basic human rights and constitutional law, that it warrants special scrutiny. The operative section gives the state health officer the following power over individuals in a public health emergency:

> *Ordering an individual to be examined, tested, vaccinated, treated, or quarantined for communicable diseases* that have significant morbidity or mortality and present a severe danger to public health. Individuals who are unable or unwilling to be examined, tested, vaccinated, or treated for reasons of health, religion, or conscience may be subjected to quarantine.
> *Examination, testing, vaccination, or treatment may be performed by any qualified person authorized by the State Health Officer.*
> If the individual poses a danger to the public health, the State Health Officer may subject the individual to quarantine. If there is no practical method to quarantine the individual, the State Health Officer *may use any means necessary to treat the individual.*
> Any order of the State Health Officer given to effectuate this paragraph shall be *immediately enforceable by a law enforcement officer* . . . .[9] (emphasis added)

This section of the Florida statute can be contrasted to a Minnesota statute on the same subject, which, rather than trading off civil liberties for security, takes a human rights and health approach. The Minnesota statute provides, for example, that even in a public health emergency, "individuals have a fundamental right to refuse medical treatment, testing, physical or mental examination, vaccination, participation in experimental procedures and protocols, collection of specimens, and preventative programs."[10]

All four provisions of the Florida statute are extreme. Each provision shows how public health can drastically overreact to a perceived threat in ways that are counterproductive to public health and devastating to human rights. The first part, relating to "ordering an individual to be examined," makes no public health sense, because there is no characteristic of the individual that gives rise to any suspicion or reason to believe that the individual either has the disease in question or has been exposed to the disease. Instead, the mere presence of a disease in Florida, which the state health officer declares as creating a public health emergency, authorizes anyone designated as qualified by the state health officer to order anyone to be "examined, tested, vaccinated, treated, or quarantined." Mere refusal can result in quarantine, without any evidence of exposure to disease, let alone that the person is a threat to others. This is not public health but a public health police state, and the police-suspect model for public health is the core mistake of the entire approach.

Americans (Floridians) are not the enemy in a bioterrorist attack. Therefore, to plan for a response that has the police seek out, confine, and forcibly inject innocent Floridians makes no scientific or public health sense. The enemy is the bioterrorist. Nonetheless, nothing in the Florida statute permits the police to take as violent action against the bioterrorist as they can against a Floridian who merely refuses quarantine or vaccination. This law not only misses the target, it shoots in the wrong direction altogether.

The "any means necessary" section of the Florida statute is the most extreme and offensive, and it is difficult to believe that anyone in the legislature actually read it. The first sentence makes perfect sense, and summarizes the law in virtually every state: "If the individual poses a danger to the public health, the State Health Officer may subject the individual to quarantine." That sentence only makes sense, however, if the phrase "provided this is the least restrictive alternative available" is inferred. The second sentence of the statute has no legal pedigree at all (at least outside of totalitarian states): "If there is no practical method to quarantine the individual, the State Health Officer may use any means necessary to vaccinate or treat the individual." This could be labeled the "torture exception." If the risk is big enough to society, we can torture bioterrorists and their victims! However, as outlined in Chapter 4, governments cannot engage in torture under any circumstances under applicable international human rights treaties.

For almost all potential bioterrorist agents, there is neither a vaccine nor an effective treatment. Nor does any approved treatment exist for garden-variety new epidemics, like SARS, that could qualify as public health emergencies under the statute. So, what can this provision possibly mean—that the state health officer can compel the use of potentially dangerous experimental drugs? This, however, would constitute a fundamental violation of not only international law but of basic US constitutional law and federal drug law. No state law can, of course, overturn any, let alone all, of these higher laws. Even assuming that an approved vaccine could also serve as a treatment if delivered quickly to an exposed person, what justification can there be for forcing the vaccination "by any means"? The state gives only one, "if there is no practical method to quarantine the individual."

The entire statute is based on the premise that state public health officials know how to respond to a public health emergency and should have the power to quarantine if needed. This provision, however, undercuts the assumption that state public health officials have done any planning at all. Instead, it assumes that the state will not be able to provide quarantine facilities when needed. The provision can also be read more cynically, to say the state need not provide quarantine for vaccination refusers since it can simply force vaccination on everyone if it is too difficult to quarantine them. Either way, there is no constitutional or human rights justification for forced treatment. Americans have a constitutional right to refuse any medical treatment, even life-saving treatment, as reaffirmed most recently in the Terri Schiavo case discussed in Chapter 11.

It is also a fundamental principle of medical ethics that patients have the right to informed choice and the right to refuse any medical intervention. An emergency may justify short periods of confinement of those individuals whom public health officials reasonably believe pose a risk to others, but nothing justifies this type of "treatment." Perhaps the only good news about the Florida statute is that even in the wake of 9/11 and the drumbeat of the threat of a possible smallpox attack, no other state passed anything like it. The Florida legislature should be ashamed.[11]

Nevertheless, the drafters of the original CDC model act have developed a mantra they repeat, with numerical modification, every time another state considers amending their public health laws. A recent one is, "Thirty-eight states have adopted the model act in whole or in part." Whether you like the model act or not, another way to describe what has happened over the past eight years is: "Forty-seven states have rejected the model act in whole or in part." While both statements are arguably correct, neither gives any indication of the substance of the law that was enacted (e.g., the Minnesota versus the Florida version), or the population of the states involved (e.g., neither New York nor California have adopted the proposal vs. the three states that arguably have, Delaware, Oklahoma, and South Carolina).

If there ever was any doubt that draconian proposals for forced vaccination and quarantine undermine public trust in government to protect it, it should have been put to rest in the fall of 2009. That was when the Massachusetts Public Health Commissioner, in response to an outbreak of Internet rumors of forced vaccination plans upon the passage of similar the model act by the Massachusetts Senate (but not adopted by the House) felt a need to respond. In a memorandum to the state legislators and all elected officials, entitled "False Rumors Regarding Mandatory Vaccination for H1N1 Influenza," he wrote: "The Department of Public Health will not call for or authorize mandatory vaccination against the pandemic flu. There are no public health officials on the state, national, or global level calling for forced vaccination for H1N1."[12] The rumors were overblown, but the public fear of arbitrary action by public health officials is not.

Proposals to grant public health officials immunity for injuring people during an emergency, even for forced treatment amounting to torture, are also counterproductive. As discussed in Chapter 4, in the context of torture, granting public officials immunity encourages unlawful and arbitrary action, neither of which have any place in public health or medicine. Public health officials should act in a transparent way and be accountable for their actions. And so should physicians. That some physicians should, for example, use their highly questionable "triage" decisions at Memorial Hospital during Katrina to endorse new laws that would help make physicians immune from lawsuit for decisions made during a declared public health emergency is shameful.[13]

At the outset of the 21st century, bioterrorism, although only one threat to public health, can be the catalyst to effectively federalize and integrate state and local public health programs, which are now uncoordinated and piecemeal. This should, I think, include a renewed effort for national health insurance; national licensure for physicians, nurses, and allied health professionals; and national patient safety standards. Federal public health leadership will also encourage us to look outward, to recognize that prevention of future bioterrorist attacks, and even naturally occurring epidemics, will require international cooperation. Universal human rights are the proper foundation for a global public health ethic.

Our fight against bioterrorism should be built on a goal of protecting liberty, not depriving people of it. There is a knee-jerk tendency in times of war and national emergencies to restrict civil liberties as the most effective way to counteract the threat. However, history has taught us that such restrictions are almost always useless, often counterproductive, and we usually wind up with deep regrets for our action. The tendency to return to the days before liberty and informed consent were taken seriously has been evident in the immediate aftermath of 9/11. Arbitrary and unlawful responses have not, however, helped make Americans safer or more secure; instead, they threaten the very liberties that make our country worth protecting. It is wrong and dangerous for our government to treat its citizens either as enemies to be controlled by force or children to be pacified with platitudes.

To be moral and effective, public planning for war and public health emergencies must be based on respecting freedom and trusting our fellow citizens. The United States should lead the world in proclaiming a new, global public health policy based on transparency, trust, science, and most importantly, respect for human rights. We do not need a new Statue of Security; the Statue of Liberty is just fine. My discussion of public health preparedness—and the role of human rights in improving health security—continues in the next chapter, which focuses on pandemic preparedness.

15

. . . .

Pandemic Fear

"**W**ill we all die?" is a question infectious disease expert John McConnell was asked at the height of the swine flu (H1N1) outbreak in 2009. His reasonable response, "Yes, we will, but probably not from flu." Fear is a normal reaction to new disease threats, and it is the role of public health officials and infectious disease experts to counter fear with facts and suggestions for reasonable precautionary measures. It is a destructive and counterproductive post-9/11 myth that countering a pandemic requires public health officials to revert to pre-World War I tactics of forced quarantine and mandatory physical examinations and vaccinations.[1]

Just as many national leaders argued that the public must barter its civil liberties for safety from terrorists attacks, so public health officials have argued that health is best protected by adopting the national security metaphor. 2001 is the excuse, but 1918 is the model. As John Barry, the author of the most definitive book on the 1918 flu pandemic, *The Great Influenza*, put it in an afterward to his book, when another flu pandemic occurs, "Public health officials will need the authority to enforce decisions, including ruthless ones ... officials might decide to order mandatory vaccination. Or, if there is any chance to limit the geographical spread of the disease, officials must have in place the legal power to take extreme quarantine measures." At the outset of the 2009 swine flu outbreak, Barry (wisely I think) reconsidered this extreme advice and argued instead that public compliance with public health advice rests on "trust," not compulsion. He continued, "Only by knowing the truth can imaginary horrors be transformed into concrete realities. And only then can people start to deal with those realities, and do so without panic."[2]

Barry has modernized his advice, but our leaders often seem trapped in 1918. For example, if "extreme" and "brutal" measures are seen as reasonable, no one should be surprised that the military come naturally to mind. President George Bush, for example, reacted to the 2005 threat of a bird flu pandemic by almost immediately suggesting the use of the US military to quarantine "parts of the country" experiencing an "outbreak."[3] The first Obama administration White House press conference on the 2009 swine flu outbreak threatened to be a repeat. The lead was taken by Secretary of Homeland Security Janet Napolitano who declared the outbreak an "emergency." No one should have been surprised when the press asked her questions like, "Should we seal our border with Mexico?" And, "Do you think this could be bioterrorism?"

I give the Obama administration generally high marks for keeping the public informed during the spring 2009 outbreak, but its message was not helped by CDC spokesperson Ann Schuchat, who consistently appeared on television in her Public Health Corps Rear Admiral's uniform. This, of course, gave the impression that the government's reaction to the outbreak was military, since few Americans know anything about the Commissioned Corps of the Public Health Service. Nor was she alone: The acting Surgeon General, Steven Galson, also appeared in his Admiral's uniform. He, like Schuchat, is in the Department of Health and Human Services (HHS), and has nothing to do with the "real" military in the Department of Defense. It is at least worth considering whether use of military ranks and military uniforms in HHS makes any sense at all anymore, or whether it is an anachronism that misleads both HHS and the public into thinking that the military metaphor in public health is real, that the public health corps really is, as their website puts it, "fighting" invaders on the "front lines." Neither Schuchat nor Galson believes, I'm sure, that being an admiral makes them anything like the chair of the Joint Chiefs of Staff, Admiral Michael Mullen. But then what is the purpose of playing "dress up" on television? This type of fake militarism, which seems to make national security a natural justification for action, has plagued post-9/11 public health and arguably made the public much less willing to trust governmental messages and advice.

It probably should surprise no one, however, that the Obama administration has continued the Bush administration's enchantment with the military. In this regard, Andrew Bacevich of Boston University has persuasively argued that the United States has a "deep infatuation with military power" that has resulted in almost constant wars and catastrophes for our country.[4] This infatuation was clearly on display on the 8th anniversary of 9/11 when the US Coast Guard conducted an anti-terrorist "training exercise" on the Potomac River while President Obama was presiding over anniversary ceremonies at the Pentagon and the White House. These exercises involved four 25 foot speedboats armed with mounted machine guns. Their actions, including fake gun shots, set off a scare that was even greater than that set off earlier in the year when the president's plane buzzed the Statue of Liberty in New York for a publicity photo. I think the Coast Guard's mission should be to prevent a terrorist attack, not to simulate one. I also think that the White House should have assured the public that this type of game-playing will never again be permitted either on an anniversary of 9/11, or while the president is in the area. Instead, spokesperson Robert Gibbs blamed the media for overreaction, and said the White House would not "second guess" those charged with national security. Who's in charge, and how are they making their decisions?[5]

The August 2009 Report of the President's Council of Advisors on Science and Technology on the 2009-H1N1 Influenza was noteworthy for its level-headed reliance on science, and its refusal to speculate about worst case scenarios, and instead to examine only plausible ones. Nonetheless, the report too struck a discordant note when it recommended that responsibility for coordinating all "important" H1N1 related decisions be placed in the hands of the White House Homeland Security Advisor—seeming to make the flu a matter of national security rather than public health. In this regard, the SARS epidemic, which together with the 1918 influenza pandemic, appears to be the government's model for the 2009 flu outbreak, merits attention.

SARS

The SARS epidemic was our first and only (unless H1N1 proves much worse than it has so far) post-9/11 contagious disease epidemic. In some respects it also returned us to late 19th-century Ellis Island days; its cause and mode of transmission were initially unknown, there was no diagnostic test; there was no vaccine; and there was no effective treatment. However, SARS appeared in a society equipped with instant global communication that made management of people through information much more important than management of people through police actions. With the Internet and television, information spreads like a virus, but even faster.

Since the epidemic ended relatively quickly in all 30 countries in which suspected SARS cases were reported, and only a few countries used quarantine (detained individuals who showed no symptoms), it is reasonable to conclude that quarantining "contacts" or even "close contacts" was unnecessary to contain the spread of the disease, and certainly unnecessarily harmful to those quarantined. It is a public health myth, the equivalent of an urban legend, that quarantine was necessary to stop the SARS epidemic. It was not, and where it was used it probably did more harm than good. This is because not only liberty is at stake in deciding to quarantine, but the effectiveness of public health itself. To be effective in preventing disease spread from either a new epidemic or a bioterrorist attack, public health officials must also prevent the spread of fear and panic—and, as importantly, must not panic themselves. Maintenance of public trust is essential to achieve this goal.

When any new contagious disease appears, public health officials must, as best they can, base their advice to the public on science, not fear and prejudice. China was rightly criticized for failing to promptly alert the international community to the existence of a possibly new and contagious virus. Had information about the initial outbreak been properly shared, SARS might never have spread beyond China. Nonetheless when, with the active intervention of the World Health Organization (WHO), the epidemic was publicly recognized, China reacted vigorously, even harshly, especially in Beijing and Hong Kong. Mass quarantines were initiated involving two universities, four hospitals, seven construction sites, and other facilities, like apartment complexes. Sixty percent of the approximately 30,000 people quarantined in mainland China were detained at centralized facilities; the remainder were permitted to stay at home. Those quarantined were "close contacts," defined as someone who has shared meals, utensils, place of residence, a hospital room, or a transportation vehicle with a probable SARS patient, or visited a SARS patient or been in contact with the secretions of a SARS patient within 14 days before the SARS patient developed symptoms.[6]

Based on the evidence available, it seems reasonable to conclude that these mass quarantines in China had little or no effect on the epidemic. Moreover, the imposition of quarantine led to panic that could have spread the disease even wider. When a rumor spread that Beijing itself might be placed under martial law, for example, China News Service reported that 245,000 migrant workers from impoverished Henan province fled the city to return home.[7] Even when officials came to relocate residents to a quarantine facility in Hong Kong's Amoy Gardens, the site of the initial cluster of SARS cases in Hong Kong, they found no one home in more than half of the complex's 264 apartments.[8] Whether the residents fled because they were afraid of the disease or afraid of the quarantine, their fleeing made the quarantine ineffective and vastly increased the number of potential contacts. People were able to evade the police even though the police were working closely with public health officials.

Canada had the only major outbreak of SARS outside of Asia, and it was limited to the Toronto area. Canada had about 440 probable or suspect SARS cases, resulting in 40 deaths, but many more lives were directly affected.[9] Approximately 30,000 people were quarantined, although unlike in China, almost all Canadians who were quarantined were confined to their own homes. Staying home, or "sheltering in place," seems to have become the new standard for quarantining individuals in public health emergencies, at least in democracies.

Canadian officials were generally level-headed in their advice to the public but seem to have overreacted on two occasions. In mid April 2003, before Easter, Ontario health officials published full-page newspaper ads asking anyone who had even one symptom of SARS (severe headache, severe fatigue, muscle aches and pains, fever of 38° Celsius or higher, dry cough, or shortness of breath) to stay home for a few days.[10] Ontario's health minister said, "This is a time when the needs of a community outweigh those of a single person."[11] Again, in June, during the second wave of infections in Ontario, the health minister, responding to reports that some people were not completing their ten-day home quarantines, said, "I don't know how people will like this, but we can chain them to a bed if that's what it takes." The initial request may have been reasonable. The threat was not. At a June 2003 WHO meeting on SARS, Health Canada's senior director general, Paul Gully, noted that intra-hospital transmission was the "most important amplifier of SARS infections" and wondered aloud about the utility of the widespread home quarantines during the Canadian epidemic.[12] His reasoning was that very few of those quarantined wound up exhibiting symptoms of SARS.

Few cases of SARS occurred in the United States, and no deaths. The CDC worked with the WHO and other countries to identify the SARS virus and issued guidelines and recommendations in press conferences and on its Web site. Perhaps the most important recommendations involved travel. In this category, the CDC issued both travel alerts (which consist of a notification of an outbreak of a specific disease in a geographic area, suggest ways to reduce the risk of infection, and give information on what to do if you become ill) and travel advisories (which include the same information, but further recommend against nonessential travel because the risk of disease transmission is considered too high). No attempt was made to prohibit

Americans from traveling anywhere, although the federal government probably has the authority to do this for international travel (e.g., through passport restrictions) should the risk of disease become extreme. No attempts were made by public health officials to quarantine asymptomatic contacts of SARS patients.

The CDC also issued reasonable guidance to businesses with employees returning from areas affected with SARS, recommending that while in areas with SARS those "with fever or respiratory symptoms should not travel and should seek medical attention" and, upon return, asymptomatic travelers "should be vigilant for fever . . . and respiratory symptoms . . . over the 10 days after departure." Most importantly, the CDC noted "these persons need not limit their activities and should not be excluded from work, meetings, or other public areas, unless fever or respiratory symptoms develop."[13] In bold letters on its guidelines, it underlined the point: "At this time, CDC is not recommending quarantine of persons returning from areas with SARS." The president did, nonetheless, add SARS to the outdated federal list of "quarantinable communicable diseases" on April 4, 2003, and customs and immigration officials were given the authority to detain those entering the United States who were suspected of having SARS. This authority was not exercised.

Of course, the public can overreact on its own, and in some cases clearly did—Chinatown's restaurants in both New York and Boston were virtually empty for a time. The worst offenders were not the uninformed public, however, but academic institutions, some of which forbade their faculty and students to travel to areas that had SARS cases or required them to spend ten days, after they returned, in self-imposed quarantine and obtain a physician's certificate that they did not have SARS before returning to campus. Academic institutions with such policies included both Harvard and Boston University, even though the Boston Public Health Commission had reasonably advised: "At this time there is no evidence that a person without symptoms may infect others with SARS. Anyone without symptoms who has traveled to high-risk areas or who has been in close contact with a SARS case may attend school, meetings, or large gatherings."[14] Anita Barry, director of communicable disease control at the Boston Public Health Commission, had warned only four days earlier, "The biggest challenge for now with SARS is fear and rumor and panic."[15]

As a general matter, local public health officials acted responsibly, even under extreme pressure. Although there were no quarantines in the United States, there were cases in which isolation of symptomatic individuals was advised or mandated by local public health departments. In

New York, the Department of Health advised 23 people to stay home for a period of ten days after their SARS fever had returned to normal. In addition, two individuals in New York City and one in Dallas were ordered to be isolated in hospitals because it was suspected they had SARS. The first of these was a foreign tourist who sought medical care in a New York City hospital and was diagnosed as a suspect case. Typically, a local resident would have been quarantined at home for ten days. However, since the tourist had no residence in New York City, and his US hosts could not provide space where he could be isolated, the New York City Department of Health ordered him to remain in the hospital for ten days after his fever abated. An unarmed security guard was posted at his door to enforce the order. Diplomats in his country's consulate advised the tourist of his legal right to counsel, who would advise him about fighting the order, but he refused. Ten days after the resolution of his fever, he left town and has not been heard of since. The second case in New York City involved a person who was voluntarily in the hospital, but who became restless and wanted to leave before the ten days. He was ordered to stay and put under guard as well.[16]

The third involuntarily detained individual, from Dallas, also sought care in a hospital and was diagnosed as a suspect case. He gave a false address. The Dallas County Department of Health and Human Services sought and obtained a court order requiring him to remain in the hospital for ten days. At the hearing, all in attendance (including the judge) were provided with protective gear to wear "to avoid any possible exposure to the disease while in the presence of the patient." This precaution alone made it virtually certain that the judge would find the patient a potential danger to the public and order continued isolation, which he did.[17]

In the midst of the SARS epidemic, New York City changed its health code to permit the city's health commissioner to order the quarantine of individuals who "may" endanger the public health because of smallpox, pneumonic plague, or other severe communicable disease. In addition, a possible contact may also be quarantined: someone who "[has] been or may have been" in "close, prolonged, or repeated association with a case or carrier." This change in the code from permitting the quarantine of people who actually pose a danger to the public health and who have actually been in close contact with infected individuals, to those who "may" pose a danger and those who "may" have been in close contact with them is breathtaking in its invitation to arbitrariness. Given this, it is very disturbing that not one person showed up to testify at the April 2003 public hearing on this change.

In the case of SARS, which the revised New York City rules specifically reference in a section on "post publication changes,"[18] the new regulation would have permitted the department to quarantine New York's entire Chinatown area since all residents there "may" have been in contact with someone who "may" have SARS. No one seems to have recognized how this replicated the totally arbitrary 1900 San Francisco Chinatown quarantine, which was allegedly for plague, and was struck down as violating the US Constitution. Nonetheless, it is worth noting that even 19th-century US courts, while granting extremely broad powers to public health agencies, condemned the arbitrary use of quarantine, even for plague and smallpox, and required public health officials to have reasonable cause for any isolation.[19]

SARS may return, but the CDC is to be commended for providing the United States with a credible official (this time, unlike with smallpox vaccination, CDC director Julie Gerberding performed well) who informed Americans about what they could voluntarily do to avoid contracting or spreading the disease.[20] (Acting CDC Director Richard Besser acted equally well during the spring 2009 swine flu outbreak, as did the president). Nationally, encouragement of sensible voluntary responses became policy, and no state invoked any public health emergency powers, including quarantine, in response to SARS. As a general rule, sick people seek treatment and accept isolation to obtain it. People do not want to infect others, especially their family members, and will voluntarily follow reasonable public health advice to avoid spreading disease. SARS, like the threat of a bird flu or swine flu pandemic, emphasizes that effective public health today must rely on actions taken at the national and international level, and that public health should be seen primarily as a global issue. Virtually every country in the world took some action to limit the exposure of its people to SARS, as they did again with regard to H1N1 swine flu.

SARS was a major public health challenge, but it was no less a medical challenge. Sick people seek medical care. In hospitals, physicians and nurses care for each individual they believe to be infected with the disease. In fact, one of the salient aspects of the SARS epidemic is that many (in some countries, most) infections were actually acquired in hospitals, and many of those infected—and some who died—were physicians and nurses who cared for SARS patients. The dedication of the physicians and nurses who treated SARS patients was exemplary. Neither public health nor medicine alone could have effectively dealt with SARS. The old distinctions between medicine and public health are blurring, and perhaps the most important message of SARS is that public health and medicine must work together to be effective.[21]

Of course, SARS is not HIV/AIDS, which is not smallpox, which is not plague, or tuberculosis, or bioterrorism. Each infectious disease is different, and epidemiology provides the key to any effective public health and medical response to a new disease. The rapid exchange of information, made possible by the Internet and an interconnected group of laboratories around the world (set up primarily for influenza identification and tracking), were critical to overcoming fear with knowledge. Information really does travel faster than a virus, and managing information is the most important task of modern public health officials. People around the world, provided with truthful, reasonable information by public health officials who are interested in both their health and human rights, will follow their advice.

Isolating sick people seems to have been critical to containing SARS, but better infection-control techniques in hospitals, and adherence to them, are equally necessary. Quarantining contacts, where it was attempted, seems to have been both ineffective (in that many, if not most, contacts eluded quarantine) and useless (in that almost none of those quarantined developed SARS). Mass quarantine is a relic of the past that seems to have outlived its usefulness. Attempts at mass quarantine, as evidenced by the experience in China, are now likely to create more harm than they prevent by imposing unnecessary liberty restrictions on those quarantined and by encouraging potentially infected people to flee from public health officials.

In the midst of concern over bioterrorism, but after the SARS epidemic, the New York Academy of Medicine did a survey of the American public asking how they would respond to two types of terrorist attacks: smallpox and a dirty bomb. Published in 2004, the results of the surveys support two lessons that were apparent on 9/11: (1) the primary concern Americans have in a crisis is the safety of their family members; and (2) the most important predictor of whether they will follow the advice of public officials is if the public trusts the officials to tell the truth and to be guided in issuing recommendations by the publics' welfare. Specifically, the survey found that roughly 40% would go to a vaccination site in a smallpox outbreak if told to do so, and fewer than 60% would shelter in place for as long as they were instructed in the event of a dirty bomb explosion.[22]

The reasons given for not following official advice are instructive. In the smallpox scenario, more than 60% of respondents had serious worries about the safety of the smallpox vaccine, which was double the number worried about getting the disease itself. The respondents also suggested ways to make them more likely to cooperate. For smallpox, an overwhelming majority of respondents wanted to speak with someone who knew a lot about smallpox (94%) and whom they trusted to want what was best for them (88%). A physician not working for the government would fit the bill. In the dirty bomb case, the primary concern respondents had was the safety of their family members. Many respondents said they would shelter in place if they could communicate with people they care about or if they knew their family was safe. Overall, the study concluded, "people are more likely to follow [official] instructions when they have a lot of trust in what officials tell them to do and are confident that their community is prepared to meet their needs if a terrorist attack occurs."

These survey results are consistent with past bioterrorist exercises. As former Senator Sam Nunn, who played the part of the President in the smallpox exercise, Dark Winter (the same exercise that persuaded Dick Cheney that we needed to vaccinate the population against smallpox), said "There is no force on earth strong enough to get Americans to do something that they do not believe is in their own best interests and that of their families."

Given the evidence from real world events, public opinion surveys, and mock exercises, it is quite remarkable that some public health officials still advocate draconian 19th-century quarantine and compulsory treatment strategies. This is likely because public health officials, who believe all their actions are designed to protect the public, are much more concerned with false negatives (failing to treat or detain someone who actually has a communicable disease) than with false positives (detaining someone who actually does not have a communicable disease), and believe that brute force can effectively control the behavior of Americans in an epidemic or a bioterrorist attack. To the extent that this militaristic faith in coercion remains alive in the public health community, it is predictable that public health officials with the power to arbitrarily quarantine large numbers of people in an emergency will use it immediately, whether it is warranted or not. From their perspective, protecting public health, which they often see as their only job, is much more important than protecting liberty. Therefore, public health officials may really believe that they have "nothing to lose" by being arbitrarily draconian.

Post-SARS Fears

The world's success in the SARS epidemic has been attributed mostly to luck, yet the trend to treat epidemic disease like a bioterrorist attack and prepare for it militarily continues virtually unabated. In 2007, for example, WHO explicitly adopted a militarized (inter)national security model for public health. Its 2007 World Health Report is titled, *A Safer Future: Global Public Health Security in the 21st Century*, WHO also termed the prospect of a pandemic flu "the most feared security threat" in the world. Safety and security are now apparently seen as more important public health goals than health itself, and preparedness for all emergencies has become the new public health mantra. The phrases "better safe than sorry," and "we must exercise an abundance of caution" and "err on the side of caution" are heard over and over, as if these chants could themselves ward off evil. Sometimes we even hear a phrase that is absurd on its face: We took this action (e.g., closing the schools, screening airplane passengers for fever) in an "overabundance of caution." Caution is fine, overreaction—in this case "over caution"—is not, since it is an oxymoron that invites arbitrary action.

Sacrificing human rights for safety under the rubric of national security is almost never necessary and almost always counterproductive in a free society. Benjamin Franklin went further in expressing an American thought from "the land of the free and the home of the brave," saying, "Those who would give up an essential liberty to purchase temporary security deserve neither liberty nor security." And President Obama has rightly characterized this way of thinking as presenting a "false choice."

Why did public health so eagerly embrace the national security model for itself after the terrorist attacks on the Twin Towers and the Pentagon? *Newsweek* commentator Fareed Zakaria accurately identified the reason well before either the Obama presidency or the swine flu scare from Mexico: The United States had "become a nation consumed by fear, worried about terrorists and rogue nations, Muslims and Mexicans, foreign companies and free trade, immigrants and international organizations. The strongest nation in the history of the world, we see ourselves besieged and over-whelmed."[23] What Zakaria did not say, but could have, is that just as the choice between liberty and safety is a false one, so is the choice between being safe and being sorry. As our preemptive war with Iraq taught almost all Americans, actions based on false premises can cause a nation to be both unsafe and sorry.

Dick Cheney, who declared the nation "less safe" shortly after President Obama took office (on the basis that our safety is wholly depen-dent upon maintaining a cadre of trained torturers), set the national security agenda for public health in the United States. His now well-known anti-terrorist standard has come to be labelled, as in the title of Ron Suskind's book on the subject, *The One Percent Doctrine*. Simply put, the doctrine is, "even if there's just a one percent chance of the unimaginable coming due, act as if it is a certainty. It's not about our analysis [of the threat], it's about our response."[24] This, of course, is a prescription to ignore scientific facts and develop "action plans" completely unrelated to the real world—or at least two orders of magnitude away from reality.

A legal insider in the Bush administration, Jack Goldsmith, former head of the Office of Legal Counsel (and the person primarily responsible for withdrawing many of the original torture memos), describes the feelings in the Bush administration in his own book, *The Terror Presidency*. He notes that reading the daily threat matrix that summarizes every known new threat easily makes one paranoid. He continues, "the most level-headed person I knew in government" told him that "reading about plans for chemical and biological and nuclear attacks over days and weeks and years causes you to 'imagine a threat so severe that it becomes an obsession."[25] As Philip Larkin's put in "*Aubade*", in a way that applies to many worst case scenarios, "This is a special way of being afraid."

Using this mode of fear-driven paranoia, the threat of bioterrorism has been hyped beyond all scientific or historic reality, even in the public health community, which should know better. And the "one percent doctrine" has morphed into an even more extreme "greater than zero" probability doctrine of an epidemic, which states in effect: unless you can prove there is absolutely no risk, you must act as if the risk of catastrophe is 100%. WHO director general Margaret Chan rightly saw the swine flu outbreak as an opportunity to encourage global responses, but, I think simultaneously overstated the actual risk to the peoples of the world from swine flu when she said in April 2009: "This is an opportunity for global solidarity as we look for responses and solutions that benefit all countries, all of humanity. After all, it really is all of humanity that is under threat during a pandemic."[26]

As previously noted, exaggerated risks produce extreme responses that themselves produce unintended consequences. An example of a gross exaggeration is the phrase often used by former CDC director Julie Gerberding, "A threat anywhere is a threat everywhere." Preparedness officials often seem to be acting as if they believe the converse is also true: "Preparedness for anything is preparedness for everything." There is no more powerful illustration of the wrong-headedness of this approach than the global spectacle of a government completely incompetent to respond to a real emergency following hurricane Katrina. The person in charge of "all-hazards" emergency federal response in the Bush administration, Homeland Security Secretary Michael Chertoff, shockingly wasn't paying attention to the hurricane disaster. Instead, he was at CDC headquarters in Atlanta making preparations for a possible bird flu pandemic. Our "all-hazards" approach, combined with a one percent doctrine predictably produced two interrelated epidemics in the United States: epidemics of fear and incompetence.

It also explains the response to US tuberculosis patient Andrew Speaker, who flew to Greece to be married and then to Rome for his honeymoon. Speaker had been treated for TB for more than four months and was not thought to be a danger to anyone. Nonetheless, when health authorities (mistakenly) determined that he had extensively drug resistant TB (XDR-TB), they contacted him in Rome and told him to go to an Italian TB hospital for treatment. When he did not, they reacted as if he were a terrorist, putting him on the no-fly list and issuing the first federal mandatory isolation order in the past 40 years (the last one was for smallpox in 1963). The order was enforced when he and his wife returned to the United States and voluntarily reported to a New York City hospital. This antiterrorism, law enforcement operation was totally unnecessary, as Speaker had returned to the United States to seek treatment voluntarily, and the detention order seems to have been issued primarily to punish him, to make him look like the bad guy and the CDC look like the good guys.

Other officials used Speaker to make their own points. WHO's director of TB, Mario Raviglione said that the Speaker incident showed that TB "Respects no border. No one should feel safe in this world." Senator Hillary Clinton said the case "exposed a disturbing picture of the federal government's ability to respond to a known public health incident and protect our homeland security." And Emory's Henry M. Blumberg, a TB expert, said "TB is a weapon of mass destruction . . . ."[27] In reality, Speaker seems to have put no one in danger—including his wife. And even his diagnosis of XDR-TB turned out to be mistaken (he had the more easily treatable multidrug-resistant TB [MDR-TB]), but the CDC under President Bush did not admit any mistakes and so told the press, absurdly, that the mistaken diagnosis didn't matter. The proper lesson from the Speaker case is not that we need more draconian laws to isolate TB patients—although such new laws have been proposed and are widely supported—but that we need better and faster TB diagnostic tests, better treatments, and better communication with patients. Gerberding did, nonetheless, properly distinguish Speaker from a terrorist in testimony before Congress, although in terms that seemed to justify the CDC's failure to prevent his leaving the United States in the first place: "There is a difference between a terrorist and an infected person. Our medical approach is to give the patient the benefit of the doubt." Speaker was not given the benefit of the doubt, but treated like a contemporary Typhoid Mary, who was forced to star in a now-standardized epidemic threat narrative.

The New York Academy of Medicine published a follow-up study to its dirty bomb and smallpox study discussed earlier. Their new study identified what members of the public needed to successfully "shelter in place" during a pandemic or other emergency. None of the measures suggested involved new laws or more police; all required the voluntary and active cooperation of the public and their neighbors and their communities. Of current federal and state plans to deal with emergencies the report concluded: "Currently, planners are developing emergency instructions for people to follow *without* finding out whether it is actually possible for them to do so or whether the instructions are even the most protective action for certain groups of people to take."[28] As Katrina illustrated, such uninformed and unaware instructions simply makes things worse.

Some public health experts remarkably advocated adoption of the Bush/Cheney Iraq war model in the wake of SARS, suggesting that public health officials take "preemptive actions" against "reasonably foreseeable threats, even under conditions of uncertainty."[29] Although they described their prescription as an application of the precautionary principle, it is actually a perversion of the precautionary principle (an analog of the Hippocratic precept, first do no harm), which is designed to maintain the status quo in the presence of scientific uncertainty. The argument is not for precaution, but for preemptive action—like our war with Iraq—apparently believing that draconian actions against civilian populations are the status quo (which could be true, if one sees the status quo as a police state). But abuse of power predictably destroys public trust and instills resistance. Even totalitarian dictatorships like China cannot control an epidemic in the 21st century by fear alone.

Wendy Mariner, Wendy Parmet, and I have suggested that the beginning of a new presidential administration—and with the lessons of SARS and the swine flu in mind—presents a reasonable opportunity to set a new, nonmilitary, non-national security agenda for public health law.[30] Six principles should guide this health law reform agenda:

1. It should emphasize the ordinary, leaving behind its obsession with one percent solutions and public health emergencies, and concentrate on promoting the publics' health in ordinary times by, for example, strengthening immunization programs, ensuring access to medical care, and improving public health education.
2. It should recognize that law alone cannot solve complex public health problems, nor can emergency powers make up for the lack of resources or trusting relationships between public health personnel and the public. Cries of plague and bald assertions of authority must be replaced with recommendations based on science and respect for the rule of law.
3. It should recognize that public health law must be grounded in the communities that public health serves. Top-down draconian authority is antidemocratic and likely to prove counterproductive. Persuasion and reasonable recommendations based on facts are much more likely to be effective.
4. It should value transparency and accountability, instead of granting broad legal immunity to officials, workers, volunteers,

and drug companies for abusing their authority. The public is the client, not the enemy, and is much more likely to trust those who take responsibility for their actions.

5. It should recognize that legal rights can themselves promote public health protection—the Constitution is not an obstacle to effective public health planning, it expresses our deepest-held values that should guide all official actions.

6. Law should be used to enable people to be healthy, not to coerce their actions, both every day and in emergencies. Instead of empowering officials to treat people against their will, for example, it should emphasize the rights of people to have access to the treatments they need. In this respect, developing an equitable system of healthcare available to all Americans would be a much more effective public health intervention than, for example, having the legal authority and military ability to quarantine every man, woman, and child in America.

This vision rejects a "biosecurity future" that seeks to fuse public health with national security and instead projects a future public health agenda that can realistically protect the health of Americans, and ultimately the people of the world. It recognizes that the threat of bioterrorism exists, but that the most powerful tools to prevent it from materializing are not after-the-fact counterattacks on our own citizens, but before-the-fact, open sharing of scientific research and the promotion of a healthy population, backed up by a strong and accessible healthcare system. The goal should be not to produce an autoimmune national security response in America's "homeland," but to bolster our national immune system so that we can both live better and respond resiliently to infectious invaders.

The final two chapters of *Worst Case Bioethics* deal with issues related to genetics—the hottest subject in modern medicine and public health. The first examines what may be termed a biosecurity tactic—the use of physical or "bio" markers that can be used to identify individuals, sometimes referred to as bioidentifiers. The most prominent of these is the DNA profile, and the question of whether it should become routine for governments to collect the DNA of all its citizens for criminal law and biosecurity purposes is the focus of my human rights discussion. The final chapter deals with my own worst case scenario: genetic genocide, the prospect that genetic enhancements could lead to dramatically destructive unintended consequences, as well as the much more likely unintended consequence of genetic screening: genism.

16

. . . .

Bioidentifiers

Post-9/11 pandemic fear has led to an overemphasis on security, including biosecurity. Government actions are routinely justified as "for security reasons", including ritualistic liquid checks at the airport. Even before 9/11, governments were intent on using DNA in criminal investigations. Likewise, privacy advocates have long sought to limit the use of DNA, and more recently of other bioidentifiers as well, and not just in the United States.[1] But 9/11 raised the stakes.

The oversimplified and often phony security versus civil liberties debate gets played out in the DNA identification debate. Even when no security justification for DNA collections exists, privacy protections are challenged as simply incompatible with scientific progress that could cure diseases and save lives. In this chapter, I examine two legal cases from Europe that explore the privacy problems—including family privacy—inherent in collecting DNA samples for use in large databanks: one involving the use of DNA in police investigations, the other involving the use of DNA in medical research. The first case is from the European Court of Human Rights, the second from Iceland's Supreme Court.

In late 2008, the European Court of Human Rights ruled that the United Kingdom's laws governing the collection and retention of DNA profiles and samples by law enforcement officials violate the human rights of members of the Council of Europe.[2] It is the most important court decision involving the privacy limits on police use of bioidentifiers by any court in the world to date.

The Council of Europe, founded by ten countries in 1949, currently has 47 member countries. The Council adopted the European Convention for the Protection of Human Rights and Fundamental Freedoms, modeled after the Universal Declaration of Human Rights, in 1950. The European Convention is the foundational document of the most comprehensive regional system of human rights protection in the world. Remarkably, the court's opinion was unanimous—signed by all 17 judges who were sitting as a Grand Chamber of the court. The court ruled that the United Kingdom's DNA profile retention policy "constitutes a disproportionate interference with the ... right to respect for private life and cannot be regarded as necessary in a democratic society."

The United Kingdom has been the world leader in collecting and using DNA profiles for criminal investigations since its first DNA dragnet, recounted vividly in Joseph Wambaugh's 1989 book, *The Blooding*. The book recounts how the application of Alex Jeffreys' then new DNA profiling technique was used to conduct a DNA dragnet that included the collection of blood samples from more than 5,000 men who lived in the vicinity where two teenage girls had been brutally raped and murdered in 1983 and 1986.[3] Collection and use of DNA by the police for identification was initially justified to help in the identification of rapists and child molesters. Predictably, use has expanded gradually to include more and more criminal suspects, even though its usefulness in improving crime detection remains contested.[4] Since 9/11, preventing terrorism has been added to crime detection to justify larger bioidentification databases.[5] Because of its pioneering work on using DNA for identification, the rules the United Kingdom adopts and the procedures it follows have had significant influence, especially in the United States, where the current trend is to collect and retain DNA samples from all persons arrested for felonies.[6]

The constitutionality of police taking and using biometric data for identification and investigation, including ordinary fingerprint impressions, has never been examined by our Supreme Court. One recurring question is whether DNA information is so unique that it requires special legislation and regulation, or whether the privacy laws that protect private information, including medical information, are sufficient. If general privacy rules are sufficient, of course, then we need not adopt new genetic privacy laws under the rubric of what has been dismissively termed "genetic exceptionalism." This remains an open and contested question in the United States. Europe may take privacy more seriously than we do in America, but this too is open to debate.[7] And whether the European opinion will influence judicial decisions in the States depends both on the respect US judges accord to non-US judicial opinions, as well as on the interpretation of the differing language of the European Convention and the less specific language in the US Constitution.

S. and Marper in the European Court of Human Rights

S., a minor (whose name was protected by the court) was arrested and charged with attempted robbery when he was 11, and later acquitted. Michael Marper, an adult, was arrested and charged with harassment of his partner. The couple was reconciled before a pretrial review, and the case was formally discontinued. Both arrests occurred in 2001. In each case, the police took both fingerprints and DNA samples. S. and Marper both asked that their fingerprints and DNA samples be destroyed, and in both cases the police refused. An administrative court refused to reverse this decision, and it was upheld in a Court of Appeal decision on a 2-to-1 vote.

One of the judges in the majority, Lord Justice Waller, argued that, although there was a major difference between fingerprints and DNA profiles on the one hand, and the actual DNA sample on the other, retention of the DNA samples themselves (instead of just the profile information that had been derived from them) could be justified for five reasons that outweighed any risk to privacy:

> Retention of samples permits (a) the checking of the integrity and future utility of the DNA database system; (b) a reanalysis for the upgrading of DNA profiles where new technology can improve the discriminating power of the DNA matching process; (c) reanalysis and thus an ability to extract other DNA markers, and thus offer benefits in terms of speed, sensitivity and cost of searches of the data base; (d) further analysis in investigations of alleged miscarriages of justice; and (e) further analysis so as to be able to identify any analytical or process errors.[8]

An appeal to the House of Lords was dismissed, with Lord Steyn giving the lead judgment. He argued, among other things, that the reason UK law permitted the retention of DNA profiles and samples was to prevent cases in which those who had been acquitted of rape or murder go on to commit these crimes and escape prosecution because their samples had not been retained. He said that evidence suggested that almost 6,000 DNA profiles that had been linked with crime-scene stain profiles, involving 53 murders and 94 rapes, would have been destroyed under the rules requiring destruction after acquittal.

Lord Steyn concluded that any interference with "private life" (what US courts would likely simply label as one aspect of privacy) was proportionate to the goal of crime investigation, in view of the fact that profiles and samples were kept only for the limited purpose of detection, investigation, and prosecution of crime; were not made public; and were not identifiable by a nonexpert. He also did not believe that retention of a sample in any way stigmatized the individual whose sample was retained by treating them as a suspect in future crimes, or that there was any difference between retaining a DNA profile and retaining a DNA sample.

S. and Marper thereafter brought a complaint to the European Court of Human Rights, arguing that the actions of the United Kingdom in retaining their fingerprints, DNA profile, and DNA samples for criminal investigation purposes violated their rights under Article 8 (Right to respect for private and family life) of the Convention:

> 1. *Everyone has the right to respect for his private and family life,* his home and his correspondence.
> 2. *There shall be no interference by a public authority with the exercise of this right except* such as is in accordance with the law and is *necessary in a democratic society in the interests of national security, public safety or the economic well-being of the country,* for the prevention of disorder or crime, for the protection of health or morals, or for the protection of the rights and freedoms of others. (emphasis added)

The court observed that at least 20 member states (of the 47 countries in the Council of Europe) allow the compulsory taking of DNA information and storing of it in national databases. Of these, the United Kingdom is the only member state "expressly to permit the systematic and indefinite retention of DNA profiles and cellular samples of persons who have been acquitted or in respect of whom criminal proceedings have been discontinued," and also is the only member state "expressly to allow the systematic and indefinite retention of both profiles and samples of convicted persons."

S. and Marper argued that retention of their fingerprints, DNA profiles, and tissue samples interfered with their right to respect for private life because they were linked to personal identity and were the types of personal information they were entitled to keep within their control. DNA samples were of particular concern because they "contained full genetic information about a person including genetic information about his or her relatives." The government agreed that all three were personal data but disagreed that any fell within the provisions of Article 8 of the Convention because, unlike the actual taking of the information, the retention of it "did not interfere with the physical and psychological integrity of the person, nor did it breach their right to personal development or to establish and develop relationships with other human beings."

The court began its assessment by noting that the concept of private life is a broad one, covering not only physical and psychological integrity of a person, but gender identification, name and sexual orientation, health information, and ethnic identity, as well as other elements "relating to a person's right to their image." Most importantly, "the mere storing of data relating to the private life of an individual amounts to an interference within the meaning of Article 8." The court reviewed the retention of DNA samples, profiles, and fingerprints separately.

As to DNA samples, the primary concern of S. and Marper was that the samples could be used in novel and currently unknown ways in the future. The court agreed that such a concern, although speculative and not yet realized, "is legitimate and relevant to a determination of the issue of whether there has been an interference." The court continued:

> *[DNA samples] contain much sensitive information about an individual, including information about his or her health.* Moreover, samples contain *a unique genetic code* of great relevance to both the individual and his relatives.... Given the nature and amount of personal information contained in cellular samples, their retention per se must be regarded as interfering with the right to respect for the private lives of the individuals concerned. (emphasis added)

Next is the DNA profile, which the United Kingdom argued was "nothing more than a sequence of numbers or a barcode containing information of a purely objective and irrefutable character...." The court had little sympathy for this argument, noting that, while the information itself may be considered objective, the way it is used undercuts this description. In particular, the court noted that the profiles have been used for "familial searching with a view to identifying a possible genetic relationship between individuals" and that this use alone "is sufficient to conclude that their retention interferes with the right to the private life of the individual concerned." The court also noted that police use the DNA profiles to assess the likely ethnic origin of a perpetrator, "which makes their retention all the more sensitive and susceptible of affecting the right to private life."

Fingerprints obviously do not contain any the type of personal, familial, ethnic, and health information contained in DNA. In prior cases, the court had concluded that retention by the police of fingerprints and their closest analog, photographs, following an arrest did not present a privacy problem because they did not contain any subjective information "which called for refutation." For example, the court had previously found that retention of photographs taken at a demonstration did not interfere with private life, at least if authorities had not tried to identify the persons photographed by entering the photos into a data processing system. Similarly, the court found that retention of the recording of a person's voice did amount to interference with the right to respect for private life if it was used to try to identify the person "in conjunction with other personal data."

Applying these cases to fingerprints, the court found that, although fingerprints are neutral, objective, and unintelligible to the untutored eye, they "contain unique information about the individual concerned allowing his or her identification with precision in a wide range of circumstances." Because of this, they are capable of affecting private life, and therefore their blanket and indefinite retention "without the consent of the individual concerned cannot be regarded as neutral or insignificant."

The only remaining issue was whether the United Kingdom had a sufficient justification for retaining the fingerprints, DNA profiles, and DNA samples under Article 8 of the Convention. S. and Marper argued that prevention or detection of crime was too vague and open to abuse, and that indefinite retention could not be regarded as necessary in a democratic society for the purpose of preventing crime, and was, in any event, disproportionate and particularly detrimental to children and members of certain ethnic groups over-represented in the database.

The United Kingdom defended its indefinite retention as of "inestimable value in the fight against crime and terrorism and the detection of the guilty," and the elimination of the innocent from suspicion. The United Kingdom also cited examples of successful prosecutions involving the retention of samples from people who had not been convicted, and argued that the retention could not be regarded as excessive because they were only kept for specific limited statutory purposes and stored securely. In the government's view, there was no stigmatization and "no practical consequences for the applicants unless the records matched a crime-scene profile."

The court found that the justification of preventing crime was so general that it could "give rise to extensive interpretation," saying:

> It is as *essential, in this context, as in telephone tapping, secret surveillance and covert intelligence-gathering, to have clear, detailed rules* governing the scope and application of measures, as well as minimum safeguards concerning, inter alia, duration, storage, usage, access of third parties, procedures for preserving the integrity and confidentiality of data and procedures for its destruction, thus *providing sufficient guarantees against the risk of abuse and arbitrariness.* (emphasis added)

The court agreed that prevention and detection of crime, particularly organized crime and terrorism, is both legitimate and increasingly reliant on modern scientific techniques, including DNA analysis. Nonetheless, the court was concerned that, in the United Kingdom, no distinctions are made on the basis of the gravity of the offense charged or the age of the suspect, there are no time limits on retention, few opportunities are presented to have the material destroyed, and no opportunity is available for independent review if a request for destruction is denied.

The court found especially troubling the risk of stigmatization from indefinite storage, which it believed undercut the presumption of innocence to which people who had not been convicted of any crime are entitled. Instead, these innocents were treated exactly the same as convicted criminals. The court also found the retention of DNA samples to be "particularly intrusive given the wealth of genetic and health information contained therein."

The court's ultimate conclusion, nonetheless, made no distinctions among ordinary fingerprints, DNA profiles, and DNA samples because of the "blanket and indiscriminate nature of the powers of retention," and the failure of the United Kingdom to strike a "fair balance between the competing public and private interests." The court accordingly held that blanket and indefinite retention of all three identifiers constituted a disproportionate interference with the applicants' right to respect for private life and cannot be regarded as necessary in a democratic society. Therefore, the practice was in violation of Article 8 of the Convention.

DNA Databanks and Privacy

The numbers are impressive. With more than five million DNA profiles and samples, the UK's criminal DNA database is the second largest in the world.[9] Of these, almost a million are from individuals who were never convicted of any crime, and about half a million are taken from juveniles. The response to the court's decision in the United Kingdom has been largely positive. Alec Jeffreys himself agreed with the decision, telling the *Guardian* newspaper that DNA samples should not be kept and that the DNA profile of innocent people should not be in the criminal databank.[10] And the United Kingdom's government issued a responsive set of proposals to reform its practices, including a proposal to destroy all DNA samples after the profile has been created. As for the DNA profiles, as well as for ordinary fingerprints, these would be retained for six years for those not convicted, and for twelve years for those not convicted, but charged with a serious violent, sexual, or terrorism-related crime. There would be separate but similar rules for minors. The proposal to destroy all DNA samples is stunning, goes well beyond the court's requirements, and deserves to be applauded (and will hopefully be implemented). The six and twelve year retention times, on the other hand, seem excessive, and depending on public reaction, could be reduced.

The Marper opinion should also serve as an opportunity to reevaluate biometric identification policies in the United States. Fingerprinting, for example, has long been limited to arrestees and some federal employees, leaving nongovernmental "law-abiding" Americans alone, although since 9/11 there have been many additional uses of fingerprints, even for visitors at the Statue of Liberty. New federal regulations also permit the storing of DNA data from arrestees from the states that collect their DNA, and from all noncitizens detained by authorities for any purpose, even if no charge is made or conviction obtained. These regulations will permit the US National DNA Index System, the largest DNA databank in the world, with almost seven million genetic profiles, to grow even larger.

It has been accurately observed that all three identifiers collected in the United States "reflect arrest patterns, policing patterns, policing practices, and biases in judicial outcomes and as such are likely to reflect race, class, and geographic inequities."[11] Nonetheless, once inscribed in a databank, they take on the appearance of objective, even scientific, data. Perhaps this is why their use in law enforcement has been widely supported in the United States, even though there is no independent, comprehensive, scientific, peer-reviewed study of the overall effectiveness of DNA data banks in solving crimes.[12] Instead we have simple assertions, such as that of a

Senator from Arizona, one of the authors of the 2005 federal DNA act, that "We know from past experience that collecting DNA at arrest or deportation will prevent rapes and murders that would otherwise be committed."[13]

The question of family privacy is critical in the United States, where some states, like California, want to use DNA profiles to do so-called family searches to see whether a close relative might be implicated in a crime through a partial-DNA match. Law professor Jeffrey Rosen, who was invited to speak at a recent FBI conference on genetic privacy, has noted that the "family members of offenders have done nothing to reduce their expectation of privacy, and the state is investigating new crimes, not stopping repeat offenders" by using this tool. Moreover blatant discrimination against African Americans is inherent in family searches:

> If the legal implications [of familial DNA searches] are murky, the political implications are clear. Given the dramatic racial disparities of family searches, African American families might be four times as likely to be put under genetic surveillance as white families. For this reason . . . a national decision [by the FBI] to begin familial searches without congressional approval might cause a political firestorm that would imperil political support for the entire CODIS [the FBI's Combined DNA Index System] system.[14]

Only the 47 member states of the Council of Europe are bound by *Marper*, but the ruling could nonetheless cause other countries, including the United States and its individual states, to reexamine their policies. Most relevant in this regard are the conclusions of the Human Rights Court that simple assertions of the effectiveness of DNA profiles or samples in solving or preventing crime, or even terrorism, are not sufficient justification for the privacy invasion inherent in the bioidentifier databank. Second, the collection and indefinite retention of fingerprints requires justification itself—and thus it should no longer be sufficient (if it ever was) to simply justify retention of DNA profiles as the same or substantially similar to fingerprints.[15] Third, juveniles are a special case, and it will be extremely difficult to justify retention of any of their biomarkers, although there may be convictions of specific violent crimes that can provide that justification. Fourth, no matter how one comes out on the collection, storage, and use of fingerprints, photographs, and DNA profiles, there seems to be insufficient justification to ever retain DNA samples.

Requiring the routine destruction of a DNA sample after a profile is created seems to be a case of genetic exceptionalism, but it's not really. It is simply a recognition that the DNA molecule itself can be considered a medical record, and like an electronic medical record, it can be read by a machine to disclose significant private information about an individual and their family members, unrelated to anything relevant to the criminal justice system. My genetics colleague Robert Green and I have suggested, for example, that presidential candidates deserve special privacy protection, so that their DNA information is not used in the next election cycle as a kind of "genetic McCarthyism" to suggest that they have specific physical or mental health problems that could compromise their ability to serve effectively as president of the United States.[16]

Biometric identifiers have complex privacy implications that demand much more rigorous analysis than they have received. Former Homeland Security Secretary Michael Chertoff, for example, may have been trying to deflect close analysis of the privacy aspects of fingerprints when he said during a Canadian press conference: " A fingerprint is hardly personal data because you leave it on glasses and silverware and articles all over the world, they're like footprints. They're not particularly private."[17] Of course, the same could be said about DNA samples; you shed them inadvertently and leave them on glasses and silverware. In this respect, fingerprints should be treated, as did the European court, more like DNA samples than footprints. Jennifer Stoddart, the Privacy Commissioner of Canada, also responded that under Canadian law (as well as under the privacy policy of the US Department of Homeland Security)[18] fingerprints are personal information, and she worried that the increasing reliance by the United States on the collection of biometric data in the name of national security and identifying suspected terrorists might lead Canada to lessen its standards of safeguarding personal information.[19]

All of these issues should be subject to wide-ranging debate in the United States. It has, for example, been suggested that one way to do away with the racial and ethnic inequalities inherent in the current method of taking biometric information only from arrestees is to have a universal criminal database that collects biometric information from everyone.[20] This suggestion, if implemented, could be viewed as converting a free country into a "nation of suspects."[21] It would not automatically make us a *1984* society in which all of our conversations were monitored and deviation from the government's line was grounds for punishment, but it could radically alter the way we view ourselves and our relationship to our government. Nonetheless, whether such a universal system of DNA profiling would be acceptable to the Human Rights Court was not specifically decided.

The European Human Rights Court is, I think, correct to emphasize the differences between democracies and police states as reflected in the types of personal information police are permitted to collect and retain about citizens. Each individual point of data may seem insignificant, but when data sets are merged, privacy is effectively destroyed. No one, I think, ever made the privacy point better than Aleksandr Solzhenitsyn in his novel *Cancer Ward*, in which he writes that in a totalitarian state people are obliged to answer questions on a variety of forms, and each answer "becomes a little thread" permanently connecting him to the local government center:

> There are thus hundreds of little threads radiating from every man.... They are not visible, they are not material, but every man is constantly aware of their existence.... Each man, permanently aware of his own invisible threads, naturally develops a respect for the people who manipulate the threads...and for these people's authority.

Some commentators seem to believe that reference to the old Soviet-style police state surveillance is excessively gloomy in the DNA context. But mainstream scientists seem to agree that it is critical to protect privacy in this context. Writing in support of the European Court's opinion, under the headline "Watching Big Brother," for example, *Nature* editorialized that the decision was especially timely, coming as it did just before the 60th anniversary of the UDHR. The editorial noted that "Technology can be a powerful force for human rights," specifically identifying the use of observation satellites for providing evidence of ethnic atrocities and DNA samples to free wrongly convicted individuals. The editorial concluded:

> The idea that the identity of a human can be revealed from [DNA] samples of any cell in his or her body is a symbol of the fact that *every person is unique. The declaration of human rights* [UDHR] *asks us to treasure and honor all these unique individuals with respect for their autonomy*—not to simply look for better ways to barcode them.[22] (emphasis added)

Bioidentifiers implicate privacy even more than answers on forms—such as tax forms—because they identify us directly and can be seen as an integral part of us. When the police have and use DNA in their investigation of criminal activity, the European Court of Human Rights is correct to conclude that privacy is being invaded, and if the sources of that DNA are innocent of any crime, this use cannot be easily justified in a democratic society.

DNA Databanks and Medical Research in Iceland

When DNA is used for non–law enforcement reasons, privacy may not be seen as so central an issue, but it should be, and consent to DNA data-banking remains an important privacy safeguard. The reasons are outlined in another legal case from Europe, this one from Iceland. Research on genetic variation is a constantly growing field, one that was pioneered in Iceland by the private biotechnology firm deCODE Genetics in a private–public genetics project to develop and link three databanks (one consisting of electronic medical records, a second of DNA samples, and a third of genealogic data) in an effort to locate disease-related genes. The project has been controversial since 1998, when Iceland's legislature approved the creation of an electronic Health Sector Database for deCODE's use for research, and the legal rules regarding privacy of the database took center-stage again in 2009 when deCODE put the database up for sale to try to avoid bankruptcy.[23]

One of the important privacy concerns has been the failure of the Iceland legislature to require informed consent; instead, patients were given the opportunity to opt out of having their medical records included in the database. In late 2003, the Iceland Supreme Court dealt with the issue of informed consent from the perspective of family privacy, asking whether families have a privacy interest in the medical records of deceased relatives sufficient to permit them to opt out of the national database on the behalf of the deceased relative.[24]

Guomundur Igolfsson died in 1991, and in 2000 his daughter, then 15 years old, through her guardian, sought to prevent the transfer of informa-tion from her father's medical records to the national Health Sector Database. In January of that year, the minister of health had formally authorized the deCODE Genetics project to create and operate the data-base. The custodian of her father's medical records denied the daughter's request, stating, among other things, that it was not the intention of the enabling legislation that people should be able to refuse on behalf of their deceased parents. The daughter, joined by her two brothers, appealed the ruling, and the case was ultimately heard by Iceland's Supreme Court.

The court, after observing that the Health Sector Database had not yet come into use and that there was "some doubt this will happen," none-theless decided to deal directly with the question of family medical privacy. The court noted, first, that, as in the United States, under Icelandic law "the personal rights of individuals lapse on their death insofar as legislation does not provide otherwise" and that the law creating the Health Sector Database did not provide for any right of descendants to exercise the privacy rights of the deceased. Thus, the only privacy rights the daughter could assert were her own (which, in fact, was what she was asserting). Specifically, she argued that she had a personal interest in preventing the transfer of her father's records to the database, because "it is possible to infer, from the data, information relating to her father's hereditary characteristics which could also apply to herself."

Medical records, the court observed, contain significant amounts of private information, including about patients' "medical treatment, lifestyles, social circumstances, employment and family.... Information of this kind can relate to some of the most intimately private affairs of the person concerned, irrespective of whether the information is seen as derogatory for the person or not." The court had no difficulty concluding that Article 71 of the Constitution of Iceland (according to which "Everyone shall enjoy the privacy of his or her life, home, and family," language similar to Article 8 of the European Convention on Human Rights) guarantees protection of the privacy of medical information, requiring the legislature to ensure, among other things, "that legislation does not result in any actual risk of information of this kind involving the private affairs of identified persons falling into the hands of parties who do not have any legitimate right of access to such information . . . ."

The mere possibility that someone might obtain "information from medical records without the explicit consent of the person whom the information concerns" does not necessarily violate the Icelandic constitution, the court ruled, but that constitution does require the legislature "to ensure to the furthest extent that the information cannot be traced to specific individuals." The court was unequivocal in declaring that "the achievement of this stated objective is far from being adequately ensured by the provisions of statutory law." This means that the law creating the Health Sector Database is unconstitutional. This ruling killed whatever was left of deCODE's original project to create a country-wide electronic database of medical records, and the project was able to continue only after it adopted an explicit consent model.[25]

With regard to the petition before it, the Supreme Court of Iceland ruled that the daughter "may herself have an interest in preventing the transfer of information from her father's medical records into the Health Sector Database because of the risk that inferences could be made from such information which could concern her private affairs." Since the enabling legislation does not adequately protect the constitutional privacy rights of individuals by making health data untraceable, the right of the daughter to prohibit the use of her father's medical data is recognized as part of her own right of privacy.

We have become accustomed to thinking about privacy as a personal right. We have also become accustomed, especially in the United States, to seeing the right of privacy applied in healthcare settings, including making decisions about one's medical treatment, in the privacy of information within the doctor–patient relationship generally, and in the use of medical information and DNA samples for research. These two cases support an individualistic view of privacy. They also indicate, however, that the concept of privacy is being broadened to protect the family unit from unwanted and unwarranted intrusion by both government and private actors. How powerful this trend is remains to be seen, but these examples suggest that both the public and the courts support it. One implication of the trend is that families will probably continue to be protected against proposals such as "presumed consent," which would permit the routine harvesting of tissues and organs from their dead relatives without the family's consent, a relatively remarkable conclusion since these organs could be used to "save lives."[26] DNA is a family matter because DNA provides direct information not only about the person from whom the sample is taken but also about siblings, parents, and children.[27]

Use of DNA for identification has required attention to both individual and family privacy, and privacy will ultimately determine the limits of governmental use of our DNA for biosurveillence. Likewise, use of DNA for research is requiring the adoption of new legal regimes to obtain consent and protect privacy. In this regard, the United Kingdom is also attempting to set standards, although, as with their use of DNA for police investigations, their use of DNA for medical research may also require changes. For example, similar to the original deCODE proposal, UK Biobank aims to enlist 500,000 British citizens aged 40 to 69 to not only provide DNA samples, but also medical records and answers to 250 personal questions, all in the cause of medical research. This is fine, at least as long as the consent process is open and fair. Current rules that require research subjects to "relinquish all rights to their blood and urine samples, and give permission for access to their medical records at any time, even after death" seem extreme and unfair without a clear provision to discontinue participation at any time.[28]

It should escape no one's attention that to the extent that our future is focused on biosecurity rather than public health and medical research, there will be increasing pressure to permit security forces, including police, to have open access to the data contained in medical research biobanks, and to de facto merge them into the state's security system. This would, of course, be the end of genetic privacy (perhaps better denoted "bioprivacy" in this context, since it will include medical records as well), and is another reason to credibly separate security databanks from health databanks.

Some researchers, including Frederick Bieber, have suggested that DNA databanks can be used in what might be termed a new eugenics regime to demonstrate that crime clusters in families.[29] But the new eugenics is likely to appear in the form of research projects to modify DNA to produce better babies. It is to this worst case scenario that I turn in the next and final chapter.

17

. . . .

Genetic Genocide

G enetics tends to be discussed in extremes, in best case and worst case scenarios, and so provides a fitting subject for the final chapter. It brings us back to the first chapter on healthcare reform because of a best case scenario in which genomic or personalized medicine is seen as the future of US healthcare. I also use genetics to summarize my own worst case bioethics scenario: the creation of better humans, which would bring with it the prospect of what I have termed "genetic genocide," and to consider whether this worst case scenario has been more distracting than illuminating in what has been termed the "genetically enhanced human" or germline genetic alteration debate.

Genetics is often viewed as a potential medical savior not just through personalized medicine in the developed world,[1] but also by applying genetic technology in the resource poor world.[2] There is an extensive literature on the bioethical issues involving genomics in both Europe and the United States. Bioethics has been used to frame the relationship between *Genomics and World Health* by the World Health Organization as well. Although, as previously noted, the WHO has adopted a health and human rights perspective, in their 241-page report on genomics and world health, human rights are mentioned only once, and then in the context of genetic enhancements; that is, using genetic manipulations to try to make better babies or simply better humans:

> Societies have a moral obligation grounded in equity or justice and human rights to ensure access to health care for their citizens. A fundamental part of *the moral imperative of health care is its role in maintaining normal function*, and in turn helping to secure equality of opportunity for persons that serious disease and disability undermine. *Genetic enhancements of normal function, on the other hand, do not serve justice* in this way and if and when they become possible, will almost certainly not be regarded as part of the social obligation to provide health care to all members of society.[3] (emphasis supplied)

Put another way, the Commission concluded that it is ethically acceptable that only some members of society, the elites, have access to the new genetics, and physicians who care for this elite can do so without worrying about bioethics. Whether one finds appeals to the norm of humanity or normal species functioning persuasive as a bright line that circumscribes the right to health or not, genetic technologies will change the way we think about ourselves and our species, and thus how we think about the rights of humans, including rights to health and healthcare, and even how we think about bioethics.

The overall question I address in this chapter is: Why do genetics and bioethics seem to be naturally paired in the context of both national healthcare and global health, and why, nonetheless, could a human rights framework—one focusing more directly on equality and the right to health itself—prove more useful than either a bioethics or a social justice frame in attaining global health?

As has been discussed in other contexts in this book, bioethics has dealt primarily with decisions made in the doctor–patient relationship (and secondarily with the researcher–subject relationship), whereas human rights doctrine has been more prominent, as reviewed especially in Chapter 13, in the global health arena. It is also in this latter context that bioethics and genomics have been most widely discussed. The risks of genomic research, for example, are highlighted in the WHO report. The report identifies three areas that present special risks: germline genetic alterations, the establishment of genetic databases, and the application of genomics to biowarfare.

The WHO authors conclude that it is premature and dangerous to attempt germline genetic alterations, that nothing can stop the establishment of population-based gene banks (but that rules to protect privacy and guard against discrimination are required), and that the scientific community should take the risk of biowarfare applications of the new genomics seriously. The report concludes on mixed notes of hope and caution: The "new and rapidly evolving" field of genomics "offers considerable possibilities for the improvement of human health" but "the full extent of its possible hazards are not yet fully appreciated."

A Canadian group followed up the WHO report with an exercise designed to identify the new biotechnologies most likely to be helpful to improving the health of people living in developing countries. Their report, based on expert assessment using a Delphi methodology, put two genomic technologies at the top of their final list, and a related technology third: First, modified molecular technologies for affordable, simple diagnosis for infectious diseases; second, recombinant technologies to develop vaccines against infectious diseases; and third, technologies for more efficient drug and vaccine delivery systems.

The thesis of the Canadian report is that "biotechnology can help to bridge rather than deepen existing divides between the developed and developing world."[4] On the other hand, the authors recognize that there is no technological fix for health, and that we will require a balanced approach, "Biotechnology will never be a panacea to current health inequities, but the evidence demonstrates that it is rightly considered part of the solution." WHO's Commission arrived at a similar conclusion, emphasizing the central role of primary care in delivering any advanced medical technology: "None of these advances will be of any value unless the developing countries can evolve the healthcare systems on which these new advances can be based."

All this is pretty vague. It is uncontroversial to hope that the new genetics will help bridge the gap between the rich and the poor, and the developed world and the resource poor world, as it improves the lives and health of those it touches directly. But none of this will be automatic, and the WHO Commission was right to acknowledge the dark side of genetics to both health and development. I think the Commission could have gone much further in this regard, and would have had the Commission employed a human rights framework instead of the more limited bioethics-social justice framework in their analysis. Here's how, I think, it should be examined in the contexts of equality and the right to health.

Equality and Genomics

Equality based on human dignity (sometimes denoted simply as the principle of nondiscrimination) is at the core of a health and human

rights approach to health. For example, a country's obligation to respect
and protect the right to health requires governments to "refrain from
denying or limiting equal access to all persons" and to ensure "equal
access to healthcare . . . ." The new genetics can be seen as scientific
validation of human equality in that it demonstrates that we all share
substantially identical genomes; but it can also be used to foster prejudice
and discrimination and thus to undercut the right to health. The human
tendency is to create divisions, which I'm sure at least some people would
describe as genetic. This tendency is well-illustrated by James Watson,
the co-discoverer of the structure of DNA, who scandalously told a
British newspaper, "I'm inherently gloomy about the prospect of Africa
because all our social policies are based on the fact that their intelligence
is the same as ours, whereas all the testing says not really." Watson later
apologized and acknowledged that no scientific evidence supports his statement about innate or genetic differences of intelligence among races. *Nature*
magazine editorialized that Watson's remarks were "rightly . . . deemed
beyond the pale," but also warned: "There will be important debates in
the future as we gain a fuller understanding of the influence of genetics on
human attributes and behavior. Crass comments by Nobel laureates
undermine our very ability to debate such issues, and thus damage science
itself."[5]

Our superficial perceptions of each other often foster racism. Simply
defined, racism is "the theory that distinctive human characteristics and
abilities are determined by race." The hunt for genes, especially in groups
labeled by racial classifications, could lead to "genism" (a term I define as
"the theory that distinctive human characteristics and abilities are determined by genes") based on DNA sequence characteristics. The resulting
discrimination could be as pernicious as racism. In this context, Watson's
ignorant remark can be seen not as one of an old-time racist, but the remark
of a new-style "genist."

The great human rights hope of genetics has been that it will
scientifically demonstrate that humans are all essentially the same, and
that this demonstration will inhibit our penchant for drawing arbitrary
distinctions among humans. And genetics has already accomplished
much of the science part. After the draft of the human genome was
announced in 2000, for example, Chris Stinger of London's Natural
History Museum observed, "We are all Africans under the skin." The
same point was made by other geneticists in different words, one noting
that "race is only skin deep" and another, that "there is nothing scientific
about race: no genes of any sort pattern along racial lines." Craig Venter,
the leader of the private genome mapping effort, concluded: "Race is a

social concept, not a scientific one. We all evolved in the last 100,000 years from the same small number of tribes that migrated out of Africa and colonized the world."

Geneticists deserve high praise for getting this antiracism message out to the public early. Unfortunately, the message of genetics, while under-cutting racism, can simultaneously make old-fashioned racism seem scien-tifically-based by invigorating its evil brother, genism. This is how it works. As geneticists have observed, although we humans are all more than 99.5% genetically identical, that less than .5% of difference is made up of 15 million spelling variations in our genomes. Each of these genetic variations could be used as a pseudoscientific basis for discrimination based on genetic endowment.

Genome leaders have recognized this, and this recognition is one reason they helped to successfully lobby for enactment of the Genetic Information Nondiscrimination Act of 2008, which seeks to prohibit genetic discrimination by employers and health insurers.[6] This is reasonable, but as suggested in the preceding chapter on bioidentifiers, antidiscrimination legislation itself provides no effective genetic privacy protection. This is because genetic discrimination can only occur if private genetic information is shared—and to protect genetic privacy, we must not only ban the result of sharing information, genetic discrimination, but also regulate the collection, analysis, and storage of DNA samples and genetic information in the first place.[7] There is some irony in the fact that James Watson's genome is one of the few that has been sequenced. After his offensive remarks, an analysis of Watson's own genome was published. Watson's genome disclosed that he has, according to Kari Stefansson of deCODE Genetics, 16 times the number of genes considered to be of African origin than the average white European, or about the same amount of African DNA that would show up if one great-grandparent were African.[8] This does not, except perhaps to a genist, mean that Watson is African—but it does help demon-strate that genes alone tell us very little about the social construct we call race, and little about full-bodied humans—even about genetic predisposi-tion to disease, which remains largely an area dominated by a handful of predictive genes for rare diseases. In the arena of common diseases, such as diabetes and heart disease, in which multiple genes—as well as multiple environmental factors—are involved, most scientists believe we have yet to discover any genetic variants of clinical significance.[9]

The WHO Commission was also right to worry about the proliferation of DNA banks and the lack of agreement on how to protect the genetic privacy of those whose DNA is stored and analyzed in these DNA banks. In addition to biosecurity and police DNA databanks, discussed in the preceeding chapter, an especially disturbing example of a human rights violation spurred by genetics is provided by the now defunct Human Genome Diversity Project, which sought to collect DNA samples from some 700 isolated ethnic groups, sometimes referred to as the world's "vanishing tribes." In the project's view, it was more important that science seize the opportunity to collect DNA from these peoples than that action be taken to help the peoples themselves. The indigenous peoples around the world properly and forcefully rejected this project, and insisted that their human rights be placed above this dubious and reductionistic DNA collection project.[10] A variation of this project has reemerged in another guise under the rubric of the Genographic Project which is sponsored by *National Geographic*.[11]

It is true that "we are all Africans under the skin." It is also true, however, that if we decide to search for genetic differences in the .5% of our DNA that is different, we will find them and likely wind up using them against each other. Philosopher-bioethicist Eric Juengst put it well: "No matter how great the potential of population genomics to show our interconnections, if it begins by describing our differences it will inevitably produce scientific wedges to hammer into the social cracks that already divide us."[12]

Preventing genism from displacing or supplementing racism by substituting molecular differences for skin color differences will not be easy. Two actions, however, seem necessary. First, genetic privacy must be protected. No one's genes should be analyzed without express authorization, and, of course, no "genetic identity cards" should be permitted. In this regard, the decision of the European Court of Human Rights, discussed in the preceeding chapter, is directly on point in ruling against human rights violations of governments holding genetic samples from individuals who have not been convicted of crimes. Second, pseudoscientific projects that purport to identify genetic differences between races should be rejected.[13]

Genetic Genocide

The WHO Commission may seem to have spent too much time and emphasis on describing the use of genetics to enhance human beings by making changes at the embryo level that could produce better babies. But I don't think so. Even though altering the genome of an embryo to create specific characteristics in the resulting child is not currently possible, it is a subject that deserves far wider attention, especially in the human rights community. James Watson, this time from statements he made at a 1998 conference on *Engineering the Human Germline*, again provides a useful introduction:

> It seems to me the question we are going to have to face is, what is going to be the least unpleasant? Using abortion to get rid of nasty genes from families? Or developing germline procedures with which.... you can go in and get rid of a bad gene.... And the other thing, because no one has the guts to say it, *if we could* make *better human beings by knowing how to add genes, why shouldn't we do it?* What would be wrong with it? .... *If you could cure* what I feel is a very serious disease— *stupidity—it would be a great thing* for people who are otherwise going to be born seriously disadvantaged.[14] (emphasis supplied)

Watson's comment on curing stupidity through genetics led him to accept an invitation from Steven Colbert to say more on Jon Stewart's *Daily Show*. Colbert showed Watson all the respect he deserved for his suggestion in the filmed interview, in which Watson said, among other things, "If you want smart children, don't marry a bimbo." Screening genomes to detect differences creates more opportunities for discrimination. Using the new genetics to try to make a better human by genetic engineering, I have previously suggested, goes beyond discrimination and genism to elimination, raising the prospect of genetic genocide. I have also suggested that both cloning and inheritable genetic alterations "can be seen as crimes against humanity of a unique sort: techniques that can alter the essence of humanity itself by taking human evolution into our own hands and directing it toward the development of a new species, sometimes termed the posthuman."

Is this inflammatory, apocalyptic, worst case scenario language justified? I think it is, but only as a counterpoint to what I take to be the implausible best case utopian scenarios of Watson and his followers, who sell genetic manipulation as the cure for all our human problems. The project to make a better baby by genetic engineering begins with attempts to cure or prevent genetic diseases, but inevitably leads to the eugenic agenda of improving or "enhancing" genetic characteristics to create the super-human or posthuman.

Posthuman proponents Lee Silver and John Harris, for example, have used as their central vision genetic manipulation of a human embryo that will create a child who is immune from HIV or cancer, and ask, who could object to this? They are correct that few, if any, would object to the prevention of a serious disease, including HIV and cancer. Nonetheless, we might wonder whether performing a genetic experiment on an embryo that could have unknown deleterious consequences to the soon-to-be child, or consequences we might not see for generations, is ethically justifiable. We might also wonder who, if anyone, has the moral authority to consent to this extreme human experiment. Our questioning seems especially appropriate when the same result might be obtained with a safe alternative, such as vaccination—as it has been in the cases of smallpox and polio—without requiring every future child born to have undergone a genetic modification at the embryo stage to attempt to prevent or eradicate a serious disease.

But even if we think embryo modification to confer immunity to particular diseases should be a choice for prospective parents to make, it seems unlikely that the project would end there. Instead, the next phase would be to attempt to make not just a disease-resistant baby, but a "better baby" by attempting to improve traits like eye color, hair color, height, or even intelligence, strength, and beauty. This type of genetic manipulation of the embryo, if successful in creating a large number of significantly better babies (a large scientific "if") creates with it the future prospect of genetic genocide as a reasonably possible, if not likely, conclusion. This is because, given the history of humankind, it is extremely unlikely that we will see the better babies or posthumans as equal in rights and dignity to us, or that they will see us, the "naturals," as their equals. Instead, it seems reasonable to conclude that we will see them as a threat to us, and seek to imprison or simply kill them before they kill us. Alternatively, the posthumans could come to see us naturals as an inferior subspecies without human rights, to be enslaved or slaughtered preemptively, much as Europeans once viewed "uncivilized" peoples, the way we Americans viewed the Japanese in World War II, or the way the Germans viewed the Jews.

My pessimistic view is shared by many, if not most, of those who welcome a posthuman future. In a survey of members of the World Transhumanist Association, released in 2008, for example, only a minority (46%) agreed with the statement that "humans and posthumans will be able to coexist in one society and polity." The transhumanists might see simple geographic separation as a solution. And we might get lucky. John Stuart Mill had great faith in our ability to use freedom to foster progress. But as Gertrude Himmelfarb has noted, Mill "looked to liberty as a means of achieving the highest reaches of the human spirit; he did not take seriously enough the possibility that men would also be free to explore the depths of depravity."[15] But we must.

It is the potential for genocide based on genetic difference that makes species-altering genetic engineering a potential weapon of mass destruction, and makes the unaccountable genetic engineer a potential bioterrorist.

Is this assertion an overblown worst case scenario that could lead us to forfeit the potentially life-saving benefits of genetic manipulation? British bioethicist John Harris certainly thinks so, and has characterized the end of my first sentence in this paragraph as "rather strained huffing and puffing" based on "mere speculation about future possible effects" that "would deny millions of people and eventually the entire population of the planet access to possible life-saving and life-enhancing therapies."[16] Harris also argues that I am wrong to suggest that the problem lies with the unaccountable genetic engineer. Rather, he believes, the problem lies with the parents (who are "all unaccountable"), and that blaming parents for their super-enhanced progeny is the equivalent of blaming Jewish parents for being the instigators of the Holocaust.

This is, I think, a silly—but nonetheless telling—argument. It is silly because it substitutes parents (who engineer nothing) for "unaccountable genetic engineers." This is a serious category error: holding Mengele accountable for his lethal genetic experiments on twins in the Nazi concentration camps is not to blame his victims (or their parents—almost all of whom were murdered in the concentration camps) in any way. The genetic engineer (Nazi doctor) does bear responsibility for his crimes; the parents (Holocaust victims and their children) are blameless. Of course, if unlike the Jews in the concentration camps, contemporary parents consent to and encourage genetic engineering experiments on their future children, they would be complicit in this project, and also responsible for them. It is telling that by choosing the Nazi concentration camps for his example, Harris highlights the racial hygiene agenda of National Socialism, and its goal of creating a super race of superior Nordic stock that would treat all other humans as inferior, proper objects of German subjugation and even extermination. The ultimate goal was to carry out this project by eugenics. Thus, it appears that even Harris recognizes that genetic enhancement researchers, at least those in the category of the unaccountable experimenters, can produce an unacceptable risk of genocide.

The Nazi doctors were tried for murder and torture at Nuremberg, rather than genocide. But this was a historical anomaly, as the crime of genocide had not yet been accepted by the international community as a war crime or crime against humanity. Nonetheless, in their state sponsorship, their concentration camp murders did qualify as war crimes and crimes against humanity. Also, as discussed in Chapter 13, the Nuremberg Doctors' Trial and the resulting Nuremburg Code set international human rights norms of human experimentation that apply globally.

Harris is, however, correct in arguing that if the real problem is racism and genism, or, as he puts it, "mindless prejudice," the solution should be to eliminate the prejudice, not eliminate the genetic engineering project. Here we agree on the goal, but not the efficacy of genetic engineering in achieving it. I doubt even Harris believes that there is a gene for prejudice, the way Watson has suggested that there is a gene for stupidity. To the extent that our view of human rights—including the principle of nondiscrimination—is based on our view of human nature, including human dignity, the human rights problem is that changing the characteristics of what it is to be human (and thus a member of the human species) could undermine both the concept of inherent human rights generally and the principle of nondiscrimination specifically.

What really seems to be in dispute then, as it is in virtually all the worst case scenarios explored in this book, is the probability of the worst case scenario actually occurring, and how high that probability must be to justify actions today to try to avoid it. Here we both engage is speculation. The issue is whether this is speculation informed by past experiences, or simply speculative fiction as cautionary tale. My own view is that given the frequency of human genocides in the past century, the probability of a future genocide based on genetically engineered differences (again, assuming germline genetic alterations become possible and predictable) is closer to 50% than Dick Cheney's 1%. This is why I have proposed application of the precautionary principle to germline genetic alteration experiments, which would shift the burden of proof to those who want to try to alter humans, rather than placing it, as it is now, on those who oppose it.[17]

A treaty outlawing replication cloning and germline genetic engineering does this directly by making the proponents of these technologies repeal the treaty before proceeding. This strikes many as an over-reaction, but shifting the burden of proof to corporations and scientists in this case is similar to what we currently do with new drugs and devices through the FDA. As discussed in Chapter 7, before a company is permitted to market a drug or device in the United States, it has the burden to demonstrate to the FDA, through scientific studies, that its product is "safe and effective." As argued in that chapter, with the exception of anti–government-regulation libertarians who worry about access to experimental cancer drugs, few people seriously contest this Hippocratic allocation of the burden of proof.

Overly optimistic commentators believe that simply failing to distribute the fruits of human genetics equitably could itself lead to the same "two species" result. James Evans, for example, has suggested that depriving the poor of personalized genomic medicine "runs the risk of creating a genetically defined underclass which, because of inheriting more than a fair share of disease-susceptibility genes, is unable to afford adequate [medical] care." Others think that the prospect of humans ever being able to engineer a genetic elite is remote because of the difficulty of identifying genes for intelligence, for example, and using those genes to make more than minimal changes in offspring. As biologist Christopher Wills put it, arguing that environmental factors will continue to overwhelm genetics in the foreseeable future: "*The Boys from Brazil* notwithstanding, it seems likely that if clones of Adolf Hitler were to be adopted into well-adjusted families in healthy societies they would grow up to be nice, well-adjusted young men."[18] Maybe Wills is right. But is the entire world obligated to take this chance because one genetic scientist decides to do the experiment?

What Future for Our Species?

Bioethics has been called on to help us regulate the research, distribute the benefits, and save us from the potential harms of the new genetics. With its focus on individual decisions made in the context of the doctor–patient relationship (and the researcher-subject relationship), however, it cannot, at least by itself, confront either global or species-wide issues. UNESCO's Universal Declaration on Bioethics and Human Rights is a step in the right direction of integrating human rights and bioethics. This attempted synthesis nonetheless suggests, as I argued in Chapter 13, that the language and practice of international human rights provides the most powerful approach to global governance of the new genetics.

In 2001, I suggested, with my colleagues Lori Andrews and Rosario Isasi, that the threat by cults and others operating on the margins of human society to clone a human being created an opportunity for the world to act preventively in ways that have been characterized as either extremely difficult or impossible. We believed that UNESCO's Universal Declaration on the Human Genome and Human Rights and the overwhelming repulsion of peoples and governments around the world to plans to clone humans made it reasonable and responsible to propose a formal treaty on The Preservation of the Human Species[19] (see box at p. 262). This proposed treaty would ban human replication cloning and germline genetic alterations. It is important to underline that adoption of this treaty would not mean that these techniques could never be legally used. What it would mean is that no individual, corporation, or government could lawfully experiment with these techniques without a worldwide discussion, followed by modification of the treaty to permit such experimentation.

To the extent that treaty negotiators and neutral scientists conclude that the prospect of genetic genocide is overblown, the treaty could be time-limited and expire automatically after the human species has gone for a period of time, perhaps 50 years, without a genocide. Because few people who have criticized the proposed treaty seem to have read it, it is also worth emphasizing that nothing in the treaty is concerned with "preserving the human genome" in its current form. Rather its authors see no compelling reasons to either eliminate the need for sexual reproduction through cloning, or to attempt to take evolution into our own genetic engineering hands. The rationale for the prohibition is that those who make such attempts are potentially putting all humans at a worst case risk of extermination and therefore should reasonably have the burden of proving to a representative international body that the benefits of their experiments are more likely to be beneficial to the human species than lethal.

Convention on the Preservation of the Human Species

Article 1: Parties shall take all reasonable action, including the adoption of criminal laws, to prohibit anyone from initiating or attempting to initiate a human pregnancy or other form of gestation using embryos or reproductive cells which have undergone intentional inheritable genetic modifications.

Article 2: Parties shall take all reasonable action, including the adoption of criminal laws, to prohibit anyone from utilizing somatic cell nuclear transfer or any other cloning technique for the purpose of initiating or attempting to initiate a human pregnancy or other form of gestation.

Article 3: Parties shall implement a system of national oversight through legislation, executive order, decree, or other mechanism to regulate facilities engaged in assisted human reproduction or otherwise using human gametes or embryos for experimentation or clinical purposes to ensure that such facilities meet informed consent, safety, and ethical standards.

Article 4: A Conference of the Parties and a Secretariat shall be established to oversee implementation of the Convention.

Article 5: Reservations to this Convention are not permitted.

Article 6: For the purpose of this Convention, the term "somatic cell nuclear transfer" shall mean transferring the nucleus of a human somatic cell into an ovum or oocyte. "Somatic cell" shall mean any cell of a human embryo, fetus, child, or adult other than a reproductive cell. "Embryo" shall include a fertilized egg, zygote (including a blastomere and a blastocyst), and a preembryo. "Reproductive cell" shall mean a human gamete and its precursors.

Our treaty proposal has not been acted on, and a similar treaty proposed by France and Germany was ultimately redrafted and adopted by the General Assemby of the United Nations as a declaration with no binding force. Unlike our proposal, the Declaration calls on countries to outlaw not just cloning to make a baby, but also cloning to produce stem cells to make medicine. Three events that occurred in 2009 may make it reasonable to reconsider our proposed treaty. The first is the inauguration of President Barack Obama and his rejection of the Bush administration's ban on stem cell research, at least research using surplus or "left over" IVF embryos. The United States would no longer insist, as it did during the Bush administration, that a treaty that bans human cloning and germline genetic engineering also bans the use of human embryos in research.

The second event is the first successful germline modification of a primate, a New World marmoset.[20] Japanese investigators reported that they had inserted a foreign gene into the marmoset embryo, and had thereby produced marmosets that incorporated the foreign gene (the gene coded for green florescent protein, GFP, into at least some of their tissues).[21] This had been done before (see Chapter 2 on the bunny named Alba and the monkey named ANDi). What was novel is that sperm was taken from one of the transgenic marmosets and used to create an embryo. The embryo was gestated by a "surrogate mother" who gave birth to a transgenic marmoset—the first time a transgenically altered primate had been able to have an offspring that also exhibited the added gene. This marmoset could have an impact on the discussion of possible human application of this technique second only to that of Dolly, the cloned sheep. Science commentators in the same issue of *Nature* in which the experiment was announced, have already warned that application of this technique to human gametes and embryos for reproductive purposes would be "unwarranted and unwise." They also wrote that the risks inherent in the technique demonstrated "the very real need for existing guidelines framed by professional societies and regulatory authorities which prevent germline genetic modifications in humans."[22]

The scientists are correct, but as demonstrated by the irresponsible actions of a few to try to make human babies by cloning, professional and regulatory action alone will not prevent attempts to modify the human germline.[23] This is apparent from the third example, the transfer of the nuclear genetic material from an egg with mutant or defective mitochondrial DNA to an egg with healthy mitochondrial DNA, and the subsequent birth of healthy rhesus macaque monkeys.[24] This germline genetic engineering technique, which results in a monkey with three genetic parents (with genes from the sperm, nucleus of one egg, and mitochrodrial DNA from another egg), was suggested for almost immediate research application in humans both by the monkey researchers and scientific commentators. *Nature* editorialized, for example, that using this technique at least "has the potential to give more couples the chance of having a healthy baby" and that "blanket bans can impede progress and encourage unethical practices."[25]

Is it too much to suggest that the births of the transgenic marmoset and the rhesus monkeys with three genetic parents provide the world with another opportunity to consider outlawing human germline genetic alterations by treaty?

Species-endangering experiments (including the creation of new genetically based bioweapons, as discussed in Chapter 2) directly concern all humans and should only be authorized by a body that is representative of everyone on the planet. These are arguably the most important decisions our species will ever make (although a reasonable case can be made that climate changes poses a more immediate survival problem for our species). And they are of special concern to the human rights community. It is not that the combination of birth, human DNA, and a human form are necessary conditions for human rights; but they are sufficient conditions for human rights. Nor is it that the human species can or should remain just the way it is (we can't), or that changes in humanity driven by evolution are not inevitable (they are). But these species changes are the result of adaptation to a new or changing environment, rather than the normative application of one particular view of human betterment or improvement. Moreover, to the extent that human rights law is grounded in our understanding of what it means to be human, changing the characteristics of the human species destabilizes that understanding and provides new tools that could encourage discrimination at best, and put the survival of the species itself at risk at worst. Cloning, for example, not only removes sexual reproduction from the definition of what it is to be human, but also seeks to eliminate human evolution by duplicating existing genomes. We have a tendency to simply let science take us wherever it will. But science has become so powerful, both in terms of making our lives better and raising the risk of worse case scenario species suicide, that we can no longer abdicate our protection responsibility to each other as members of the human species.

It is illusory to believe either that the new genetics is likely to do more good than harm to people in resource poor countries, or to believe that either bioethics or concepts of social justice alone provide sufficient guidance to deal with genetics research globally. We need a much wider, global framework and a more inclusive language—human rights—to both promote social justice and inhibit discrimination. We must work together to promote genetic privacy, prevent the genetic engineering of humans, and promote and protect universal human rights based on dignity and equality. Without action on the species level there is at least a possibility of a worst case scenario species suicide.

This is, I think, about as much as can be said—and like all worst case scenarios, probability matters. If the probability of genetic genocide really can only be roughly quantified as "at least a possibility" then it is worth spending time, money and effort to deal with it only if no other more plausible "bad case scenarios" exist. Of course, there are many more plausible problems to work on in the reproductive genetics realm, including defining the limits of prenatal genetic screening, and deciding what pre-implantation embryo experiments, including mitochondria alterations, should be permissible and who should make this determination. I leave it to the reader to decide whether the prospect of genetic genocide is a distracting, science fiction scenario, or a plausible basis for motivating public policy; whether it has more in common with H.G. Wells and his *Time Machine*, Olaf Stapledon's *Last and First Men*, or even Margaret Atwood's *The Year of the Flood*, than with current scientific and medical developments in primate reproduction research.

At the conclusion of *Worst Case Bioethics* some broad conclusions seem reasonable. The first is that there are three basic rationales that governments (and private entities) consistently employ to justify almost anything they want to do: the action will save lives; promote national security and/or promote progress. These are powerful rationales (the fourth, reliance on free markets rather than government regulation lost much of its appeal during the global financial meltdown, but will likely make a comeback in the future), and are usually simply asserted without any factual or scientific basis. What they have in common is that they all embody an implicit worst case scenario: if we don't do "X", (hundreds, thousands, or millions of) people will die, our country will be attacked (by terrorists or others), and/or we will remain ignorant (and reject all the good things more science and technology could bring the human race).

It has been frequently argued that "rights talk," including the assertion of human rights, is a conversation stopper because rights are often used as trump cards to win arguments. This is, at best, an over statement. More commonly the three rationales, individually or together, act as conversation stoppers and sufficient justification for action. As best case scenarios they can usually only be countered by worst case scenarios – which can be either plausible or entirely fictional. There are three major counter-scenarios to those that promise to save lives, protect us and our country from harm, or simply help civilization progress: war crimes and crimes against humanity, including human experimentation without consent, risk to the planet, and risk to the human species. When any of these are plausibly at stake, most people will listen to an argument for precautionary measures to limit risks, at least if it has a reasonable probability of occurring in the near future. Keynes after all was correct, "In the long run, we're all dead."

It is also worth underlining that all of our current concepts of human rights, including all of the major human rights documents, were developed and adopted in direct reaction to horrible human abuses of fellow humans—specifically those inflicted during World War II. It has been asserted that it is a paradox that recognition of human rights follows their gross abuse. It may be more accurate to say, however, that humans are able to understand and recognize human dignity only by witnessing it being violated. It takes the horrors of slavery, murder, torture, and genocide, to name just a few war crimes and crimes against humanity, for us humans to try to prevent these acts from being repeated. If this is so, then it is also reasonable to believe that compelling worst case scenarios, informed by historical precedent and scientific plausibility, could cause humans to take precautionary action before catastrophy strikes us. But maybe that's just too much to hope for.

Kurt Vonnegut, through one of his most compelling characters, science fiction writer Kilgore Trout, made this same point a different way. In *Breakfast of Champions* Vonnegut writes that as an "old, old man" Trout was asked by the Secretary General of the United Nations if he "feared the future." Trout responded, "Mr. Secretary-General, it is the *past* which scares the bejesus out of me."[26]

Acknowledgments

Worst Case Bioethics follows the path set out in my *American Bioethics*, in which I proposed a synthesis of bioethics, health law, and human rights. The interlocking webs woven by spiders representing each of these three fields is also suggested by the renaming of my Department at the Boston University School of Public Health: the Department of Health Law, Bioethics & Human Rights (previously the Health Law Department). The new designation is thanks to Dean Robert Meenan, former Boston University President Aram Chobanian, and current President Robert Brown. All have been consistent and strong supporters of my Department's scholarly and advocacy work, and it is a pleasure to acknowledge their support.

As with almost all of my work, I have my long-time department colleagues, Leonard Glantz, Wendy Mariner, Michael Grodin, and Winnie Roche to thank for the many conversations, debates, critiques, and outright disagreements we have had over the past 30 years on almost all of the subjects covered in *Worst Case Bioethics*. Leonard and Wendy are two of the nation's most prominent academic health lawyers, and Winnie is one of the nation's most knowledgeable experts on genetics and the law.

I especially want to thank one of the world's leading bioethicists and human rights activists, Michael Grodin, with whom I founded our department's NGO, Global Lawyers and Physicians (GLP). Michael has been the heart and soul of the Boston Center for Refugee Health and Human Rights at Boston Medical Center. Together we have taught a course in Human Rights and Health for the past decade, a course in which we stress the interrelationships of bioethics, health law, and human rights, and how acting in all of these arenas simultaneously increases the likelihood of successful public health action at home and abroad. Supportive advisers to GLP who died while this book was being written—and whose work helped inspire much of it—are Jay Katz of Yale (who introduced me to the Nuremberg Doctors' Trial), and Robert Drinan of Georgetown (who introduced me to international human rights law).

My family has also been deeply involved in my work. My wife Mary is not only my most insistent critic, but has also helped me learn from the refugees she teaches English to at the Boston Center for Refugee Health and Human Rights, and from the medical students we co-teach (with Michael Grodin) in our Literature and Medicine seminar. My daughter Katie is a health lawyer who works to promote patient safety in hospital settings, and my son David is in the midst of his psychiatry residency training. Both give me faith that their generation will restore much of what mine has squandered and improve upon what they have inherited. Special thanks are also due to my students at the School of Public Health, the Law School, and the Medical School—especially those in my Health Law, Bioethics, and Human Rights seminar.

Early versions of most of the chapters in *Worst Case Bioethics* appeared in the *New England Journal of Medicine* in my "Health Law, Ethics, and Human Rights" feature, and I want to acknowledge the *Journal*'s editor-in-chief, Jeffrey Drazen (who also approved changing the feature's name from "Legal Issues in Medicine" to its current title), and the feature's editor, Mary Beth Hamel. Of course, I would not be writing for the *Journal* at all were it not for the support of prior editors-in-chief Arnold Relman, Jerome Kassier, and Marcia Angell. Of the chapters that did not originally appear in the *Journal* in some form (in Health Law, Ethics, and Human Rights, as Sounding Boards, or as Perspectives), Chapters 6 and 13 were written for this book, Chapters 14 and 15 are adapted from three law reviews articles and Chapter 17 is adapted from a chapter in *Realizing the Right to Health*. Earlier versions of material contained in each chapter are referenced in the first note of the chapter.

Abbreviations

ACOG	American College of Obstetricians and Gynecologists
AMA	American Medical Association
CIA	US Central Intelligence Agency
CAT	Convention Against Torture
CDC	US Centers for Disease Control and Prevention
CEDAW	Convention on the Elimination of all Forms of Discrimination Against Women
CFR	Code of Federal Regulations
CPR	Cardiopulmonary Resuscitation
CRC	Convention on the Rights of the Child
CSA	Controlled Substances Act
D&E	Dilation and Extraction (abortion)
DEA	US Drug Enforcement Administration
DOD	US Department of Defense
DNAR	Do Not Attempt Resuscitation
DNR	Do Not Resuscitate
FBI	US Federal Bureau of Investigation
FEMA	US Federal Emergency Management Agency
HHS	US Department of Health and Human Services

HIV/AIDS	Human Immunodeficiency Virus/Acquired Immunodeficiency Disease
ICCPR	International Covenant on Civil and Political Rights
ICESCR	International Covenant on Economic, Social and Cultural Rights
ICRC	International Committee of the Red Cross
ICU	Intensive Care Unit
IMT	International Military Tribunal
IOM	Institute of Medicine
IVF	In vitro fertilization
JAG	Judge Advocate General (US military)
MSF	Medecins sans Frontieres (Doctors without Borders)
MDR-TB	Multidrug Resistant Tuberculosis
NGO	Nongovernmental Organization
NORAD	North American Aerospace Defense Command
NRC	National Research Council
NICU	Neonatal Intensive Care Unit
NORAD	North American Aerospace Command
PHR	Physicians for Human Rights
PVS	Permanent Vegetative State (also Persistent Vegetative State, based on context)
SARS	Severe Acute Respiratory Syndrome
SSRIs	Selective Serotonin Reuptake Inhibitors
TB	Tuberculosis
UDHR	Universal Declaration of Human Rights
UN	United Nations
USA	US Army
USAID	US Agency for International Development
WHO	World Health Organization
WMA	World Medical Association
XDR-TB	Extensively Drug Resistant Tuberculosis

Notes

Introduction, Scared to Death

The sources for the quotations in the introduction are mostly referenced with enough detail so they will be relatively easy to find. But a few sources used deserve more documentation. On Hiroshima, Robert Jay Lifton and Greg Mitchell, *Hiroshima in America: A Half Century of Denial*, New York: Avon Books, 1995, and John Coster-Mullen, *Atom Bomb: The Top Secret Inside Story of Little Boy and Fat Man*, 2009 (self-published by Coster-Mullen, available through Amazon).

On Cheney and doomsday exercises, Jane Mayer, *The Dark Side*, New York: Doubleday, 2008.

On the psychology of terrorism, Tom Pyszczynski, Sheldon Solomon, and Jeff Greenberg, *In the Wake of 9/ll: The Psychology of Terror*, Washington, D.C.: American Psychological Association, 2002; and Elizer Yudkowsky, Cognitive Biases Potentially Affecting Judgment of Global Risks (in) Nick Bostrom and Milan Cirkovic, editors, *Global Catastrophic Risks*, New York: Oxford University Press, 2008; and Brian Michael Jenkins, *Will Terrorists Go Nuclear?*, Amherst, NY: Prometheus Books, 2008 (the quotation from Thomas Schelling is taken from the preface).

The two prominent public health lawyers are David Fidler and Lawrence Gostin, *Biosecurity in the Global Age: Biological Weapons, Public Health, and the Rule of Law*, Stanford: Stanford University Press, 2008.

The name of the Institute of Medicine Committee mentioned is the Committee on Medical Preparedness for a Terrorist Nuclear Event, *Assessing*

Medical Preparedness to Respond to a Terrorist Nuclear Event: Workshop Report, Washington, D.C.: National Academies Press, 2009.

For more on the "end of humanity" *see* Damien Broderick, ed., *Year Million: Science at the Far Edge of Knowledge*, New York: Atlas & Co., 2008, and for an excellent introduction to the uses of worst case scenarios in public policy *see* Cass Sunstein, *Worst-Case Scenarios*, Cambridge: Harvard University Press, 2007, and Cass Sunstein, *Laws of Fear: Beyond the Precautionary Principle*, New York: Cambridge University Press, 2005.

Chapter 1, American Healthcare

1. Lyndon Johnson, *The Vantage Point*, New York: Holt, 1971 (quoted by Blumenthal, D. and Morone, J., The Lessons of Success: Revisiting the Medicine Story, *New England Journal of Medicine* 2008; 359: 2384–89). This chapter is adapted from my McDonald-Merrill-Ketcham Memorial Lecture, published as Annas, G.J., Health Care Reform in America: Beyond Ideology, *Indiana Health Law Review* 2008; 5: 441–59, and Annas, G.J., Reframing the Debate on Health Care Reform by Replacing Our Metaphors, *New England Journal of Medicine* 1994; 332: 745–748.

2. Blumenthal and Morone, Id. at 2388. *See also* David Blumenthal and James Morone, *The Heart of Power: Health and Politics in the Oval Office*, Los Angeles: University of California Press, 2009.

3. Brown, L.D., The Amazing Noncollapsing U.S. Health Care System – Is Reform Finally at Hand?, *New England Journal of Medicine* 2008; 358: 325–327.

4. Sage, W.M., Legislating Delivery System Reform: A 30,000-Foot View of the 800-Pound Gorilla, *Health Affairs* 2007; 26: 1553–1556.

5. Annas, Reframing, supra note 1.

6. Martin, A., Damien Hirst Unveils his Jewels in the Crown, a 50-Million British Pound Diamond-Studded Skull, *Daily Mail*, June 1, 2007. An argument could also be made that we like imitation or make-believe better than reality. Damien Hirst's skull, for example, was said to sell for about $100 million; an imitation, "For the Laugh of God" skull by Peter Fuss, with imitation diamonds, was priced to sell at about $10,000. Crow, K., Doubling Down on the Art Market, *Wall Street Journal*, September 10, 2009, W14.

7. Susan Sontag, *Illness as Metaphor,* New York: Farrar, Straus and Giroux, 1977.

8. Ricks, C., A Successful Defiance, *New York Review of Books*, March 20, 2008. *See generally* on selling sickness, Lynn Payer, *Disease-Mongers: How Doctors, Drug Companies, and Insurers Are Making You Feel Sick*, New York: John Wiley, 1992, and T.R. Reid, *The Healing of America: A Global Quest for Better, Cheaper, and Fairer Health Care*, New York: Penguin Press, 2009 (a contemporary comparison of the US response to a complaint of a "sore shoulder" to that of nine other countries, including the United Kingdom, Canada, France, Germany, India, and Japan).

9. Gawande, A., The Cost Conundrum, *New Yorker*, June 1, 2009, 36–43.

10. Clymer, A., Clinton's Health Plan: The Overview, *New York Times*, September 23, 1993, Al. Physician-bioethicist (and now in the White House's Office of Management and Budget) Ezekiel "Zeke" Emanuel has suggested his own list of healthcare goals: guaranteed coverage; effective cost controls; high-quality, coordinated care; choice; fair funding; reasonable dispute resolution; and economic revitalization. It is worth noting that the first three are the old access, quality and cost trio in a different order; the fourth is the all-American "choice"; and of the final three, fair funding seems a restatement of responsibility. The last two are new and it remains to be seen if they have any traction at all. Ezekiel Emanuel, *Healthcare, Guaranteed: A Simple, Secure Solution for America*, New York: Public Affairs, 2008. Some reviewers of this book have also used metaphors to describe its suggested solution. For example, Tom Miller has remarked, "The underlying theory of health cost containment in *Healthcare Guaranteed* appears to be that we first need to load everyone into the same leaky boat of basic coverage and then hope that someone later figures out how to row it back to the shoreline of fiscal balance with acceptable health care quality." *Health Affairs* 2008; 27: 1738–39.

11. McCain, J., Access to Quality and Affordable Health Care for Every American, *New England Journal of Medicine* 2008; 359: 1537–41.

12. Collins, S.R. and Kriss, J.L., *Envisioning the Future: The 2008 Presidential Candidates' Health Reform Proposals*, New York: The Commonwealth Fund, 2008, (available at http://64.251.193.200/BriefingMaterials/CMWF-EnvisioningFuture%28full%29-1114.pdf).

13. Obama, B., Modern Care for All Americans, *New England Journal of Medicine* 2008; 359: 1537441.

14. Al Gore, *An Inconvenient Truth: The Planetary Emergency of Global Warming and What We Can Do About It*, New York: Rodale, 2006.

15. Mongoven, A., The War on Disease and the War on Terror: A Dangerous Metaphorical Nexus?, *Cambridge Quarterly of Healthcare Ethics* 2006; 15: 403–16.

16. George Lakoff and Mark Johnson, *Metaphors We Live By*, Chicago: University of Chicago Press, 1980, and http://www.rockridgeinstitute.org.

17. Torry, J. and Candisky, C., Clinton's Anecdote Grounded in Error: Campaign, Media Didn't Check out Ohio Deputy's Story, *Columbus (Ohio) Dispatch*, April 11, 2008, 1A. Confusion about the facts in individual cases is common and certainly not limited to Hillary Clinton. President Obama, for example, opened his healthcare speech to a joint session of Congress with two anecdotes, both of which did involve real people, but the facts in each were different than he relayed them. For example, Otto Raddatz was dropped from his insurance while receiving chemotherapy, but did not "die because of it." Instead his sister and the state attorney general were able to get his policy reinstated within three weeks, he got the treatment he needed, and lived another four years. *See* Weisman, J., Obama Used Faulty Anecdote in Speech to Congress, *Wall Street Journal*, September 17, 2009, A4.

18. George J. Annas, *The Rights of Patients*, 3rd ed., New York: NYU Press, 2004.

19. Thomas Ricks, *The Gamble*, New York: Penguin, 2009, 3–8, *and see* Jeremy Scahill, *Blackwater*, New York: Nation Books, 2007, 3–9.

20. Goode, E., Toddler Returns to Iraq after Life-saving Surgery, *New York Times*, March 10, 2008, A6.

21. Fuchs, V., Three 'Inconvenient Truths' about Health Care, *New England Journal of Medicine* 2008; 359: 1749–51. *See also* Smith, S., Newhouse, J., and Freeland, M., Income, Insurance, and Technology: Why Does Health Spending Outpace Economic Growth?, *Health Affairs* 2009; 28: 1276–83 ("Real per capita health spending grew roughly by a factor of 9 during 1960–2007—an annual growth rate of 4.8 percent. Spending on new medical technologies accounted for 27 to 48 percent of this amount."), and Daniel Callahan, *Taming the Beloved Beast: How Medical Technology Costs are Destroying our Health Care System*, Princeton: Princeton University Press, 2009.

22. Leff, B. and Finucane, T.E., Gizmo Idolatry, *Journal of the American Medical Association* 2008; 299: 1830–1832.

23. Zeleny, J., Obama Addresses the Opposition on Health Care, *New York Times*, September 19, 2009, A10.

24. David Rieff, *Swimming in a Sea of Death*, New York: Simon & Schuster, 2008.

25. *See* Chapter 7, Cancer.

26. Markus Kornprobst, Vincent Pouliot, Nisha Shah, and Ruben Zaiotti, eds. *Metaphors of Globalization: Mirrors, Magicians and Mutinies*, New York: Palgrave MacMillan, 2008.

27. Leonhardt, D., After the Great Recession: An Interview with President Obama, *New York Times Magazine*, May 3, 2009, 37, 76. *See also*, Marmor, T., Oberlander J., and White, J., The Obama Administration's Options for Health Care Cost Control: Hope Versus Reality, *Annals of Internal Medicine* 2009; 150: 485–89 ("In short, if medical costs are to be controlled, no substitute exists for constraining prices and capping expenditures…painless savings [is an illusion].")

28. Goodman, E., A Rational Talk About Rationing Care, *Boston Globe*, May 8, 2009, A19.

29. Ivan Illich, *Medical Nemesis: The Expropriation of Health*, London: Calder & Boyars, 1975, 149.

30. Hugh Thomas, *Rivers of Gold*, New York: Random House, 2003.

Chapter 2, Bioterror and Bioart

1. This chapter is adapted from Annas, G.J., Bioterror and "Bioart" – A Plague o' both your Houses, *New England Journal of Medicine* 2008; 354: 2715–20. The report of the Commission is entitled simply *World at Risk* and was published in December 2008 as a trade paperback (New York: Vintage Books); it is also available at www.preventwmd.gov/report/. *See also* Packer, G., Risk Factors, *New Yorker*, December 15, 2008, 29–30, noting that the report suggests that every problem has a "common-sense solution" but also note that a chapter entitled Pakistan suggests that the "nation itself is a kind of W.M.D"; *see also* National Research Council, Committee on Methodological Improvements to the

Department of Homeland Security's Biological Agent Risk Analysis, *Department of Homeland Security Biological Risk Assessment: A Call for Change*, Washington, D.C.: National Academies Press, 2008 ("The threat posed by biological agents employed in a terrorist attack on the United States is arguably the most important homeland security challenge of our era.")

2. Committee on Advances in Technology and Prevention of Their Application to Next Generation Biowarfare Threats, Institute of Medicine. *Globalization, Biosecurity, and the Future of the Life Sciences*, Washington, D.C.: National Academies Press, 2006.

3. Roger Shattuck, *Forbidden Knowledge*, New York: St. Martin's Press, 1996, 224.

4. Broad, W.J. and Shane, S., For Suspects, Anthrax Case Had Big Costs, *New York Times*, August 10, 2008, A1.

5. Shane, S., Troubled Life of an Anthrax Suspect, *New York Times*, January 4, 2009, A1. A number of programs were developed during the anthrax investigations to help determine the trustworthiness of scientists employed in biosafety labs. In one scenario played in 2007 by the Office of the Director of National Intelligence, group members were divided into red and blue teams. The red teams devised 3 bioterrorist attack scenarios, while the blue teams identified points at which the attacker could be stopped or the attack foiled. One scenario involved a trained biologist plotting an attack from within a sophisticated lab. In the words of one of the participants: "The key judgment we arrived at was that if such an individual was truly intent on carrying out an attack, they would succeed . . . It scared the crap out of us." Bhattacharjee, Y., The Danger Within, *Science* 2009; 323: 1282–83.

6. Hafer, N., How Scientists View Law Enforcement, *Science Progress*, December 22, 2008 (available at www.scienceprogress.org/2008/12/science-and-law-enforcement/print/).

7. *U.S. v. Butler*, 429 F.3d 140 (5th Cir. 2005).

8. Murray, B.E., Anderson, K.E., Arnold, K., et al., Destroying the Life and Career of a Valued Physician-Scientist Who Tried to Protect Us from Plague: Was It Really Necessary?, *Clinical Infectious Diseases* 2005; 40: 1644–48.

9. Gold, R., With Plague Fears on Rise, An Expert Ends up on Trial, *Wall Street Journal*, April 14, 2003, A1. When another researcher, Malcolm Casadaban, who was working on a plague vaccine, actually died of plague in 2009, the event barely merited mention in the national press. Fitzsimmons, E.G., Researcher had Bacteria for Plague at his Death, *New York Times*, September 22, 2009, A13.

10. Enserink, M. and Malakoff, D., The Trials of Thomas Butler, *Science* 2003; 302: 2054–20.

11. The Case Against Dr. Butler, *60 Minutes* (transcript), October 19, 2003.

12. Turner, C., Culture: 'This is Right Out of Hitler's Handbook': Steve Kurtz Was Just Another Subversive U.S. Artist Until the FBI Accused Him of Bioterrorism, *The Guardian* (London), October 20, 2005, 18.

13. *U.S. v. Steven Kurtz and Robert Ferrell*, Grand Jury Indictment 0-CR-155E, W.D.N.Y., June 2004.

14. Tansey, B., Serratia Has Dark History in Region: Army Test in 1950 May Have Changed Microbial Ecology, *San Francisco Chronicle*, Oct. 31, 2004, A7.

15. Hauser, J., Genes, Genius, Embarrassment, (in) Jens Hauser, ed., *L'art Biotech*, Nantes: Editions Filigranes, 2003. *See also* Andrews, L., Tissue Culture: The Line Between Art and Science Blurs When Two Artists Hang Cells in Galleries, *Journal of Life Sciences*, September 2007, 68–73.

16. Quoted in Pool, B., From Horror to Art: Re-creating One 'Beautiful' Atomic Bomb, *Boston Globe*, July 26, 2006, A5.

17. Somerville, M.A. and Atlas, R.M., Ethics: A Weapon to Counter Bioterrorism, *Science* 2005; 307: 1881–1882.

18. Gaudioso, J. and Salerno, R.M., Biosecurity and Research: Minimizing Adverse Impacts, *Science* 2004; 304: 687.

19. Committee on Research Standards and Practices to Prevent the Destructive Application of Biotechnology. National Research Council, *Biotechnology Research in an Age of Terrorism*, Washington, D.C.: National Academies Press, 2004.

20. Bhattacharjee, Y., Army Bans Pathogen Work at Lab after Security Lapse, *Science* 2009; 324: 707.

21. Kwik, G., Fitzgerald, J., Inglesby, T.V., and O'Toole, T., Biosecurity: Responsible Stewardship of Bioscience in an Age of Catastrophic Terrorism, *Biosecurity & Bioterrorism: Biodefense Strategy, Practice and Science* 2003; 1: 27.

22. See Chapter 14, The Statue of Security.

23. Laura K. Donohue, *The Cost of Counterterrorism: Power, Politics, and Liberty*, New York: Cambridge University Press, 2008, 330–32.

24. Supra note 2.

25. Relman, D.A., Bioterrorism – Preparing to Fight the Next War, *New England Journal of Medicine* 2006; 354: 113–15.

26. *See, e.g.*, Kennedy, D., Science and Security, Again, *Science* 2008; 321: 1019 (editorial arguing against the use of the elusive "Sensitive But Unclassified" label, but seeming to accept the classification of basic research under National Security Decision Directive 189).

27. Supra note 3.

Chapter 3, State of Emergency

1. Major portions of this chapter are adapted from Annas, G.J., Extremely Preterm Birth and Parental Authority to Refuse Treatment: The Case of Sidney Miller, *New England Journal of Medicine* 2004; 351: 2118–23.

2. *See, e.g.*, McCartney, S., Crash Courses for the Crew, *Wall Street Journal*, January 27, 2009, D1, and McFadden R.D., All 155 Aboard Safe as Crippled Jet Crash-Lands in Hudson, *New York Times*, January 16, 2009, Al.

3. *See* Chapter 2, Bioterror and Bioart.

4. *E.g*, the nonderrogable provisions of the International Covenant of Civil and Political Rights.

5. *See, e.g.*, Hoffman, S., Responders' Responsibility: Liability and Immunity in Public Health Emergencies, *Georgetown Law Journal* 2008; 96: 1913–69.

6. Annas, G.J., Negligent Samaritans Are No Good, *Medicolegal News* 1979; 7: 4. *See also*, Annas, G.J., Beyond the Good Samaritan: Should Doctors Be Required to Provide Essential Services?, *Hastings Center Report* April, 1978, 16–17.

7. Id.

8. Although utilitarianism is generally not seen as a proper decision-making rule for medical treatment decisions, it is almost universally cited as the basis for triage decisions in mass emergencies, as in doing "the best we can for the most people."

9. *Miller v. HCA*, 47 Tex. Sup. J. 12, 118 S.W.3d 758 (2003).

10. Atkinson. J., A Houston Couple Says a Hospital Is Responsible for Their Daughter's Severe Disabilities, *Texas Monthly*, December 2002: 88–90.

11. *HCA v. Miller*, 36 S.W.3d 187 (Tex. App. 2000).

12. *Moss v. Rishworth*, 222 S.W. 225 (Tex. App. 1920).

13. Linden, D.W. and Doron, M.W., Eyes of Texas Fasten on Life, Death and the Premature Infant, *New York Times*, April 30, 2002, F5.

14. Cole, F.S., Extremely Preterm Birth—Defining the Limits of Hope, *New England Journal of Medicine* 2000; 343: 429–30.

15. Wood, N.S., Marlow, N., Costeloe, K., Gibson, A.T., and Wilkinson, A.R., Neurologic and Developmental Disability after Extremely Preterm Birth. *New England Journal of Medicine* 2000; 343: 378–38. *See also* Geoffrey Miller, *Extreme Prematurity: Practices, Bioethics, and the Law*, New York: Cambridge University Press, 2007.

16. George J. Annas, *The Rights of Patients*, 3rd ed., New York: NYU Press, 2004, 273–97. On Schiavo, *see* Chapter 10, Culture of Death.

17. *See, e.g.*, McGraw, M. and Perlman, J.M., Attitudes of Neonatologists Toward Delivery Room Management of Confirmed Trisomy 18: Potential Factors Influencing a Changing Dynamic, *Pediatrics* 2008; 121: 1106–10.

18. Fink, S., The Deadly Choices at Memorial, *New York Times Magazine*, August 30, 2009, 28–49. *See also*, Richard Deichmann, *Code Blue: A Katrina Physician's Memoir*, Bloomington, IN: Rooftop Publishing, 2007, 39–40 ("These DNR patients would continue to be cared for, but would be evacuated after the rest of the patients.").

19. President's Commission for the Study of Ethical Problems in Medicine and Biomedical and Behavioral Research, *Deciding to Forego Life-Sustaining Treatment*, Washington D.C.: President's Commission, 1983, 218–19.

20. *Bowen v. American Hospital Association*, 476 U.S. 610 (1986).

21. Robertson, J.A., Extreme Prematurity and Parental Rights After Baby Doe, *Hastings Center Report* 2004; 34: 32–39. *See also* Robert F. Weir, *Selective Nontreatment of Handicapped Newborns: Moral Dilemmas in Neonatal Medicine*, New York: Oxford University Press, 1984.

22. Hansmann, G., Neonatal Resuscitation on Air: Is It Time to Turn Down the Oxygen Tanks? *Lancet* 2004; 364: 1293–94.

23. Supra notes 15 and 21.

24. Supra note 19.

Chapter 4, Licensed to Torture

1. Portions of this chapter are adapted from Annas, G.J., Unspeakably Cruel: Torture, Medical Ethics, and the Law, *New England Journal of Medicine* 2005; 352: 2127–32.

2. Bob Woodward, *State of Denial*, New York: Simon & Schuster, 2006. According to Woodward, Rumsfeld was from the beginning of his tenure as Secretary of Defense against having the generals at the Pentagon rely on the JAGs, and instead wanted them to rely on his civilian lawyers. In talking to one candidate for chairman of the Joint Chiefs of Staff, Admiral Vern Clark, the following exchange was summarized:

> The Joint Staff is a national treasure, Clark said, and the secretary tended to undervalue it, even malign it. Clark said he believed Rumsfeld was dead wrong on that score. Rumsfeld scoffed again. What they provided was not worth the paper it was written on . . . *Why does the chairman need a* head of policy, or a spokesman, a liaison to the Congress, or a *lawyer?* Rumsfeld asked repeating his earlier comments to Shelton [Army General Henry H. "Hugh"]. "*Why shouldn't he use my lawyer?*" (*State of Denial* at 67, emphasis supplied)

This version is confirmed by General Myers, *see* Richard B. Myers, *Eyes of the Horizon: Serving on the Front Lines of National Security*, New York: Simon & Schuster, 2009, 197–208.

3. *See* Chapter 1, American Healthcare, and Annas, G.J., Reframing the Debate on Health Care Reform by Replacing Our Metaphors, *New England Journal of Medicine* 1995; 332: 744–48.

4. Even before the president used the phrase "new kind of war" to characterize the "global war on terror," he had characterized the 9/11 attacks as an "acts of war" and had characterized the war as "a monumental struggle between good and evil," concluding, "But good will prevail." Bob Woodward, *Bush at War*, New York: Simon & Schuster, 2002, 45.

5. Reprinted in Karen J. Greenberg and Joshua L. Dratel, eds., *The Torture Papers: The Road to Abu Ghraib*, New York: Cambridge University Press, 2005, 134–35.

6. Winston S. Churchill, *The Second World War: The Grand Alliance*, Boston: Houghton Mifflin Co., 1950; Vol. 3, at 329. *See* Horton, S., Through a Mirror, Darkly: Applying the Geneva Conventions to 'A New Kind of Warfare,' in Karen J. Greenberg, ed., *The Torture Debate in America*, New York: Cambridge University Press, 2006, 136–50. *Compare* George Washington's orders for the treatment of British prisoners of war during our war of independence: "Treat them with humanity, and Let them have no reason to Complain of our Copying the brutal example of the British army in their Treatment of our unfortunate brethren . . . Provide everything necessary for them on the road." Quoted in David Hackett Fischer, *Washington's Crossing*, New York: Oxford University Press, 2004, 379.

7. The Trial of German Major War Criminals, Part 11, April 4, 1946 to April 15, 1946, 16 (1947).

8. The Trial of German Major War Criminals, Part 6, February 2, 1946 to February 13, 1946, 310–311 (1946).

9. The ignorance of history on the part of Bush's legal team has been widely commented on. *See e.g.,* Mayer, J. The Hidden Power: The Legal Mind Behind the White House's War on Terror, *New Yorker,* July 3, 2006, 44.

10. The text of Common Article 3 (called "common" because it appears in all four of the 1949 Geneva Conventions) is:

> In the case of armed conflict not of an international character occurring in the territory of one of the High Contracting Parties, each Party to the conflict shall be bound to apply, as a minimum, the following provisions:

> (1) Persons taking no active part in the hostilities, including members of armed forces who have laid down their arms and those placed *hors de combat* by sickness, wounds, detention, or any other cause, shall in all circumstances be treated humanely, without any adverse distinction founded on race, color, religion or faith, sex, birth or wealth, or any other similar criteria. To this end the following acts are and shall remain prohibited at any time and in any place whatsoever with respect to the above-mentioned persons:
>> (a) Violence to life and person, in particular murder of all kinds, mutilation, cruel treatment and torture;
>> (b) Taking of hostages;
>> (c) Outrages upon personal dignity, in particular, humiliating and degrading treatment;
>> (d) The passing of sentences and the carrying out of executions without previous judgment pronounced by a regularly constituted court affording all the judicial guarantees which recognized as indispensable by civilized peoples.
> (2) The wounded and sick shall be collected and cared for.
> An impartial humanitarian body, such as the International Committee of the Red Cross, may offer its services to the Parties of the conflict.
> The Parties to the conflict shall further endeavour to bring into force, by means of special agreements, all or part of the other provisions of the present Convention.

> The application of the preceding provisions shall not affect the legal status of the Parties to the conflict. The Geneva Conventions of August 12, 1949.

11. Elaine Scarry, *The Body in Pain: The Making and Unmaking of the World*, New York: Oxford University Press, 1985, 42. ("Brutal, savage, and barbaric, torture [even if unconsciously] self-consciously and explicitly announces its own nature as an undoing of civilization, acts out the uncreating of the created contents of consciousness.").

12. Taylor, T. Opening statement of the prosecution, *United States v. Karl Brandt et al.*, December 9, 1946 reprinted in George J. Annas and Michael A. Grodin, eds., *The Nazi Doctors and the Nuremberg Code*, New York: Oxford University Press, 1992, 67, 68.

13. Id. at 180–181, n. 2.

14. Miles, S., Abu Ghraib: Its Legacy for Military Medicine, *Lancet* 2004; 364: 725. Steve Miles expanded and updated this article in his book, *Oath Betrayed*, New York: Random House, 2006.

15. Lewis, N., Red Cross Finds Detainee Abuse in Guantanamo, *New York Times*, November 30, 2004, A1.

16. Bloche, G. and Marks, J., When Doctors Go to War, *New England Journal of Medicine* 2005; 352: 3–5.

17. Lifton, R.J., Doctors and Torture, *New England Journal of Medicine* 2004; 351: 415–17.

18. Wiesel, E., Without Conscience, *New England Journal of Medicine* 2005; 352: 1511–13.

19. The Siracusa Principles were developed to help signatory states determine when derogable rights could be derogated, and what actions were permitted under emergency circumstances, with specific reference to a public health emergency.

20. *Hearing on the Nomination of Alberto Gonzales to be Attorney General,* January 6, 2005 (Federal News Service Transcript).

21. Weisman, S.R. and Brinkley, J., The Condoleezza Rice Hearing, *New York Times*, January 19, 2005, A1. Even after leaving the administration, Rice continued to justify waterboarding because she was told it was "legal." MacGillis, A., 4th-Grader Questions Rice on Waterboarding—Ex-Secretary of State Stresses Legality, *Washington Post*, May 4, 2009, A1.

22. Bob Woodward, *State of Denial*, New York: Simon & Schuster, 2006; and *see* supra note 2.

23. *See, e.g.*, Mayer, J., supra note 9. ("Rear Admiral Donald Guter, who was the Navy's chief JAG until June 2002, said that he and the other Judge Advocate Generals [JAGs], who were experts on the laws of war, tried unsuccessfully to amend parts of the military-commission plan when they learned of it, days before the order was formally signed by the President. 'But we were marginalized,' he said. 'We were warning them that we had this long tradition of military justice, and we didn't want to tarnish it. The treatment of detainees was a huge issue. They didn't want to hear it.'" at 52). The marginalization of the JAGs was planned and vigorously pursued. Even when Congress acted in the Ronald Reagan National Defense Authorization Act of 2005 (H.R. 4200), President Bush wrote the following in his signing statement of October 29, 2004:

> Section 574 of the Act amends sections 3037, 5046, 5148, and 8037 of title 10, United States Code, to prohibit Department of Defense personnel from interfering with the ability of a military department judge advocate general, and the staff judge advocate to the Commandant of the Marine Corps, to give independent legal advice to the head of a military department or chief of a military service or with the ability of judge advocates assigned to military units to give independent legal advice to unit commanders. *The executive branch shall construe section 574 in a manner consistent with*; (1) the President's constitutional authorities to take care that the laws are faithfully executed, to supervise the unitary executive branch, and as Commander in Chief;

(2) the statutory grant to the Secretary of Defense of authority, direction, and control over the Department of Defense (10 U.S.C.113(b)); (3) *the exercise of statutory authority by the Attorney General* (28 U.S.C. 512 and 513) *and the general counsel of the Department of Defense as its chief legal officer* (10 U.S.C. 140) *to render legal opinions that bind all civilian and military attorneys within the Department of Defense;* and (4) the exercise of authority under the statutes (10 U.S.C. 3019, 5019, and 8019) by which the heads of the military departments may prescribe the functions of their respective general counsels. (emphasis supplied)

24. Convention Against Torture (1975). *See also Sosa v. Alvarez-Machain,* 540 U.S. 1160 (2004), and Torture Victim Protection Act, 28 USCS sec.1350; and Nowak, M., What Practices Constitute Torture?: US and UN Standards, *Human Rights Quarterly* 2006; 28: 809.

25. 18 U.S.C. sections 234—2340A.

26. Memorandum for Alberto R. Gonzales, Counsel to the President, from Jay S. Bybee. Re: Standard of Conduct for Interrogation under 18 U.S.C. sections 2340-2340A. August 1, 2002. Reprinted in *The Torture Papers,* supra note 5, 172–217.

27. Memorandum for James B. Comey, Deputy Attorney General, from Daniel Levin, re: *Legal Standards Applicable Under* 18 U.S.C. secs. 2340-2340A, December 30, 2004.

28. Jehl, D. and Johnston, D., White House Fought New Curbs on Interrogations, Officials Say, *New York Times,* January 13, 2005, A1. Elaine Scarry notes persuasively that giving torture techniques names (like "waterboarding") "is to make language and civilization participate in their own destruction." She continues: "The nomenclature for torture is typically drawn from three spheres of civilization. First...the prolonged, acute distress of the body is in its contortions claimed to be mimetic of a particular invention or technological feat: the person's pain will be called 'the telephone' in Brazil, 'the plane ride' in Vietnam, 'the motorola' in Greece, and the 'San Juanica Bridge' in the Philippines. The second sphere is the realm of cultural events, ceremonies, and a games: there is 'the dance' in Argentina, 'the birthday party' in the Philippines . . . and 'the tea party' in Greece . . . The third realm is nature or nature civilized . . . the 'little hare' of Greece, 'the parrot's perch' of Brazil and Uruguay, and 'the dragon's chair' of Brazil. In all of these cases the designation of an intensely painful form of bodily contortion with a word usually reserved for an instance of civilization produces a circle of negation: there is no human being in excruciating pain; that's only a telephone . . ." (supra note 11 at 44).

29. Cheney had asserted in a radio interview that dipping a terrorist in a tub of water to obtain information of a pending attack was a "no brainer."

Question: "Would you agree a dunk in the water is a no-brainer if it can save lives?"

Cheney: "It's a no-brainer for me." Hendrik Hertzberg has commented on this exchange: "The 'dunk in the water' they were talking about is waterboarding. It has been used by the Gestapo, the North Koreans, and the Khmer Rouge. After the Second World War, a Japanese soldier was sentenced to 25 years' hard labor for using it on American prisoners. It is torture, and torture is not a no-brainer. It is a no-souler. The no-brainer is the choice on Election Day." Hertzberg, H., Hearts and Brains, *New Yorker,* November 6, 2006, 47, 48. *See also* Lewis, N., Furor Over

Cheney Remark on Tactics for Terror Suspects, *New York Times*, October 28, 2006, A8. In his "exit interviews" in January 2009, Cheney repeated his belief that waterboarding was not torture, that it was a very effective technique, and that in any event it was only used on 3 suspects and had not been used since 2003.

30. *See* John W. Dean, *Conservatives Without Conscience*, New York: Penguin Group, 2006, 162–67.

31. Luban, D., Liberalism, Torture, and the Ticking Bomb, *Virginia Law Review* 2005; 91: 1425. Jonathan Schell has persuasively argued as well that "The power of the state that tortures may be increasingly fictional, but the degradation of its civilization is real." Schell, J., Torture and Truth, *Nation*, June 15, 2009, 15–18.

32. Alan M. Dershowitz, *Why Terrorism Works: Understanding the Threat, Responding to the Challenge*, New Haven: Yale University Press, 2002, 131–63. Kenneth Roth has noted that "any effort to regulate torture ends up legitimizing it and inviting its repetition . . . Regulation too easily becomes license." Roth, K., Justifying Torture (in) Kenneth Roth, Minky Worken, and Amy Bernstein, eds., *Torture*, New York: The New Press, 2005, 884–201.

33. Dershowitz, Id. at 144, 144, 154. *See also* Scarry, E., Five Errors in the Reasoning of Alan Dershowitz (in) Sanford Levinson, ed., *Torture: A Collection*, New York: Oxford University Press, 2004, 281–85. ("the ticking bomb scenario . . . presents us with three major problems: (1) it assumes a population that is (against robust evidence) cowardly and self-regarding—able and willing to torture, but unable and unwilling to themselves suffer harm; (2) it assume a population that is (against robust evidence) omniscient; and (3) by providing legal immunity, it eliminates the felt-aversiveness to cruelty that acts as a way to test one's level of conviction that thousands of lives are at risk and that one is uniquely positioned to act as their savior."); *and see* Shue, H., Torture in Dreamland: Disposing of the Ticking Bomb, *Case Western Reserve Journal of International Law* 2006; 37: 231, 233–35. (The problems with the hypothetical are that it is idealized, assuming as it does that we have captured the right man, that he will make a prompt and accurate disclosure, and that this will be a rare case; second, it is grossly abstract, in the real world we will require organizations, training, research, and physician involvement. "The moderate position on torture is an impractical abstraction—it is torture in dreamland.")

34. Relying on one or two examples from police work involving kidnapped individuals [e.g., *Leon v. Wainwright*, 734 F.2d 770 (11th Cir. 1984)] does not change this. This is why it is only nonmilitary and non-CIA people, mostly in academics and the entertainment business, who argue for torture. Experienced interrogation professionals know better. As General John (Jeff) Kimmons, the US Army's deputy chief of staff for intelligence told reporters in an August 2006, press briefing about the Army's new *Field Manual*:

> *No good intelligence is going to come from abusive practices.* I think history tells us that. I think the *empirical evidence* of the last five hard years, tells us that. And, moreover, any piece of intelligence which is obtained under duress, through the use of abusive techniques, would be of *questionable credibility*, and additionally it would do more harm than good when it inevitably became

known that abusive practices were being used. And we can't afford to go there. Some of our most significant successes on the battlefield have been—in fact, I would say all of them have accrued from expert interrogators using mixtures of authorized *humane interrogation practices*, in clever ways that you would hope Americans would use them, to push the envelop within the bookends of legal, moral, and ethical, now as further refined this field manual. So we don't need abusive practices in there. (emphasis supplied)

Quoted by Packer, G., Prisoners, *New Yorker*, September 18, 2006, 25, 26.

The new *Army Field Manual* (September 6, 2006, FM 2-22.3) quieted almost all concern with military interrogations, although some still question the new Appendix M, which provides for isolation, here termed "Restricted Interrogation Technique – Separation." *See generally*, Sanford Levinson, ed., *Torture: A Collection*, New York: Oxford University Press, 2004; Symposium: Torture and the War on Terror, *Case Western Reserve Journal of International Law* 2006; 37: 145; Karen J. Greenberg, ed., *The Torture Debate in America*, New York: Cambridge University Press, 2006; Intelligence Science Board, *Educing Information: Interrogation: Science and Art, Foundations for the Future* (Phase 1 Report), Washington, D.C.: National Defense Intelligence College, 2006.

35. Memorandum for the President from Alberto R. Gonzales. Decision re: application of the Geneva Conventions on prisoners of war to the conflict with Al Qaeda and the Taliban, January 25, 2002 can be usefully contrasted with *Filartiga v. Pena-Irala*, 630 F.2d 876 (2d Cir.1980), in which the Second Circuit Court of Appeals ruled that US courts, under the Federal Alien Tort Statute (also referred to as the Alien Tort Claims Act) had jurisdiction to hear civil cases brought by noncitizen victims of torture against their torturers. In his opinion, upholding jurisdiction, Judge Kaufman summarized universally accepted principles of international human rights law, "the torturer has become—like the pirate and the slave holder before him—hostis humani generis, an enemy of all mankind."

On the other hand, it wasn't until 2004 that the Supreme Court answered the question of the reach of the Alien Tort Statute for the entire country in the case of Humberto Alvarez-Machain, a Mexican physician, *Sosa v. Alvarez-Machain*, 540 U. S. 1160 (2004). US Drug Enforcement Administration (DEA) officials believed that when a DEA agent, Enrique Camarena-Salazar, was captured in Mexico, tortured over a two-day period, and then murdered, Alvarez had been present and used his medical skills to extend the interrogation and torture. Demonstrating how strongly the US government objected to physicians participating in torture, the DEA took the extraordinary step of hiring Mexican nationals to kidnap Alvarez and bring him to the United States for trial. The kidnapping succeeded, but at trial Alvarez was found not guilty. After returning to Mexico, Alvarez himself brought an action against the United States under the Alien Tort Statute (ATS), alleging false arrest and arbitrary detention. Alvarez won at trial, and the Ninth Circuit Court of Appeals affirmed. In support of his position that his arbitrary detention was a violation of international law, Alvarez cited the UDHR and the ICCPR. The Court found that the UDHR did not have the force of law, and that "the United States ratified the Covenant [ICCPR] on the express understanding that it was not self-executing and so did not itself create obligations enforceable in the federal courts." The case thus stands for the proposition that a brief illegal detention is insufficient grounds for a claim for money damages in US courts as a violation of international law.

The decision is more important, however, for the Court's conclusion that when acts are universally condemned by international law, such as state-sanctioned piracy, torture, and murder, they can be the basis for a lawsuit under the Alien Tort Statute. In case of torture, the Supreme Court would find torture a violation of international law both because it is universally condemned in international law, and because Congress has ratified the CAT and also adopted a law authorizing individual lawsuits for torture victims. Thus, under the Alien Tort Statute, the victims of torture at Guantanamo and Abu Ghraib, for example, may bring a claim against their alleged torturers in US courts, and many undoubtedly will.

36. Memorandum from Secretary of Defense for Commander, US Southern Command. *Counter-Resistance Techniques in the War on Terrorism*, April 16, 2003. Reprinted in Karen J. Greenberg and Joshua L. Dratel, eds., *The Torture Papers: The Road to Abu Ghraib*, New York: Cambridge University Press, 2005, supra note 5 at 360–65.

37. Seymour M. Hersh, *Chain of Command: The Road from 9/11 to Abu Ghraib*, New York: Harper Collins Publishers, 2004, 31–32. *See also* Thomas E. Ricks, *Fiasco: The American Military Adventure in Iraq 2003–2005*, New York: Penguin Press, 2006, 238–40, 290–97.

38. George J. Annas, *American Bioethics: Crossing Human Rights and Health Law Boundaries*, New York: Oxford University Press, 2005, 8–10 (citing Protocol 1 to the Geneva Conventions, 1977, article 16 of which provides that "under no circumstances shall any person be punished for carrying out medical activities compatible with medical ethics, regardless of the person benefiting there from").

39. Schlesinger, J.R., Brown, H., Fowler, T.K., and Horner, C.A., *Final Report of the Independent Panel to Review DOD Detention Operations*, August 2004, reprinted in *The Torture Papers* supra note 5 at 908-84.

40. Transcript, Dick Cheney Interview with CNN's John King, Cheney says Obama Choice Create Risk, March 15, 2009 available at http://www.clipsand-comment.com/2009/03/15/transcript-dick-cheney-interview-with-cnns-john-king-cheney-says-obama-choices-create-risk/.

And compare June 10, 2004 statement of President George W. Bush: "Look, I'm going to say it one more time . . . Maybe I can be more clear. The instructions went out to our people to adhere to the law. That ought to comfort you. We're a nation of law. We adhere to laws. We have laws on the books. You might look at these laws, and that might provide comfort for you." President Obama is well aware of the damage US torture policy had done to our country's international reputation. In his first address to the UN General Assembly, on September 23, 2009, he told the assembled representatives to judge the United States by its actions, beginning with his own torture ban: "On my first day in office, I prohibited without exception or equivocation the use of torture by the United States of America. I order the prison at Guantanamo Bay closed. And we are doing the hard work of forging a framework to combat extremism without the rule of law. Every nation must know America will live its values, and we will lead by example." Full text available at www.Whitehouse.gov.

41. International Committee of the Red Cross, *Report on the Treatment of Fourteen 'High Value Detainees' in CIA Custody*, February 2007. Summarized in Danner, M., US Torture: Voice from the Black Sites, *New York Review of Books*, April 9, 2009; *see also* Danner, M., Tales from Torture's Dark World, *New York Times*, March 15, 2009, wk 13.

42. Id. Danner was nonetheless convinced that the worst case scenario, a ticking time bomb, could still carry the day, and believes that only an independent investigation that demonstrated to the American people that torture since 9/11 actually produced no life-saving information could quell its power.

43. *See* Isikoff, M. and Thomas, E., The Lawyer and the Caterpillar, *Newsweek*, April 27, 2009, 28–29.

44. *Rasul v. Bush*, 542 U.S. 466 (2004).

45. *Gherebi v. Rumsfeld*, 374 F. 3d 727, 738 (9th Cir. 2003).

46. *Hamdi v. Rumsfeld*, 542 U.S. 507 (2004).

47. Henri Alleg, *The Question* (Calder, trans.), preface by Jean-Paul Sartre, London: John Calder Publisher's Ltd., 1958 (quoted in Page duBois, *Torture and Truth*, New York: Routledge, Chapman and Hall, Inc. 1991, 5).

48. The Abu Ghraib photos, most taken by Charles Graner and turned over to the Army's Criminal Investigation Division by Sergeant Joseph Darby, are available at http://www.thememoryhole.org/war/iraqis_tortured/ [Images from Abu Ghraib]. Fernando Botero's paintings are available in book form, which includes an essay on them by David Ebony, *Botero: Abu Ghraib*, New York: Prestel Publishing, 2006. *See also* Forero, J., 'Great Crime' at Abu Ghraib Enrages and Inspires an Artist: Botero Depicts Torture of Prisoners by Americans, *New York Times*, May 8, 2005, 8; and Danto, A.C., The Body in Pain, *The Nation*, November 27, 2006, 23.

49. As of November 2009 the Obama administration continued to resist the publication of additional photographs from Abu Ghraib, following the example of the Bush administration.

50. Remarks by President George W. Bush at a Media Availability at the United States-European Union Summit, June 21, 2006. ("And obviously they brought up the concern about Guantanamo. And I understand their concerns, but let me explain my position. First, I'd like to end Guantanamo. I'd like it to be over with . . . And so I understand the concerns of the leaders. They expressed the concerns of the European leaders and the European people about what Guantanamo says. I also shared with them my deep desire to end this program, but I also assured them that we will—are not going to let people out on the street that will do you harm.")

Less than three months later, on September 6, 2006, Bush announced that he had moved 14 terror suspects from CIA black locations to Guantanamo for war crimes trials. Sanger, D., President Moves 14 Held in Secret to Guantanamo, *New York Times*, September 7, 2006, A1.

Chapter 5, Hunger Strikes

1. Bukovsky, V., Account of Torture, October 1986; lecture at the University of Chicago. Portions of this chapter are adapted from Annas, G.J., Hunger Strikes at Guantanamo: Medical Ethics and Human Rights in a 'Legal Black Hole,' *New England Journal of Medicine* 2006; 355: 1377–82.

2. President's Council on Bioethics, *Being Human: Readings from the President's Council on Bioethics*, 2003.

3. Golden, T., Tough U.S. Steps in Hunger Strike at Camp in Cuba, *New York Times*, February 9, 2006, Al.

4. E.R.C. Inc. *See* http://www.restraintchair.com.

5. Schmitt, E. and Golden, T., Force-feeding at Guantanamo Is Now Acknowledged, *New York Times*, February 22, 2006, A5.

6. Al-Shehri's name was first made public by *Time* in June 2006, immediately after the three suicides there. Zagorin, A. and Corliss, R., Death Comes to Guantanamo, *Time*, June 19, 2006, 38, 39 ("According to medical records obtained by *Time*, a 20-year-old named Yusuf al-Shehri, jailed since he was 16, was regularly strapped into a specially designed feeding chair [sic] that immobilizes the body at the legs, arms, shoulders, and head. Then a plastic tube, sometimes as much as 50% bigger than the type commonly used for feeding incapacitated patients, was inserted through his nose and down his throat—a procedure that can trigger nausea, bleeding, and diarrhea.") Medical records confirm his force-feeding, but his case is hardly the worst. Up to five prisoners have endured this "treatment" for months. In an affidavit for one of them, his lawyer, Julia Tarver Mason, says he told her, when she was finally allowed to see him on September 8, 2006, that he had been strapped into the emergency restraint chair and force-fed twice a day for more than seven months. In the chair, he was "incapable of movement, as nurses and corpsmen rammed tubes up his nose, pumped five to ten cans of liquids into his fragile and emaciated body, and then left him there to urinate and defecate on himself for hours at a time, ignoring his pleas to use the bathroom" (dated September 19, 2006).

7. *E.g.*, Nicholl, D., et al., Force-feeding and Restraint of Guantanamo Bay Hunger Strikers, *Lancet* 2006; 367: 811; Sherman, N., Holding Doctors Responsible at Guantanamo?, *Kennedy Institute of Ethics Journal* 2006; 16: 199. *See also* U.N. Commission on Human Rights, *Economic and Social Council, Situation of Detainees at Guantanamo Bay*, New York: United Nations, February 15, 2006, and Mitchell, L., God Mode, *Harper's*, August 2006, 9–11.

8. Center for Constitutional Rights, *The Guantanamo Prison Hunger Strikes and Protests: February 2002–August 2005*, 2005 (available at http://www.ccr-ny.org).

9. Transcript, Defense Department News Briefing, Secretary Donald Rumsfeld, *Federal News Service*, November 1, 2005.

10. *See, e.g., Singletary v. Costello*, 665 So. 2d 1099 (Fla. Dist. Ct. App. 4th Dist. 1996) (not acceptable for force-feed if no suicidal intent and hunger strike doesn't undermine prison security); *In re Caulk*, 125 N.H. 226, 480 A.2d 93 (1984) (acceptable to force-feed if prisoner is suicidal); *Zant v. Prevatte*, 286 S.E.2d 715 (Ga. 1982) (competent prisoner may refuse tube feeding); *Von Holden v. Chapman*, 87 A.D.2d 66, 450 N. Y.S.2d 623 (1982) (acceptable to force-feed a prisoner to prevent suicide [citing three trial court decisions in accord with this holding]); *Thor v. Superior Court*, 855 P.2d 375 (Cal. 1993). (competent prisoner has the right not to eat) *Cf. Commissioner of Corrections v. Myers*, 379 Mass. 255, 399 N.E. 452 (1979) (prisoner may not refuse kidney dialysis in an attempt to be transferred). Prison hunger strikes are dangerous for both prisoner and jailers, but are often the only way, or the last

resort, for a prisoner to protest the conditions of his confinement. *See generally,* Sharman Apt Russell, *Hunger: An Unnatural History,* New York: Basic Books, 2005.

The best known force-feeding cases have to do with comatose patients and patients in persistent or permanent vegetative states, like Karen Ann Quinlan, Nancy Cruzan, and Terri Schiavo, but these have nothing to do with competent prisoners on a hunger strike except that they all affirm a common law and/or constitutional right on the part of competent adults to refuse any medical treatment, including tube feeding, regardless of a likely lethal outcome. The Terri Schiavo case, which was specifically used by Winkenwerder to justify force-feeding hunger strikers, is discussed in detail in Chapter 11, Culture of Death.

11. Annas, G.J., Prison Hunger Strikes: Why Motive Matters, *Hastings Center Report* December, 1982, 21–22.

12. *Media Roundtable with Department of Defense Assistant Secretary for Health Affairs William Winkenwerder,* News Transcript, June 7, 2006 (available at http://www.defenselink.mil/transcripts/transcript.aspx?transcriptID=33).

13. Reyes, H., *Medical and Ethical Aspects of Hunger Strikes in Custody and the Issue of Torture,* 1998 (available at http://www.icrc.org/). *See generally,* Ryan Goodman and Mindy Jane Roseman, eds., *Interrogations, Forced Feedings, and the Role of Health Professionals,* Cambridge: Harvard Human Rights Program, 2009 (especially Allen, S. and Reyes, H., New Perspectives: Operational Guidance on Interrogations and Hunger Strikes, 189–204, and Welsh, J., Responding to Food Refusal: Striking the Human Rights Balance, 143–71).

14. Oguz, N.Y. and Miles, S., The Physician and Prison Hunger Strikes: Reflecting on the Experience in Turkey, *Journal of Medical Ethics* 2005; 31: 169, and Fessler, D.M.T., The Implications of Starvation Induced Psychological Changes for the Ethical Treatment of Hunger Strikers, *Journal of Medical Ethics* 2003; 29: 243.

15. World Medical Association, *Declaration on Hunger Strikers (Declaration of Malta),* 1991, revised 1992, and revised again in 2006.

16. *See, e.g.,* Winkenwerder, supra note 12.

17. Okie, S., Glimpses of Guantanamo – Medical Ethics and the War on Terror, *New England Journal of Medicine* 2005; 353: 2529–34.

18. Hunger Strikes, Inmate, 28 CFR sec. 549.60 et seq. (1994).

19. Okie, supra note 17.

20. Royal Dutch Medical Association, *Assistance in Hunger Strikes: A Manual for Physicians and Other Health Personnel Dealing with Hunger Strikers* (1995).

21. Annas, G.J., Hunger Strikes: Can the Dutch Teach Us Anything? *British Medical Journal* 1995; 311: 1114, 1115.

22. *See generally,* George J. Annas and Michael A. Grodin, *The Nazi Doctors and the Nuremberg Code,* New York: Oxford University Press, 1993.

23. *See generally,* Thomas E. Bean and Linette R. Sparacino, eds., *Military Medical Ethics,* 2 vols., Office of the Surgeon General, U.S. Army, 2003 (described in Annas, G.J. and Grodin, M.A., Book Review: Military Medical Ethics, *New England Journal of Medicine* 2005; 352: 312–14.

24. Department of Defense, Medical Program Support for Detainee Operations, No. 2310.08E, June 6, 2006 (available at http://www.dtic.mil/whs/directives/corres/html/231008.htm).

Edmund (Randy) Howe, who teaches medical ethics at the Uniformed Services University of the Health Sciences in Bethesda, Maryland, told a conference on "War, Torture and Terrorism" in Philadelphia on November 17, 2006, that he had just returned from a visit to Guantanamo and there were now only two prisoners who remained on hunger strike and who were being force-fed. The rationale for force-feeding, Howe was told, now being used is twofold: (1) there is peer pressure on the hunger-striking prisoners who are therefore not fasting voluntarily; and (2) the prisoners have been trained not to eat to win over others around the world to their cause (i.e., it is a tactic to further their war effort). If these are, in fact, the two rationales, they remain deficient. Force-feeding only plays into the enemies' hands by confirming our ruthlessness, and even if there is peer pressure, it does not justify involuntary medical feeding until the prisoner begins to deteriorate and requires it from a medical point of view. More recently, Howe has reviewed all of the rationales for force-feeding at Guantanamo, seeming to believe that "saving lives" is the most supportable from a medical ethics viewpoint. Nonetheless he concedes, "New analyses of force-feeding may go against the present practice . . . [and conclude] if detainees are competent, they should not be force-fed at all." And even if it doesn't, Howe suggests, "greater transparency may be helpful, particularly by moving all these questions more to an 'outside arena.'" Howe, E., Further Consideration Regarding Interrogations and Forced Feeding (in) Goodman and Roseman, supra note 13 at 75–102.

25. *See* Joseph Margulies, *Guantanamo and the Abuse of Presidential Power*. New York: Simon & Schuster, 2006. *And see* Raban, J., The Prisoners Speak, *New York Review of Books*, October 5, 2006, 25 (reviewing Margulies as well as the film "The Road to Guantanamo"), and Moazzam Begg, *Enemy Combatant: The Terrifying True Story of a Briton in Guantanamo*, London: The Free Press, 2006.

26. *Hamdan v. Rumsfeld*, 546 U.S. 1002 (2006). The JAGs, both active duty and retired, had unanimously opposed any movement away from honoring the Geneva Conventions by the US military. *See* Zernike, K., Military Lawyers Urge Protections for Detainees, *New York Times*, July 14, 2006, A16, and Lewis, N., Military Lawyers Prepare to Speak on Guantanamo, *New York Times*, July 11, 2006, A14.

27. The complete text of Common Article 3 appears in note 10 of Chapter 4, Licensed to Torture.

28. This assessment may be overly optimistic. As of November 2009, the only official report on the hunger strikers during the Obama presidency, done by a team led by Admiral Patrick Walsh, Vice Chief of Naval Operations, was delivered to the president in late February and was highly complimentary to the force-feeders and their techniques (*Review of Department Compliance with President's Executive Order on Detainee Conditions of Confinement*). The President had specifically directed the Secretary of Defense to review the conditions at Guantanamo to ensure that all prisoners there are held "in conformity with all applicable laws governing the conditions of confinement, including Common Article 3 of the Geneva Conventions." The section of the report on the hunger strikers essentially ignores the prohibitions of Common Article 3 of the Geneva Conventions, and instead relies exclusively on DOD's own 2006 regulations, and the regulations of the US Bureau of Prisons. In summarizing current practice, however, the Walsh team did

highlight some of the major problems with physician involvement in force-feeding. The first is that the decision to force-feed is based on an undisclosed (and to date classified) medical protocol. Second, the decision is ultimately not medically made, only medically facilitated, since "a medical recommendation for intervention with involuntarily intravenous therapy or enteral feeding must be approved by the CJTF [Commander Joint Task Force]." Third, restraints are used "to protect both the detainee and staff." Fourth, "time in the feeding chair may not exceed two hours . . . ." From these observations the team concluded that (1) the policy is designed to preserve the life and health of the prisoners; (2) the policy is similar to that used by the US Bureau of Prisons; (3) the feeding program is being conducted solely as a medical procedure to sustain the life and health of hunger strikers; (4) the process is lawful and is being administered in a humane manner; and (5) is "in accordance with Common Article 3" and DOD policy.

The shortcomings in this shallow and self-serving report can be briefly summarized. It made no attempt to contest the ethical positions of the AMA and the WMA, both of which have condemned force-feeding as unethical. The Walsh team also failed to question the ethics of having a classified medical protocol, which should be a contradiction in terms; the propriety of having a nonphysician (the base commander) make what they themselves characterize as a medical treatment decision; the seeming commonsense contradiction that if a prisoner is strong enough to pose a safety and security danger to the guards it is extremely unlikely that the prisoner needs to be force-fed to save his life; and the complete failure to justify the use of restraint chairs for two-hour periods as consistent with Common Article 3 of the Geneva Conventions; and the reliance instead on the equally brutal methods used in US prisons which are not, of course, governed by the Geneva Conventions at all. The Walsh report underscores once again the difficulties posed when the Department of Defense investigates itself. *See* Rubenstien, L. and Annas, G.J., Medical Ethics at Guantanamo and in the U.S. Military: Time for Reform, *Lancet*, 2009; 374: 353–5.

29. Justice Anthony Kennedy, who joined the five-justice majority, would have postponed ruling on this issue for another day.

30. Memorandum for the President from Alberto Gonzales, *Decision Re Application of the Geneva Convention on Prisoners of War to the Conflict with Al Qaeda and the Taliban,* January 25, 2002. The JAGs were intentionally kept out of the loop on this decision, but it was strongly opposed by State Department lawyer William H. Taft, IV who wrote in a February 2, 2002 memo to Gonzales concerning his January 25 memo, "The President should know that a decision that the Conventions do apply is consistent with the plain language of the Conventions and the unvaried practice of the United States in introducing its forces into conflict over fifty years. It is consistent with the advice of DOS [Department of State] lawyers and, as far as is known, the position of every other party to the Conventions . . . The Conventions call for a decision whether they apply to the conflict in Afghanistan. If they do, their provisions are applicable to all persons involved in that conflict—al Qaeda, Taliban, Northern Alliance, U.S. troops, civilians, etc. If the Conventions do not apply to the conflict, no one involved in it will enjoy the benefit of their protections as a matter of law."

31. Quoted in Mayer, J., The Hidden Power, *New Yorker*, July 3, 2006, 44, 46.

32. Military Commissions Act of 2006.

33. *See*, e.g., September 12, 2006 letter to Chairman of the Senate Armed Services Committee John Warner and Ranking Member Carl Levin by 40 retired admirals, generals, and others, which opposed any attempt to redefine Common Article 3 or to avoid it, and praised the action of the Department of Defense, which had, in reaction to *Hamdan*, issued a directive "reaffirming that the military will uphold the requirements of Common Article 3 with respect to all prisoners in its custody."

34. General John (Jack) W. Vessey, USA (Ret.) noted in his September 12, 2006 letter to Senator John McCain (written on his four-star retired general's stationery) that it would be a serious mistake for Congress to do anything "which might relax the United States support for adherence to Common Article 3 of the Geneva Conventions." He continued:

> In 1950, three years after the creation of the Department of Defense, the then Secretary of Defense, General George C. Marshall, issued a small book, titled *The Armed Forces Officer*. The book summarized the laws and traditions that governed our Armed Forces through the years. As the Senate deals with the issue it might consider a short quote from the last chapter of the book which General Marshall sent to every American Officer. The last chapter is titled "Americans in Combat" and its lists 29 general propositions which govern the conduct of Americans in war. Number XXV, which I long ago underlined in my copy, reads as follows:
>
>> *The United States abides by the laws of war.* Its Armed Forces, in their dealing with all other peoples, are expected to comply with the laws of war, *in the spirit and the letter.* In waging war, we do not terrorize helpless non-combatants, if it is within our power to avoid so doing. Wanton killing, torture, cruelty or the working of unusual hardship on enemy prisoners or populations is not justified under any circumstances. Likewise, *respect for the reign of law, as that term is understood in the United States, is expected to follow the flag wherever it goes* . . . For the long term interest of the United States as a nation and for the safety of our own forces in battle, we should continue to maintain those principles . . . . (emphasis added)

The next day, September 13, 2006, General Colin Powell, USA (ret.), Bush's former Secretary of State who had unsuccessfully opposed him in February 2002 when Bush set aside the Geneva Conventions, wrote Senator McCain the following letter (also written on his four-star retired general's stationery):

> I just returned to town and learned about the debate taking place in Congress to redefine Common Article 3 of the Geneva Conventions. I do not support such a step . . . I have read the powerful and eloquent letter sent to you by one of my distinguished predecessors as Chairman of the Joint Chiefs of Staff, General Jack Vessey. I fully endorse his powerful argument. *The world is beginning to doubt the moral basis of our fight against terrorism. To redefine Common*

Article 3 would add to those doubts. Furthermore it would put our own troops at risk. I am as familiar with *The Armed Forces Officer* as is Jack Vessey. It was written after all the horrors of World War II and General George Marshall, then Secretary of Defense, used it to tell the world and to remind our soldiers of our moral obligations with respect to those in our custody. (emphasis added)

35. *The Armed Forces Officer*, Washington D.C.: Department of Defense, 1950, 4, 241.

36. Zagorin, A., *Time*, November 10, 2006; and Landler, M., 12 Detainees Sue Rumsfeld in Germany, Citing Abuse, *New York Times,* November 15, 2006, A17. Most notably, the case against the defendants had been expanded from Abu Ghraib to include Guantanamo, with special reference to the case of Mohammed al-Qahtani first described in Zagorin, A., One Life Inside Gitmo, *Time*, March 13, 2006, 21.

37. Id. One of the named defendants in the initial filing, General Janis L. Karpinski, the commander of Abu Ghraib during the time the photographs were taken of prisoner abuse, was dropped as a defendant and offered to testify as a witness for the prosecution.

38. These are the five lawyers most intimately involved in pushing the Bush torture policy through the White House and in the Department of Defense. *See, e.g.,* Mayer, J., supra note 31, and Alvarez, J.E., Torturing the Law, *Case Western Reserve Journal of International Law* 2006; 37: 175–223. Of this group, John C. Yoo, has been the most aggressive in defending his actions in the context of "a new kind of war against an enemy we haven't faced before." Liptak, A., Interrogation Methods Rejected by Military Win Bush's Support, *New York Times*, September 8, 2006, A1, A18; *and see* Golden, T., Junior Aide Laid the Legal Basis for White House Terror Plans, *New York Times*, December 23, 2005, A1, and John Yoo, *The Powers of War and Peace: The Constitution and Foreign Affairs after 9/11*, Chicago: University of Chicago Press, 2005; John Yoo, *War by Other Means: An Insider's Account of the War on* Terror, New York: Atlantic Monthly Press, 2006. *See also* Cole, D., The Torture Memos: The Case Against the Lawyers, *New York Review of Books*, October 8, 2009, 14–16 ("When considered as a whole, the memos reveal a sustained effort by the OLC [Office of Legal Council in the Dept of Justice] lawyers to rationalize a predetermined and illegal result . . . [the OLC lawyers] used law not as a check on power but to facilitate brutality . . .")

39. Trials of War Criminals before the Nuremberg Military Tribunals under Control Council Law No. 10, Vol. III, 31–32 (*U.S. v. Altstoetter*, "The Justice Case") (1951).

40. *See* Alvarez, supra note 38 and Cole, supra note 38.

41. Grodin, M.A., Annas, G.J., and Glantz, L.H., Medicine and Human Rights: A Proposal for International Action, *Hastings Center Report* 1993; 23(4): 8. *See also,* Annas, G.J. and Grodin, M.A., Medicine and Human Rights: Reflections on the Fiftieth Anniversary of the Doctors' Trial, *Health and Human Rights* 1996; 2: 7–21, and Annas, G.J. and Grodin, M.A., Medical Ethics and Human Rights: Legacies of

Nuremberg, *Hofstra Law & Policy Symposium* 1999; 3: 111–123; Justo, L., Doctors, Interrogation, and Torture, *British Medical Journal* 2006; 332: 1462, 1463 (urging further discussion of our proposal and noting, "An international medical tribunal could initially act by making public statements denouncing doctors who have committed documented violations of human rights, but could also use its influence to urge national medical associations to revoke such doctors' license to practice. It would be a demanding task, but it would be worth the international effort to do it").

42. Our proposal has been criticized as being unnecessary and perhaps counterproductive in the presence of the new International Criminal Court. Meier, B.M., International Criminal Prosecution of Physicians: A Critique of Professors Annas and Grodin's Proposed International Medical Tribunal, *American Journal of Law & Medicine* 2004; 30: 419–52. Although we strongly support the International Criminal Court, we do not believe a parallel court—with or without criminal sanction—which addressed itself only to professionals licensed by the state (most notably physicians, but lawyers as well) would interfere with the International Criminal Court in any meaningful way, and would be an even more powerful influence on the professions because of its more specific mandate.

43. *See*, e.g., *Thorburn v. Dept. Corrections*, 66 Cal. App. 4th 1284, 78 Cal. Rptr.2d 584 (1998) (participation by physicians in lethal injection executions under state law is not unprofessional conduct that can be used to discipline a physician by the state medical licensing board because this conduct is approved by the legislature). For discussion, *see* LeGraw, J.M. and Grodin, M.A., Health Professionals and Lethal Injection Execution in the United States, *Human Rights Quarterly* 2002; 24: 382–423.

44. The complaint against John S. Edmondson was filed with the California Medical Board on July 6, 2005 and alleged a variety of medical ethics violations in the treatment of prisoners. There are, of course, very difficult logistical problems should the Board ultimately proceed with this or any other similar complaint, most involving access to medical records and to the patient-prisoners themselves. Edmondson was reassigned in January 2006 (he had been the head of the hospital at Guantanamo since July 2003) and replaced by Captain Ronald Sollock, who had previously served in the Medical Inspectors General's Office. Buomgton, S., Sollock Takes Command of Naval Hospital, *Guantanamo Bay Gazette*, January 13, 2006, 3. And on Guantanamo from April 2005 to September 2006, *see* Golden, T., The Battle for Guantanamo, *New York Times Magazine*, September 17, 2006.

45. This is, of course, true of lawyers as well, and complaints of aiding and abetting in the commission of war crimes are equally justified. *See* Cole, supra note 38.

Chapter 6, War

1. John Keegan, *A History of Warfare*, New York: Vintage Books, 1993, 56–57.

2. Geiger, J., The Impact of War on Human Rights (in) Barry S. Levy and Victor W. Sidel, eds., *War and Public Health*, New York: Oxford, 1997, 39.

3. Jane Stromseth, David Wippman, and Rosa Brooks, *Can Might Make Rights?: Building the Rule of Law after Military Interventions*, Cambridge: Cambridge University Press, 2006.

4. Drinan, R.F., The Nuremberg Principles in International Law (in) George J. Annas and Michael A. Grodin, eds., *The Nazi Doctors and the Nuremberg Code*, New York: Oxford University Press, 1992, 174–82.

5. O'Brien, W.V. and Arend, A.C., Just War Doctrine and the International Law of War (in) Thomas E. Bean and Linette R. Sparacino, eds., *Military Medical Ethics*, Vol. 1, Bethesda, Maryland: Uniformed Services University of the Health Sciences, 2003, 221–49.

6. Editorial, *Life*, August 20, 1945, 32. The best book on America's inability to come to grips with the implications of the Hiroshima bombing is Robert Jay Lifton and Greg Mitchell, *Hiroshima in America: A Half Century of Denial*, New York: Avon Books, 1996. ("Hiroshima and Nagasaki radically altered our relationship to killing civilians from the air . . . . Almost anything was permissible if used to 'save lives.' " at 304.) *See generally* on American exceptionalism as a justification for war, Andrew J. Bacevich, *The Limits of Power: The End of American Exceptionalism*, New York: Metropolitan Books, 2008, Curtis E. LeMay, *Mission with LeMay*, New York: Doubleday, 1965 ("I have sought to slaughter as few civilians as possible." at viii), and Warren Kozak, *LeMay: The Life and Wars of General Curtis LeMay*, Washington, D.C.: Regency Publishing, 2009 ("In his firebombing campaign over Japan, LeMay ordered the deaths of more civilians than any military officer in American history— well over three hundred thousand and perhaps as many as half a million. No one else come close . . . Yet in the strange calculus of war, by killing so many human beings, LeMay saved millions more by making an invasion of Japan unnecessary." at x–xi).

7. Sven Lindqvist and Linda Haverty Rugg, *A History of Bombing*, New York: The New Press, 2003. *See also*, Donald Miller, *Masters of the Air: America's Bomber Boys Who Fought the Air War Against Nazi Germany*, New York: Simon & Schuster, 2006.

8. David McCullough, *Truman*, New York: Simon & Schuster, 1992, 458.

9. Thomas E. Ricks, *The Gamble: General David Petraeus and the American Military Adventure in Iraq, 2006–2008*, New York: Penguin Press, 2009, 5. See also *The U.S. Army-Marine Corps Counterinsurgency Field Manual* (U.S. Army Field Manual No. 3-24), Chicago: University of Chicago Press, 2007 ("This field manual directs U.S. forces to make securing the civilian, rather than destroying the enemy, their top priority. The civilian population is the center of gravity—the deciding factor in the struggle" at xxv). General Stanley McChrystal brought this civilian-sparing counterinsurgency model to Afghanistan, but as US casualties mounted, families of troops stationed there started to object that it was putting US troops in too much danger. *See, e.g.*, Tyson, A.S., Less Peril for Civilians, but More for Troops: As U. S. Toll in Afghanistan Rises, Lawmakers and Families are Questioning New Restrictions, *Washington Post*, September 23, 2009, A1.

10. Jaffe, G., Joint Probe Planned of Deadly US Strike in West Afghanistan: Red Cross Says Children, Women Died, *Washington Post*, May 7, 2009, A1, and Gall C. and Shah T., Civilian Deaths Imperil Support for Afghan War, *New York Times*, May 7, 2009, Al.

11. Margalit A. and Walzer, M., Israel: Civilians & Combatants, *New York Review of Books*, May 14, 2009, 21–22. Madelyn Hsiao-Rei Hicks and Michael Spagat have developed a "dirty war index" as an attempt to try to quantify the

"dirtiness" of war by comparing the ratio of unjustifiable civilian deaths to the total number of deaths. Hicks, M. and Spagat, M., The Dirty War Index: A Public Health and Human Rights Tool for Examining and Monitoring Armed Conflict Outcomes, *PLOS Medicine* 2008, 5: 1658–64. *See also*, Hicks, M.H., Dardagen, H., Serdan, G.G., et al., The Weapons the Kill Civilians: Deaths of Children and Noncombatants in Iraq, 2003–2008, *New England Journal of Medicine* 2009; 360: 1585–88 (arguing that data support a prohibition on aerial bombing in civilian areas unless civilians are being protected).

12. Bronner, E., Soldier's Accounts of Gaza Killings Are Raising Furor in Israel, *New York Times*, March 20, 2009, Al, and Bronner, E., Israel Fights Accusations of Abuses in Gaza War, *New York Times*, March 28, 2009, A4. On the Goldstone report *see* MacFarquhar, N., U.N. Inquiry Sees Gaza War Crimes: Israel Chastised, *New York Times*, September 16, 2009, A1. The report, *Human Rights in Palestine and Other Occupied Arab Territories* (September 15, 2009) is available at http://www2.ohchr.org/english/bodies/hrcouncil/specialsession/9/docs/UNFFMGC_Report.pdf

13. Seelye, K., For Families of the War Dead, a Mournful Ritual of Homecoming, *New York Times*, May 6, 2009, A18.

14. *JB Pictures v. Dept. of Defense*, 86 F.3d 236 (D.C. App. 1996).

15. Letter of USAF Col. Laurel A. Warish to Russ Kick, dated April 14, 2004.

16. http://www.thememoryhole.org/war/coffin_photos/dover. *See also,* Jim Sheeler, *Final Salute: A Story of Unfinished Lives*, New York: Penguin Press, 2008, and the HBO movie, *Taking Chance* (2009).

17. Davies, F., Military Families Reveal Mixed Feelings on Casket Photos, *Miami Herald*, April 24, 2004, A1. *See also* Kornblut, A.E. and Bender, B., Pentagon to Review Photo Ban, *Boston Globe*, April 24, 2004, Al. In June 2004, the Senate voted 54 to 39 to retain the press ban policy. Senator John McCain made the proper policy point, noting that "these caskets that arrive at Dover are not named; we just see them . . . . I think we ought to know the casualties of war"; Stolberg, S.G., Senate Backs Ban on Photos of G.I. Coffins, *New York Times*, June 22, 2004, A17.

18. Grady, D., In Scans, Answers for Soldiers' Survivors and Aid for Comrades, *New York Times*, May 26, 2009, A1.

19. Pelligrino, E., The Moral Foundations of the Patient–Physician Relationship: The Essence of Medical Ethics (in) *Military Medical Ethics*, supra note 5, 3–21.

20. Id.

21. *See* Annas, G.J., Protecting Soldiers from Friendly Fire: The Consent Requirement for Using Investigational Drugs and Vaccines in Combat, *American Journal of Law & Medicine* 1998; 24: 245–60, and Benedek, D., Schneider, B., and Bradley, J., Psychiatric Medications for Deployment: An Update, *Military Medicine* 2007; 172: 681–85.

22. *See also*, Annas, C.L. and Annas, G.J., Enhancing the Fighting Force: Medical Research on American Soldiers, *Journal of Contemporary Health Law and Policy* 2009; 25: 283–308.

23. US Dept. of Defense, News Transcript, William Winkenwerder, Assistant Sec'y Defense for Health Affairs, Media Roundtable (June 7, 2006) available at http://www.defenselink.mil/Transcripts/Transcript.aspx?TranscriptID=33.

24. As President Obama quoted from the "soldier's creed" at a White House ceremony pressing the Medal of Honor posthumously to Sergeant Jared C. Monti on September 17, 2009: "He embodied that creed all soldiers strive to meet: 'I will always place the mission first. I will never accept defeat. I will never quite. I will never leave a fallen comrade.' " (remarks of the president available at www.white-house.gov).

25. Bouke, J., The Complexity of Medicine and War, *Lancet* 2009; 373: 113–14. Bouke made this observation after viewing the Wellcome Collection's exhibit on War and Medicine. *See also* Judt, T., What Have We Learned, If Anything?, *New York Review of Books*, May 1, 2008, 16–20 ("In the US, at least, we have forgotten the meaning of war.... War, total war, has been the crucial antecedent condition for mass criminality in the modern era" at 18.)

Chapter 7, Cancer

1. J.M. Coetzee, *Age of Iron*, London: Seeker & Warburg, 1990. This chapter is adapted from Annas, G.J., Cancer and the Constitution: Choice at Life's End, *New England Journal of Medicine* 2007; 357: 408–13.

2. James T. Patterson, *The Dread Disease: Cancer and Modern American Culture*, Cambridge: Harvard University Press, 1987. Of course, we dread other things, like lethal epidemics, as well. *See* Philip Alcabes, *Dread: How Fear and Fantasy Have Fueled Epidemics from the Black Death to Avian Flu*, New York: Public Affairs, 2009. On current cancer experiments *see* Kolata, G., Long Drive to Cure Cancer, Advances Have Been Elusive: Forty Years' War, *New York Times*, April 24, 2009, A1; Pollack, A., Taking Risk for Profit, Industry Seeks Cancer Drugs, *New York Times*, September 2, 2009, A1 ("About 860 cancer drugs are being tested in clinical trials . . . more than twice the number of experimental drugs for heart disease and stroke combined . . ."), and Alberts, B., Redefining Cancer Research, *Science* 2009; 325: 1319 (arguing for expanding the cancer research agenda to include genomic and proteomic technologies to develop drugs to attack specific tumors).

3. *Abigail Alliance v. Von Eschenbach*, 445 F.3d 470 (D.C. Cir. 2006). *Vacated* 469 F.3d 129 (D.C. Cir. 2006).

4. *Proposed Rules for Charging for Investigational Drugs and Expanded Access to Investigational Drugs for Treatment Use*, Rockville: Food and Drug Administration, 2006. These rules were adopted on August 13, 2009: 21 CFR Part 312 and 316: *Charing for Investigational Drugs Under and Investigational New Drug Application; Expanded Access to Investigational Drugs for Treatment Use; Final Rules*, Federal Register 74: 40872–40945. There seems to have been, however, no change in the attitude of the Abigail Alliance toward the FDA or the head of its cancer drug office for the past decade, Richard Pazdur. *See* Harris, G., Where Progress is Rare, the Man Who Says No, *New York Times*, September 16, 2009, A1 (" 'Patients are right to be angry and frustrated with Richard Pazdur,' said Steven Walker, cofounder of the Abigail Alliance, a patient advocate group. 'He is a dinosaur.' ")

5. *Abigail Alliance v. Von Eschenbach*, 429 F.3d 129 (D.C. Cir. 2006).

6. Jacobson, P.D. and Parmet, W.E., A New Era of Unapproved Drugs: The Case of *Abigail Alliance v Von Eschenbach*, *JAMA* 2007; 297: 205–208.

7. *Cruzan v. Director, Missouri Dept. of Health*, 497 U.S. 261 (1990).

8. *United States v. Rutherford*, 442 U.S. 544 (1979).

9. *Washington v. Glucksberg*, 521 U.S. 702 (1997); *Vacco v. Quill*, 521 U.S. 793 (1997).

10. Annas, G.J., The Bell Tolls for a Constitutional Right to Assisted Suicide, *New England Journal of Medicine* 1997; 337: 1098–1105.

11. *Abigail Alliance v. Leavitt*, 495 F.3d 695 (App. D.C. 2007).

12. How about a "Kianna's Law"? *Wall Street Journal*, March 24, 2005, A14.

13. Kianna's Legacy. *Wall Street Journal*, March 29, 2005, Al4.

14. ACCESS Act (Access, Compassion, Care, and Ethics for Seriously Ill Patients), S. 1956, 109th Cong (2005). *See* Groopman, J., The Right to A Trial: Should Dying Patients Have Access to Experimental Drugs? *New Yorker*, December 18, 2006, 40–47.

15. Annas, G.J., Faith (Healing), Hope and Charity at the FDA: The Politics of AIDS Drug Trials, *Villanova Law Review* 1989; 34: 771–79.

16. FDA proposes rules overhaul to expand availability of experimental drugs: the agency also clarifies permissible charges to patients. Rockville, MD: Food and Drug Administration, December 11, 2006. *See* supra, note 4.

17. Alex Prud'homme, *The Cell Game: Sam Waksal's Fast Money and False Promises—and the Fate of ImClone's Cancer Drug*, New York: Harper Business, 2004.

18. Jay Katz, *The Silent World of Doctor and Patient*, New Haven: Yale University Press, 1984, 151.

19. Anand, G., Saying No to Penelope: Father Seeks Experimental Cancer Drug, but a Biotech Firm Says Risk Is Too High, *Wall Street Journal*, May 1, 2007, A1. Treating dying children may be the most difficult situation for both parents and physicians. *See, e.g.*, Gretchen Kruger, *Hope and Suffering: Children, Cancer, and the Paradox of Experimental Medicine*, Baltimore: Johns Hopkins University Press, 2008, and Harmon, A., Fighting for a Last Chance at Life: One Family's Tenacious Campaign for Access to an Unproven Drug, *New York Times*, May 17, 2009, Al (recounting one family's struggle to get access to an unproven drug to treat their son who was dying of amyotropic lateral sclerosis).

20. Robertson, J., Controversial Medical Treatment and the Right to Health Care, *Hastings Center Report*, November 2006, 15–20.

21. Michael L. Culbert, *Vitamin B17: Forbidden Weapon Against Cancer*, New Rochelle, NY: Arlington House, 1974.

22. Miller H.I., Paternalism Costs Lives, *Wall Street Journal*, March 2, 2006, A15. *See also*, Falit, B.P. and Gross, C.P., Access to Experimental Drugs for Terminally Ill Patients, *JAMA* 2008; 300: 2793–95.

23. Annas G.J., The Changing Landscape of Human Experimentation: Nuremberg, Helsinki, and Beyond, *Health Matrix Journal of Law-Medicine* 1992; 2: 119–40; Appelbaum P.S. and Lidz, C.W., Re-evaluating the therapeutic misconception: response to Miller and Joffe, *Kennedy Institute of Ethics Journal* 2006; 16: 367–73.

24. David G. Nathan, *The Cancer Treatment Revolution: How Smart Drugs and Other Therapies Are Renewing Our Hope and Changing the Face of Medicine*, New York: John Wiley, 2007; Brugarolas, J., Renal-cell Carcinoma—Molecular Pathways and Therapies, *New England Journal of Medicine* 2007; 356: 185–86. It has also been

suggested that clinical trials themselves should be considered "public health goods" and that this provides an alternative rationale for the Abigail Alliance decision. Leonard, E.W., The Public's Right to Health: When Patient Rights Threaten the Commons, *Washington University Law Review* 2009; 86: 1335–96.

25. Daniel Callahan, *False Hopes: Why America's Quest for Perfect Health Is a Recipe for Failure*, New York: Simon and Schuster, 1998.

26. Berenson, A., Hope, at $4,200 a Dose: Why a Cancer Drug's Cost Doesn't Hurt Demand, *New York Times*, October 1, 2006, BU1; Anand, G., From Wall Street, A Warning About Cancer Drug Prices, *Wall Street Journal*, March 15, 2007, A1; Abelson, R. and Pollack, A., Medicare Widens Drugs It Accepts for Cancer Care, *New York Times*, January 27, 2009. *See also* Pollack, supra note 2.

Chapter 8, Drug Dealing

1. Charles Neider, ed., *The Complete Short Stories of Mark Twain*, New York: Hanover House, 1957, 1–6. The first half of this chapter is adapted from Annas, G. J., Jumping Frogs, Endangered Toads, and California's Medical Marijuana Law, *New England Journal of Medicine* 2005; 353: 2291–96, and the second from Annas, G.J., Elephants in Mouseholes: Congress, Controlled Substances, and Physician-Assisted Suicide, *New England Journal of Medicine* 2006; 354: 1079–84.

2. 39th District Agricultural Association, *Animal Welfare Policy (Calaveras County Fair and Jumping Frog Jubilee)*, April 2003 (http://www.frogtown.org/).

3. *NLRB v. Jones & Laughlin Steel Corp.*, 301 U.S. 1 (1937).

4. *Wickard v. Filburn*, 317 U.S. 111 (1942).

5. *U.S. v. Lopez*, 514 U.S. 549 (1995).

6. *U.S. v. Morrison*, 529 U.S. 598 (2000).

7. *Gonzales v. Raich*, 545 U.S. 1 (2005).

8. *Raich v. Ashcroft*, 352 F.3d 1222 (9th Cir. 2003).

9. Annas, G.J., Glantz, L.H., and Mariner, W.K., The Right of Privacy Protects the Doctor–Patient Relationship, *JAMA* 1990; 263: 858–61.

10. Annas, G.J., Reefer Madness—The Federal Response to California's Medical-Marijuana Law, *New England Journal of Medicine* 1997; 337:435–39.

11. *GDF Realty v. Norton*, 326 F.3d 622 (5th Cir. 2003).

12. *Rancho Viejo v. Norton*, 323 F.3d 1062 (D.C. Cir. 2003); and *Rancho Viejo v. Norton*, 357 F.3d 1158 (D.C. Cir. 2003). On a request for a hearing by the entire appeals court, which was rejected, Chief Justice John Roberts—who at the time was a member of the appeals court—wrote a dissent that was not unlike Justice O'Connor's dissent in the California medical marijuana case. In it he argued that the court's conclusion seemed inconsistent with the guns-in-school and gender-violence cases, and that there were real problems with using an analysis of the Commerce Clause to regulate "the taking of a hapless toad that, for reasons of its own, lives its entire life in California." The case has since been settled. The development is going ahead in a way that protects the toad's habitat. Asked about his "hapless toad" opinion during the Senate confirmation hearings on his nomination to replace Rehnquist as chief justice, Roberts said: "The whole point of my argument in the dissent was that there was another way to look at this [i.e., the

approach taken by the Fifth Circuit Court in the Cave Species case] . . . . I did not say that even in this case that the decision was wrong . . . . I simply said, let's look at those other grounds for decision because that doesn't present this problem." Supreme Court nomination hearings provide an opportunity for all Americans to review their understanding of our constitutional government and the manner in which it allocates power between the federal government and the 50 states. To the extent that this division of power is determined by the Court's view of the Commerce Clause, a return to an expansive reading of this clause seems both likely and, given the interdependence of the national and global economies, proper.

13. Neider, supra note 1.

14. *Gonzales v. Oregon*, 546 U.S. 243 (2006).

15. *Washington v. Glucksberg*, 521 U.S. 702 (1997).

16. Oregon Death with Dignity Act. Ore. Rev. Stat. sec. 127.800 et seq. (2003).

17. *Dispensing of Controlled Substances to Assist Suicide*. Federal Register 2001; 66: 56607–08.

18. *Oregon v. Ashcroft*, 192 F.Supp. 2d 1077 (U.S. Dist. Ore. 2002).

19. *Oregon v. Ashcroft*, 368 F.3d 1118 (2004).

20. *U.S. v. Moore*, 423 U.S. 122 (1975).

21. In another 6-to-3 opinion, the Court arrived at the same conclusion in an analogous Commerce Clause case, *Wyeth v. Levine*, discussed in Chapter 12, Patient Safety.

22. *American Trucking Association v. Whitman*, 531 U.S. 457 (2001).

23. Samuel Richardson, *Clarissa: Or, the History of a Young Lady*, 1748.

24. Annas, G.J., Death by Prescription: The Oregon Initiative, *New England Journal of Medicine* 1994; 331: 1240–43.

25. Drug Enforcement Administration, *The Myth of the Chilling Effect*, available at www.justice.gov/dea/pubs/pressrel/pr103003.html (Oct. 30, 2003); *and see* Johnson, S.H., The Social, Professional, and Legal Framework for the Problem of Pain Management in Emergency Medicine, *Journal of Law, Medicine & Ethics* 2005; 33: 741–60.

26. Quill, T.E. and Meier, D.E., The Big Chill: Inserting the DEA into End-of-Life Care, *New England Journal of Medicine* 2006; 354: 1–3.

27. Joseph Fins, *A Palliative Ethics of Care*, Boston: Jones and Bartlett, 2006. *See also*, Kathleen Foley and Hellen Gelband, eds., *Improving Palliative Care for Cancer*, Washington, D.C.: National Academies Press, 2001.

Chapter 9, Toxic Tinkering

1. Michel Foucault, *Discipline and Punish: The Birth of the Prison*, Sheridan, A., trans., New York: Pantheon Books, 1977. This chapter is based on Annas, G.J., Toxic Tinkering: Lethal Injection Execution and the Constitution, *New England Journal of Medicine* 2008; 359: 1512–18.

2. Denno, D., When Legislatures Delegate Death: The Troubling Paradox Behind State Uses of Electrocution and Lethal Injection and What It Says About Us, *Ohio State Law Journal* 2002; 63: 63–99.

3. Curran, W. and Casscells, W., The Ethics of Medical Participation in Capital Punishment by Intravenous Drug Injection, *New England Journal of Medicine* 1980; 302: 226–30.

4. Robert Veatch, *A Theory of Medical Ethics*, New York: Basic Books, 1981: 293–305.

5. Truog, R.D. and Brennan, T.A., Participation of Physicians in Capital Punishment, *New England Journal of Medicine* 1993; 329: 1346–50; Gawande, A., When Law and Ethics Collide—Why Physicians Participate in Executions, *New England Journal of Medicine* 2006; 354: 1221–29.

6. *Baze v. Rees*, 128 S. Ct. 1520 (2008).

7. *Baze v. Rees*, 217 S.W.3d 207 (Ky. 2006).

8. Koniaris, L.G., Zimmers, T.A., Lubarsky, D.A., and Sheldon, J.P., Inadequate Anaesthesia in Lethal Injection for Execution, *Lancet* 2005; 365: 1412–14.

9. *Furman v. Georgia*, 408 U.S. 238 (1972).

10. Memorandum for Alberto R. Gonzales, counsel to the president: standards of conduct for interrogation under 18 U.S.C. sec. 2340-2340A, August 1, 2002 (in) Karen. J. Greenberg and Joshua L. Dratel, eds., *The Torture Papers: The Road to Abu Ghraib*, New York: Cambridge University Press, 2005, 172–217.

11. Gawande, A., Denno, D.W., Truog, R.D., and Waisel, D., Physicians and Execution—Highlights from a Discussion of Lethal Injection, *New England Journal of Medicine* 2008; 358: 448–451.

12. Id.

13. Waisel, D., Physician Participation in Capital Punishment, *Mayo Clinic Proceedings* 2007;82: 1073–82.

14. Caplan, A., Should Physicians Participate in Capital Punishment? *Mayo Clinic Proceedings* 2007; 82: 1047–48.

15. Gawande, supra note 5.

16. Annas, G.J., Unspeakably Cruel—Torture, Medical Ethics, and the Law, *New England Journal of Medicine* 2005; 352: 2127–32; Human Rights Watch, *So Long As They Die: Lethal Injections in the United States*, April 2006. (http://hrw.org/reports/2006/us0406). Gawande has also written the most powerful argument against one alternative to the death penalty often employed in the United States: confinement in a "supermax" prison, which usually means solitary confinement that Gawande persuasively labels as torture. Gawande, A., Hellhole, *New Yorker*, March 30, 2009, 36–45 ("In much the same way that a previous generation of Americans countenanced legalized segregation, ours has countenanced legalized torture. And there is no clearer manifestation of this than our routine use of solitary confinement—on our own people, in our own communities, in a supermax prison, for example, that is a thirty-minute drive from my door." at 44.)

17. Denno, D.W., The Lethal Injection Quandary: How Medicine Has Dismantled the Death Penalty, *Fordham Law Review* 2007; 76: 49–128.

18. Annas, G.J., Killing with Kindness: Why the FDA Need Not Certify Drugs Used for Execution Safe and Effective, *American Journal of the Public Health* 1985; 75: 1096–99.

19. *Heckler v. Chaney*, 470 U.S. 821 (1985).

20. Koniaris, L.G., Goodman, K.W., Sugarman, J., Ozomaro, U., Sheldon, J., and Zimmers, T.A., Ethical Implications of Modifying Lethal Injection Protocols, *PLoS Medicine* 2008; 5: e126-e126; Shah, S., How Lethal Injection Reform Constitutes Impermissible Research on Prisoners, *American Criminal Law Review* 2008; 45: 1101–46.

21. Liptak, A. and Ellick, A.B., Judge Orders Ohio to Alter Its Method of Execution, *New York Times*, June 11, 2008, A16. Ohio requires the prison warden to shake the condemned prisoner and call out to him after the anesthesia in injected to make sure he is unconscious. Its execution teams, however, have either had difficulty or been unable to start an IV. The execution of Romell Broom, for example, had to be rescheduled because even after multiple attempts the execution team failed to establish an IV line. Driehaus, B., Prisoner in Ohio Wins a Stay Against Second Attempt to Execute Him, *New York Times*, September 19, 2009, A9.

22. Davey, M., Missouri Officials Debate Executions Even as the State Prepares to Carry One Out, *New York Times*, May 19, 2009, A14; and Salter, J., Missouri Carries Out First Execution in 4 Years, Associated Press Release, May 20, 2009.

23. Curfman, G.D., Morrissey, S., and Drazen, J.M., Physicians and Execution, *New England Journal of Medicine* 2008; 358: 403–404.

24. Human Rights Watch, supra note 16.

25. Legraw, J.M. and Grodin, M.A., Health Professionals and Lethal Injection Execution in the United States, *Human Rights Quarterly* 2002; 24: 382–423; Groner, J. I., The Hippocratic Paradox: The Role of the Medical Profession in Capital Punishment in the United States, *Fordham Urban Law Journal* 2008; 35: 883–917.

26. *Callins v. Collins*, 510 U.S. 1141 (1994) (Blackmun J., dissenting).

Chapter 10, Abortion

1. *Gonzales v. Carhart*, 550 U.S. 124 (2007). This chapter is adapted from Annas, G.J., The Supreme Court and Abortion Rights, *New England Journal of Medicine* 2007; 356: 2201–07.

2. Annas, G.J., Partial-Birth Abortion, Congress and the Constitution, *New England Journal of Medicine* 1998; 339: 279–83; Remarks on Returning Without Approval to the House of Representatives Partial Birth Abortion Legislation, *Weekly Compilation of Presidential Documents*, April 10, 1996, 643–47.

3. *Stenberg v. Carhart*, 530 U.S. 914 (2000); Annas, G.J., 'Partial-Birth Abortion' and the Supreme Court, *New England Journal of Medicine* 2001; 344: 152–56.

4. Stevenson, R.W., Bush Signs Ban on a Procedure for Abortions, *New York Times*, November 6, 2003, A1.

5. Cummings, J. and Bravin, J., New Round: Choice of Alito for High Court Sets Stage for Ideological Battle, *Wall Street Journal*, November 1, 2004, A1.

6. Seelye. K.Q., A Partial-Victory Abortion Vote, *New York Times*, May 25, 1997, E5.

7. *Planned Parenthood of Southeastern Pennsylvania v. Casey*, 505 U.S. 833 (1992); Annas G.J., The Supreme Court, Liberty, and Abortion, *New England Journal of Medicine* 1992; 327: 651–54.

8. *Roe v. Wade*, 410 U.S. 113 (1973).

9. Greene, M.F. and Ecker, J.L., Abortion, Health, and the Law, *New England Journal of Medicine* 2004; 350:184–86; Drazen, J.M., Inserting Government Between Patient and Physician, *New England Journal of Medicine* 2004; 350: 178–79.

10. Garrow, D.J., Don't Assume the Worst, *New York Times*, April 21, 2007, A25.

11. *Jacobson v. Massachusetts*, 197 U.S. 11 (1905); Mariner W.K., Annas G.J., and Glantz, L.H., *Jacobson v Massachusetts*: It's Not Your Great-Great-Grandfather's Public Health Law, *American Journal of Public Health* 2005; 95: 581–90.

12. *Doe v. Bolton*, 410 U.S. 179 (1973).

13. Id.

14. Kassirer J.P., Practicing Medicine Without a License—The New Intrusions by Congress, *New England Journal of Medicine*, 1997; 336: 1747; Drazen, J.M., Government in Medicine, *New England Journal of Medicine* 2007; 356: 2195.

15. Gianelli D.M., House Affirms AMA Stance on Abortion, *American Medical News*, March 3, 1997, 3.

16. ACOG Statement on US Supreme Court Decision Upholding the Partial-Birth Abortion Ban Act of 2003, April 18, 2007.

Chapter II, Culture of Death

1. This chapter is adapted from Annas, G.J., 'Culture of Life' Politics at the Bedside: The Case of Terri Schiavo, *New England Journal of Medicine* 2005; 352: 1710–15, and "I Want to Live": Medicine Betrayed by Ideology in the Political Debate over Terri Schiavo, *Stetson Law Review* 2005; 35: 49–80.

2. The piece appeared in print in an issue of the *Journal* published on April 21: Annas, supra, note 1. Details of the case from the viewpoints of the family members involved can be found in their books, each published about a year after Terri died: Michael Schiavo, *Terri: the Truth*, New York: Dutton, 2006, and Mary and Robert Schindler, *A Life That Matters*, New York: Warner Books, 2006. The most balanced book on the case is probably Lois Shepherd's, *If That Ever Happens to Me: Making Life and Death Decisions after Terri Schiavo*, Chapel Hill: University of North Carolina Press, 2009.

3. The constitutional law on the right to refuse any medical treatment, including life-sustaining treatment, is based primarily on two landmark cases, both of which also dealt with young women in persistent vegetative states (more accurately termed "permanent vegetative states" after 12 months) like Terri Schiavo's. The first, the 1976 case of Karen Quinlan, made international headlines when her parents sought the assistance of a judge to have their daughter, who was in a persistent vegetative state, removed from a ventilator. *In re Quinlan*, 70 N.J. 10, 355 A.2d 647 (1976). The publicity surrounding the Quinlan case energized two independent developments: It encouraged states to adopt "living will" legislation and hospitals to establish "ethics committees" as forums to attempt to resolve similar treatment disputes without going to court. The second case is that of Nancy Cruzan, a young woman in a permanent vegetative state caused by an accident, essentially in identical physical circumstances to that of Karen Quinlan except that she was not on a ventilator but, like Terri Schiavo, only needed tube feeding to continue to live. The Missouri Supreme Court had ruled that the tube feeding could be discontinued

based on Nancy's right of self-determination, but that only Nancy herself should be able to make this decision. If others, including her parents, wanted to refuse on her behalf, they could only do so if they could demonstrate her wishes by "clear and convincing" evidence. *Cruzan v. Harmon*, 760 S.W.2d 408 (Mo. 1988). The Supreme Court, in a 5-to-4 decision, agreed, saying that the state of Missouri had the authority to adopt this high level of evidence because of the finality of a decision to terminate treatment. In the words of the Chief Justice, Missouri was entitled to "err on the side of life." (Judge Greer used this high "clear and convincing evidence" standard in finding that Terri Schiavo herself would refuse continued tube feeding if she were in a permanent vegetative state.) Six of the nine justices in *Cruzan* explicitly found that there was no legal distinction to be made between artificially delivered fluids and nutrition and other medical interventions, such as ventilator support, and none of the other three found a constitutionally relevant distinction. This issue is not controversial as a matter of constitutional law. Justice Sandra Day O'Connor recognized in a concurring opinion (her vote decided the case) that young people do not generally write down explicit treatment instructions. She suggested that had Nancy simply said something like, "if I'm not able to make medical treatment decisions myself, I want my mother to make them," this should be a constitutionally protected delegation of authority to decide her treatment. O'Connor's opinion is why the Cruzan case energized the health care proxy and durable power of attorney movement—encouraging people to use these documents to designate someone (usually called a healthcare agent, or simply an agent) to make decisions for them if they are not able to make them themselves. All states authorize this, and most states explicitly grant authority to a close relative, almost always the spouse first in line, if the patient has not personally made a designation. *Cruzan v. Director, Missouri Dept. of Health*, 497 U.S. 261 (1990). *See also* Allen, W., Erring too Far on the Side of Life: Deja vu All Over Again in the Schiavo Saga, *Stetson Law Review* 2005; 35: 123–45.

4. President's statement on Terri Schiavo, March 17, 2005. The president's interruption of his vacation to return to Washington to sign the legislation was not necessary (it could have been delivered to him for signature), but seems to have been done primarily to please his extreme right wing evangelical Christian base. Richard Cizik, vice president of the National Association of Evangelicals, said signing the bill in Crawford, Texas "would have been acceptable.... But this president seizes opportunities when they come his way. That's what makes him a good politician." Bumiller, E., *New York Times*, March 21, 2005, A15.

5. *Bush v. Schiavo*, 885 So.2d 321 (Fla. 2004).

6. Kirpatrick, D.D. and Stolberg, S.G., How Family's Cause Reached the Halls of Congress, *New York Times*, March 22, 2005, A1. In mid-2009, DeLay joined the "birthers," asking that President Obama produce his birth certificate to prove he was born in the United States (although on MSNBC he first said the president should produce a "gift certificate"), and shortly thereafter appeared on *Dancing with the Stars*.

7. Statement of Bill Frist on Senate floor, March 20, 2005, taken from his website.

8. Ruth, D., The Best Part? Sen. Mel's Term Is Just Starting. *Tampa Tribune*, April 11, 2005, 2; Gailey, P., The Senator Pleads Ignorance, *St. Petersburg Times*,

April 12, 2005. (Martinez has since said he did not know who wrote the memo at the time—his legal counsel Brian Darling—or that he had himself given it to Senator Tom Harkin).

9. The full text of the law is:

SECTION 1. RELIEF OF THE PARENTS OF THERESA MARIE SCHIAVO.

The United States District Court for the Middle District of Florida shall have jurisdiction to hear, determine, and render judgment on a suit by or on behalf of Theresa Marie Schiavo for the alleged violation of any right of Theresa Marie Schiavo under the Constitution or laws of the United States relating to the withholding or withdrawal of food, fluids, or medical treatment necessary to sustain her life.

SEC. 2. PROCEDURE.

Any parent of Theresa Marie Schiavo shall have standing to bring a suit under this Act. The suit may be brought against any other person who was a party to State court proceedings relating to the withholding or withdrawal of food, fluids, or medical treatment necessary to sustain the life of Theresa Marie Schiavo, or who may act pursuant to a State court order authorizing or directing the withholding or withdrawal of food, fluids, or medical treatment necessary to sustain her life. In such a suit, the District Court shall determine de novo any claim of a violation of any right of Theresa Marie Schiavo within the scope of this Act, notwithstanding any prior State court determination and regardless of whether such a claim has previously been raised, considered, or decided in State court proceedings, and regardless of whether remedies available in the State courts have been exhausted.

SEC. 3. RELIEF.

After a determination of the merits of a suit brought under this Act, the District Court shall issue such declaratory and injunctive relief as may be necessary to protect the rights of Theresa Marie Schiavo under the Constitution and laws of the United States relating to the withholding or withdrawal of food, fluids, or medical treatment necessary to sustain her life.

SEC. 4. TIME FOR FILING.

Notwithstanding any other time limitation, any suit or claim under this Act shall be timely if filed within 30 days after the enactment of this Act.

SEC. 5. NO CHANGE OF SUBSTANTIVE RIGHTS.

Nothing in this Act shall be construed to create substantive rights not otherwise secured by the Constitution and laws of the United States or of the several States.

SEC. 6. NO EFFECT ON ASSISTING SUICIDE.

Nothing in this Act shall be construed to confer additional jurisdiction on any court to consider any claim related

(1) to assisting suicide, or
(2) a State law regarding assisting suicide

SEC. 7. NO PRECEDENT FOR FUTURE LEGISLATION.
Nothing in this Act shall constitute a precedent with respect to future legislation, including the provision of private relief bills.

SEC. 8. NO EFFECT ON THE PATIENT SELF-DETERMINATION ACT OF 1990.
Nothing in this Act shall affect the rights of any person under the Patient Self-Determination Act of 1990.

SEC. 9. SENSE OF THE CONGRESS.
It is the Sense of Congress that the 109th Congress should consider policies regarding the status and legal rights of incapacitated individuals who are incapable of making decisions concerning the provision, withholding, or withdrawal of food, fluids, or medical care.

10. DeLay added during the brief floor debate, "I say again, the legal and political issues may be complicated, but the moral ones are not. A young woman in Florida is being dehydrated and starved to death. For 58 long hours, her mouth has been parched and her hunger pangs have been throbbing. If we do not act, she will die of thirst. However helpless, Mr. Speaker, she is alive. She is still one of us. And this cannot stand. Terri Schiavo survived her Passion weekend, and she has not been forsaken. No more words, Mr. Speaker. She is waiting. The Members are here. The hour has come." 151 *Congressional Record House* 1725, 109th Cong., 1st sess. (March 20, 2005). *See also* supra note 6.

11. Congressman James Sensenbrenner, who led the floor debate for the Republicans, echoed Frist's sentiments and added a distinctly religious tone in his opening remarks on the floor, "As millions of Americans observe the beginning of Holy Week this Palm Sunday, we are reminded that every life has purpose, none is without meaning. The battle to defend the preciousness of every life in a culture that respects and defends life is not only Terri's fight, but it is America's fight." 151 *Congressional Record House* 1700 (2005).

12. 151 *Congressional Record House* 1714 (2005). (Gingrey also said, "Florida law prohibits the starvation of dogs, yet will allow the starvation of Terri Schiavo.... Although I am not a neurologist, my basic courses in medical school taught me that dehydration is a horrific process.")

13. 115 *Congressional Record House* 1715 (2005). (Weldon also questioned Michael's veracity based on his medical experience, "My clinical experience has always been that the family immediately brings that up [the patient's stated wishes regarding life-sustaining treatment]. They do not wait seven years.")

14. 115 *Congressional Record House* 1716 (2005). (Price, to his credit, did not try to make a diagnosis, instead he said he prayed about the case: "As I sat in church this morning, I struggled with this and I prayed. I prayed for a lowering of the rhetoric. I prayed for a decrease in the emotion.")

15. Id. at 1717.

16. Id. at 1727.

17. Id. at 1718.

18. Id. at 1712. (Congressman Barney Frank continued, "The point is this: The gentleman [Congressman Sensenbrenner] is making specific medical arguments. He has said, in strong criticism of the entire judicial system of the state of Florida, that they did not give her a fair chance; that the entire judicial system, all of those appeals, all of those trials, all of that litigation, did not give her a fair chance and we will now vacate the judgment of Florida. And why? Not because any of us know one thing or another, but *because many Members here genuinely have a strong ideological interest*, and that is precisely why this ought to be a judicial decision and not a legislative decision (emphasis added)." Congressman Frank was their leader, but other Members of Congress who were especially eloquent in opposing the measure included Ginny Brown-Waite, John Conyers, Michael Capuano, and Debbie Wasserman Schultz.)

19. *Schiavo ex rel. Schindler v. Schiavo*, 358 F. Supp 2d 1161 (D.C. Fla. 2005). Whittemore's opinion incensed the right to life and religious communities. Burke J. Balch of the National Right to Life Committee, for example, said "Judge Whittemore has engaged in a gross abuse of judicial power." Rev. Jerry Falwell said, "Just because there is a judge somewhere in the world who would give an estranged husband like that the time of day tells you how bad the court system is." And Richard Viguerie, a conservative group direct mail advisor said, "It could be the opening shot in the Supreme Court nomination battle that we expect sooner rather than later." Quoted in Hulse, C. and Kirkpatrick, D., Casting Angry Eye on Courts, Conservative Prime for Bench-Clearing Brawl in Congress, *New York Times*, March 23, 2005, A15.

20. *See also* Kennicott, P., Symbol of Emptiness: Terri Schiavo Was a Woman, Not an Idea, *Washington Post*, April 1, 2005, C1. ("Schiavo couldn't speak for herself, and she was hidden from view, in a hospice. This silence, this absence, made her an attractive figure for people [who wanted to use her as a symbol of their cause] to speak for her . . . the creators of Terri went further. She began saying more than it was quite possible to believe . . . she even tried to say 'I want to live,' according to family members . . . . To believe in this Terri required more and more disbelief in medical science.") *See also Wall Street Journal* editorial on Schiavo entitled "I Want to Live," March 25, 2005, W 11.

21. *See, e.g.*, www.faithandaction.org.

22. Id.

23. Bell, M., Sophisticated Tactics Aid Schiavo's Parents, *Orlando Sentinel*, March 13, 2005, A1.

24. Danforth, J., In the Name of Politics, *New York Times*, March 30, 2005, A27. Danforth could have noted that Republicans have not been consistent in their anti–state interference with personal decision since they adopted the anti-abortion agenda of the right to life movement and its attempt to make abortion a crime.

25. *Report of Autopsy on Theresa Schiavo*, Date of Death, March 31, 2005, Jon R. Thogmartin, MD, Chief Medical Examiner, District Six, Pasco & Pinellas Counties, Largo, Florida, June 13, 2005. *See also*, Wijdicks, E. and Cranford, R., The Clinical Diagnosis of Prolonged States of Impaired Consciousness in Adults, *Mayo Clinic Proceedings* 2005; 80: 1037–46.

26. Oral comments, at "Schiavo Revisited: An Inside Look at the Case the Shook the Nation," June 10, 2005, D.C. Bar Association, Washington, D.C.

27. Goodnough, A., Gov. Bush Seeks Another Inquiry in Schiavo Case, *New York Times*, June 18, 2005, A1 (focusing on a possible inconsistency between the time Michael remembered calling 911 and the time the call was actually placed, Gov. Bush said, "It's a significant question that during this entire ordeal was never brought up." Michael responded immediately saying the Governor's actions were "sickening" and said he had called 911 promptly.)

28. Herbert, B., Cruel and Unusual, *New York Times*, June 23, 2005, A19. (Bernie McCabe, the state attorney for Pinellas County that Gov. Bush asked to start an investigation, told Herbert he had no indication that a crime had been committed and was conducting what he called an inquiry, rather than an investigation, only because the governor had requested it, "My purpose is simply to respond to the governor. The governor asked me to do something, and I'm going to do it.")

29. Statement of William M. Hammesfahr, Christian Communication Network posted on earnedmedia.org. A declaration of Hammesfahr was also read into the Congressional Record during the debate on the Schiavo bill. In it he declared under oath: "As a patient, Terri Schiavo is not in that bad of a condition to begin with. We treat many patients who are a lot worse. There are a lot of therapies out there that will very likely improve her condition, and they all complement each other, so if you do them all in a series, she could get a lot better. Without a doubt, I observed Terri swallow . . . ." 151 *Congressional Record House* 1712 (March 20, 2005).

30. Posted on the White House website, www.whitehouse.gov, June 15, 2005 press briefing.

31. Stewart, J., *The Daily Show*, Comedy Central, June 17, 2005.

32. Hook, J., Frist Plagued Again by Comments on Schiavo, *Los Angeles Times*, June 17, 2005.

33. Brooks, D., What Makes Bill Frist Run?, *New York Times*, June 19, 2005, WK12. Frist would like to forget the whole incident, telling the *Wall Street Journal*, "Knowing what I know now I would have done things differently, but at the time, I think I probably made the right decisions . . . I think it's left a negative aura everywhere." Rogers, D., Still an Enigma, Bill Frist Reflects a Complex Past, *Wall Street Journal*, June 27, 2005, A1.

34. Cranford, R., Facts, Lies and Videotapes: The Permanent Vegetative State and the Sad Case of Terri Schiavo, *Journal of Law, Medicine & Ethics* 2005; 33:363-78. Some nonphysician observers were, however, impressed with Cheshire. *See, e.g.*, Didion, J., The Case of Theresa Schiavo, *New York Review of Books*, June 9, 2005, 60. Cranford died on May 31, 2006, just two months after he participated in a conference on the Schiavo case at Boston University along with Congressman Barney Frank, Judge George Greer, and me.

As an expert witness in a series of the most important right-to-die cases in the United States, Ron not only strove to provide the judges with solid medical information in an understandable manner, but also to provide support for the families as an adviser to them. He was outstanding in both of these roles. For more on Ron *see* Annas, G.J., Foreword: Imagining a New Era of Neuroimaging, Neuroethics, and Neurolaw, *American Journal of Law & Medicine* 2007; 33: 163–70. Ron's presentation at the March 2006 conference is on the Boston University School of Law's website.

35. Quotes of Note, *Boston Globe*, March 26, 2005, Al.

36. George J. Annas, *American Bioethics: Crossing Human Rights and Health Law Boundaries*, New York: Oxford University Press, 2005.

37. Annas, G.J. and Elias, S., Politics, Morals and Embryos: Can Bioethics in the United States Rise Above Politics?, *Nature* 2004: 431: 19–20. *See also* Moreno, J., The End of the Great Bioethics Compromise, *Hastings Center Report*, Jan. 2005, 14; and Caplan, A., 'Who Lost China?' A Foreshadowing of Today's Ideological Disputes in Bioethics, *Hastings Center Report*, May/June 2005, 12.

38. Leon Kass, *Toward a More Natural Science*, New York: Free Press, 1985, 203.

39. Id. at 206.

40. Id. at 204.

41. Caplan was well positioned to be the unofficial spokesperson for the bioethics community not only because he has the ability to engage in sound-bite debate better than any other bioethicist in the United States, but also because his own career as a public bioethicist began when the Hastings Center started getting press inquiries about the case of Karen Ann Quinlan in 1976; because most of the bioethics staff there was away at a conference, he wound up taking the calls and hasn't looked back.

42. For example, an April 1–2 CNN/*USA Today* poll found 76% of American disapproved of congressional involvement in the Schiavo case, and only 20% approved. An earlier, March 21–22 poll by CBS News found 82% of Americans saying "Congress and the President should stay out of deciding what happens to Terri Schiavo," and only 13% thinking they should be involved. Likewise, a *Time* poll taken March 22–24 found 75% of Americans saying it was "not right" for Congress to intervene in the Schiavo case, and 20% thinking it was right.

43. An ABC News poll taken March 20 showed that the public, by a 63% to 28% margin supported the removal of the feeding tube. Similar, but closer margins were found on other polls. The *Time* poll of March 22–24 found 59% agreed with the decision to remove the feeding tube, and 35% disagreed. The CNN/*USA Today* poll of April 1–2 found the margin closer, 52% agreeing with the decision to remove the tube and 42% opposed.

44. Rosen, J., Center Court, *New York Times Magazine*, June 12, 2005, 17. *See also* Toobin, J., Bench Press: Are Obama's Judges Really Liberals?, *New Yorker*, September 21, 2009, 42–49 ("This is the paradox of the judiciary—unelected judges must protect democracy. Obama's belief that judges reflect the prevailing political environment raises a paradox of its own. He is launching his nominees into an atmosphere that is so poisoned that scarcely anyone can get confirmed.")

45. For more on slogans in this context *see* Annas, G.J., The 'Right to Die' in America: Sloganeering from Quinlan and Cruzan to Quill and Kevorkian, *Duquesne Law Review* 1996; 34: 875–97.

Chapter 12, Patient Safety

1. This chapter is adapted from Annas, G.J., The Patient's Right to Safety: Improving the Quality of Care through Litigation against Hospitals, *New England Journal of Medicine* 2006; 354: 2063–66; and Annas, G.J., Tragic Facts Make Good

Law: Congress, the FDA, and Drug Regulation Preemption, *New England Journal of Medicine* 2009; 361: 1206–11.

2. Consumers Union Safe Patient Project, *To Err Is Human—To Delay Is Deadly: Ten Years Later, A Million Lives Lost, Billions of Dollars Wasted*, New York: Consumers Union, 2009. This conclusion is also supported by the 2009 annual report of the US Agency for Healthcare Research and Quality. *See* Kuehn, B., AHRQ: US Quality of Care Falls Short: Patient Safety Declining, Disparities Persist, *JAMA* 2009; 301: 2427–28 ("This report documents that 1 in 7 Medicare patients experienced a medical adverse event in 2005 and 2006 and that overall measures of patient safety declined by nearly 1% in each of the past 6 years."), The Institute of Medicine report is, Committee on Quality of Health Care in America, *To Err Is Human: Building a Safer Health System*, Washington, D.C.: National Academies Press, 1999.

3. Pronovost, P.J. and Colantuoni, E., Measuring Preventable Harm: Helping Science Keep Pace with Policy, *JAMA* 2009; 301: 1273–75; Altman, D. E., Clancy, C., and Blendon, R.J., Improving Patient Safety: Five Years After the IOM Report, *New England Journal of Medicine* 2004; 351: 2041–43; Romano, P.S., Improving the Quality of Hospital Care in America, *New England Journal of Medicine* 2005; 353: 302–304.

4. Annas, G.J., Reframing the Debate on Health Care Reform by Replacing Our Metaphors, *New England Journal of Medicine* 1995; 332: 744–47.

5. J.M. Morath and Joanne E. Turnbull, *To Do No Harm: Ensuring Patient Safety in Health Care Organizations*, San Francisco: Jossey-Bass, 2005.

6. James Reason, *Human Error*, New York: Cambridge University Press, 1990.

7. Leape, L.L. and Berwick, D.M., Five Years After 'To Err Is Human': What Have We Learned? *JAMA* 2005; 293: 2384–90.

8. George J. Annas, *The Rights of Patients*, 3rd ed., New York: NYU Press, 2004.

9. *T.J. Hooper*, 60 F.2d 737 (2d Cir. 1932).

10. *Darling v. Charlestown Community Memorial Hospital*, 33 Ill. 2d 326, 211 N. E.2d 253 (1965).

11. *Clark v. St. Dominic-Jackson Memorial Hospital*, 660 So.2d 970 (Miss. 1995).

12. *Thompson v. Nason Hospital*, 527 Pa. 330, 591 A.2d 703 (1991).

13. Hand Hygiene Task Force, Guidelines for Hand Hygiene in Health Care Settings, *Morbidity and Mortality Weekly Report* 2002; 51:1; Gawande, A., On Washing Hands, *New England Journal of Medicine* 2004; 350: 1284–86.

14. Berwick, D.M., Calkins D.R., McCannon C.J., and Hachbarth, A.D., The 100,000 Lives Campaign: Setting a Goal and a Deadline for Improving Health Care Quality, *JAMA* 2006; 295: 324–27.

15. Hyman, D.A. and Silver, C., The Poor State of Health Care Quality in the U.S.: Is Malpractice Liability Part of the Problem or Part of the Solution?, *Cornell Law Review* 2005; 90: 893–992. Consumers Union came to a similar conclusion in their 2009 report, saying simply: "Doctors and hospitals raise concerns that public reporting of medical harm will lead to frivolous lawsuits. But the best way to prevent claims is to put systems in place to prevent harm. Experience with public reporting in the states demonstrates that the tort concerns about such disclosures is overstated." Consumers Union, supra note 2, at 1.

16. Schoen, C., Osborn, R., Huynh, P.T., et al., Taking the Pulse of Health Care Systems: Experiences of Patients with Health Problems in Six Countries, *Health Affairs* 2005; W5: 509–13.

17. Mariner, W.K. and Miller, F., *Medical Error Reporting: Professional Tensions Between Confidentiality and Liability: Issue Brief 13*, Boston: Massachusetts Health Policy Forum, 2001.

18. Patient Safety and Quality Improvement Act of 2005, P.L. 109-41.

19. Sage, W.M., Medical Liability and Patient Safety, *Health Affairs* 2003; 22: 26–36.

20. Wachter, R.M., The End of the Beginning: Patient Safety Five Years After "To Err is Human," *Health Affairs* 2004; 23: W4-534–44.

21. Board of Registration in Medicine, Commonwealth of Massachusetts, *Medical Malpractice Analysis*, Boston, 2004.

22. Bludetti, P.P., Tort Reform and the Patient Safety Movement: Seeking Common Ground, *JAMA* 2005; 293: 2660–62.

23. Mello, M.M. and Brennan, T.A., Legal Concerns and the Influenza Vaccine Shortage, *JAMA* 2005; 294: 1817–20.

24. Hallinan, J.T., Once Seen as Risky, One Group of Doctors Changes Its Ways, *Wall Street Journal*, June 21, 2005, A1.

25. Supra note 22. *See also* Wachter, R.M. and Pronovost, P.J., Balancing "No Blame" with Accountability in Patient Safety, *New England Journal of Medicine* 2009; 361: 1401–06.

26. Berwick, D., What 'Patient-Centered' Should Mean: Confessions of an Extremist, *Health Affairs*, May 19, 2006, w555–565. *See also*, Donald M. Berwick, *Escape Fire: Designs for the Future of Health Care*, San Francisco: Jossey-Bass, 2004.

27. Weinstein, R.A., Siegel, J.D., and Brennan, P.J., Infection-control Report Cards—Securing Patient Safety, *New England Journal of Medicine* 2005; 353: 225–27.

28. Editorial, A Win for Injured Patients, *New York Times*, March 5, 2009.

29. Editorial, Pre-empting Drug Innovation, *Wall Street Journal*, March 5, 2009, A16.

30. Rosen, J., Supreme Court, Inc., *New York Times Magazine*, March 16, 2008.

31. *Wyeth v. Levine*, 129 S.Ct. 1187 (2009) .

32. Curfman, G.D., Morrissey, S., and Drazen, J.M., Why Doctors Should Worry about Preemption, *New England Journal of Medicine* 2008; 359: 1–3.

33. *Northern Securities v. U.S.*, 193 U.S. 197, 400 (1904).

34. Kennedy, D., Misbegotten Preemptions, *Science* 2008; 320: 585; Editorial, Warning Signs, *Nature* 2008; 452: 254.

35. Committee on the Assessment of the U.S. Drug-Safety System, *The Future of Drug Safety: Promoting and Protecting the Health of the Public*, Washington, DC: National Academies Press, 2006; Psaty, B.M. and Burke, S.P., Protecting the Health of the Public—Institute of Medicine Recommendations on Drug Safety, *New England Journal of Medicine* 2006; 355: 1753–55. *See also* Gilhooley, M., Drug Preemption and the Need to Reform the FDA Consultation Process, *American Journal of Law & Medicine* 2008; 34: 539–61.

36. *Wyeth v. Levine*, 944 A.2d 179 (Vt. 2006).

37. Glantz, L.H. and Annas, G.J., The FDA, Preemption, and the Supreme Court, *New England Journal of Medicine* 2008; 358: 1883–85.

38. *Riegel v. Medtronic*, 128S.Ct. 999 (2008).

39. 71 *Federal Register* 3922 (2006).

40. *Geier v. American Honda Motor Co.*, 529 U.S. 861 (2000).

41. Curfman, G.D., Morrissey, S., and Drazen, J.M., The Medical Device Safety Act of 2009, *New England Journal of Medicine* 2009; 360: 1550.

42. Memorandum for the Heads of Executive Departments and Agencies on Preemption, May 20, 2009, available on White House website. In September 2009, the FDA changed Phenergan's label to require a stronger warning. Harris, G., FDA to Require Strict Warning on Anti-Nausea Drug, *New York Times*, September 19, 2009, B6.

Chapter 13, Global Health

1. Harold Koh, Oral Presentation ("Father Drinan's Revolution") at the announcement of the Robert F. Drinan, S.J., Chair in Human Rights, Georgetown University Law Center, October 23, 2006. An early version of this chapter, "Global Health and Post-9/11 Human Rights," was prepared for a May 2007, Workshop on "Values and Moral Experience in Global Health: Bridging the Local and the Global," held at Harvard University.

2. Annas, G.J., Human Rights Outlaws: Nuremberg, Geneva, and the Global War on Terror, *Boston University Law Review* 2007; 87: 427–66, and Chapters 4 and 5 in this book.

3. Benatar, S.R. and Fox, R.C., Meeting Threats to Global Health: A Call for American Leadership, *Perspectives in Biology and Medicine* 2005; 48: 344–61.

4. *See generally*, Jonathan Mann, Sofia Gruskin, Michael Grodin, and George Annas, eds., *Health and Human Rights: A Reader*, New York: Routledge, 1999; Sofia Gruskin, Michael Grodin, George Annas, and Stephen Marks, eds. *Perspectives on Health and Human Rights*, New York: Routledge, 2005; and Mann, J., Health and Human Rights, *Lancet* 1996; 312: 924–25.

5. Farmer, P. and Gastineau, N., Rethinking Health and Human Rights: Time for a Paradigm Shift, *Journal of Law, Medicine & Ethics* 2002; 30: 655–66.

6. Gruskin, S. and Tarantola, D., Health and Human Rights (in) Sofia Gruskin et al., supra note 4 at 3–57.

7. Gruskin, S., What Are Health and Human Rights?, *Lancet* 2004; 363: 329.

8. Annas, G.J., The Rich Have More Money, *Health and Human Rights* 1998; 5: 180–85.

9. Sudhir Anand, Fabienne Peter, and Amartya Sen, eds., *Public Health, Ethics, and Equity*, Oxford: Oxford University Press, 2004. *See also*, Angus Dawson and Marcel Verweij, eds., *Ethics, Prevention, and Public Health*, Oxford: Oxford University Press, 2007; and Ronald Bayer, Lawrence O. Gostin, Bruce Jennings, and Bonnie Steinbock, eds., *Public Health Ethics: Theory, Policy, and Practice*, New York: Oxford University Press, 2007.

10. Madison Powers and Ruth Faden, *Social Justice: The Moral Foundations of Public Health and Health Policy*, New York: Oxford University Press, 2006.

11. Ruger, J.P., Ethics and Governance of Global Health Inequalities, *Journal of Epidemiology and Community Health* 2006; 60: 998–1003.

12. Ruger, J.P., Toward a Theory of a Right to Health: Capability and Incompletely Theorized Agreements, *Yale Journal of Law & the Humanities* 2006; 18: 273–326. On the "right to health" *see* General Comment No. 14: The Right to the Highest Attainable Standard of Health (Article 12 of the International Covenant on Economic Social and Cultural Rights; July 4, 2000) reprinted in Sofia Gruskin et al., supra note 4 at 473–95,; Judith Asher, *The Right to Health: A Resource Manual for NGOs*, London: British Medical Association, 2004; Backman, G., Hunt, P., Khorla, R. et al, Health Systems and the Right to Health: An Assessment of 194 Countries, *Lancet* 2008; 372: 2047–85; Andrew Clapham and Mary Robinson, eds., *Realizing the Right to Health*, Zurich: Ruffer & Rub, 2009.

13. *Compare* Louis Henkin, *The Age of Rights*, New York: Columbia University Press, 1990.

14. Kennedy, D., The International Human Rights Movement: Part of the Problem?, *Harvard Human Rights Journal* 2002; 15: 101–40.

15. Kunz, J., The United Nations Declaration of Human Rights, *American Journal of International Law* 1949; 43: 316–22. For a persuasive argument that the rights set forth in the UDHR are inherent in human beings as humans *see* Johannes Morsink, *Inherent Human Rights: Philosophical Roots of the Universal Declaration*, Philadelphia: University of Pennsylvania Press, 2009.

16. Glickman, S.W., McHutchison, J.G., Peterson, E.D., et al., Ethical and Scientific Implications of the Globalization of Clinical Research, *New England Journal of Medicine* 2009; 360: 816–23. This section, on the Pfizer litigation, is based on Annas, G.J., Globalized Clinical Trails and Informed Consent, *New England Journal of Medicine* 2009; 360: 2050–53.

17. Angell, M., The Ethics of Clinical Research in the Third World, *New England Journal of Medicine* 1997; 337: 847–49. *See generally*, Adriana Pertryna, *When Experiments Travel: Clinical Trials and the Global Search for Human Subjects*, Princeton: Princeton University Press, 2009.

18. Kimmelman, J., Weijer, C., and Meslin, E.M., Helsinki Discords: FDA, Ethics, and International Drug Trials, *Lancet* 2009; 373: 13–14.

19. Stephens, J., Where Profits and Lives Hang in the Balance; Finding an Abundance of Subjects and Lack of Oversight Abroad, Big Drug Companies Test Offshore to Speed Products to Market, *Washington Post*, December 17, 2000, A1.

20. *Abdullahi v. Pfizer*, 562 F.3d 163 (2d Cir. 2009).

21. *Filartiga v. Pena-Irala*, 630 F.2d 876 (2d Cir. 1980).

22. *Sosa v. Alvarez-Machain*, 542 U.S. 466 (2004).

23. *See, e.g.*, Roberts, L., Polio: Looking for a Little Luck, *Science* 2009; 323: 702–705.

24. Powers and Faden, supra note 10.

25. Physicians for Human Rights, *The Taliban's War on Women: A Health and Human Rights Crisis in Afghanistan*. Boston: Physicians for Human Rights 1998. *See also*, Audrey Chapman and Leonard Rubenstein, eds., *Human Rights and Health: The Legacy of Apartheid*, New York: American Association for the Advancement of Science, 1998.

26. *See* the Commission's website for this and other reports, www.aihrc.org. af. *See also* Samar, S., Despite the Odds: Providing Reproductive Health Care to Afghan Women, *New England Journal of Medicine* 2004; 351: 1047–49.

27. Cook, R., Gender, Health and Human Rights. *Health and Human Rights* 1995; 1: 350–66.

28. George J. Annas, *American Bioethics: Crossing Human Rights and Health Law Boundaries*. New York: Oxford University Press, 2005, 159–66.

29. Irene Khan summarized the situation regarding transnational corporations and human rights well in her foreword to Amnesty International's 2007 Annual Report, which she titled "Freedom from Fear": "Corporations have long resisted binding international standards. The United Nations must confront the challenge, and develop standards and promote mechanisms that hold big business accountable for its impact on human rights. The need for global standards and effective accountability becomes even more urgent as multinational corporations from diverse legal and cultural systems emerge in a global market." (at 4).

30. United Nations, Human Rights Council (4th sess. It. 2), *Business and Human Rights: Mapping International Standards of Responsibility and Accountability for Corporate Acts*, Feb. 19, 2007. For a more skeptical view *see*, Adriana Petryna, Andrew Lakoff, and Arthur Kleinman, eds., *Global Pharmaceuticals: Ethics, Markets, Practices*, Durham: Duke University Press, 2006.

31. Don DeLillo,*Underworld*, New York: Scribner, 1997, 788.

32. For an account of MSF's campaign to lower drug prices for the resource poor world *see* James Orbinski, *An Imperfect Offering: Humanitarian Action for the Twenty-First Century*, New York: Walker & Company, 2008, 351–79.

33. Joseph O'Neill, *Netherland*, New York: Pantheon Books, 2008, 211.

34. Blair, T., A Battle for Global Values, *Foreign Affairs* 2007, 79–90. It is worth noting that Telford Taylor used similar language describing the Nazi atrocities in his opening statement at the Doctors' Trial at Nuremburg: "The perverse thoughts and distorted concepts which brought about these savageries are not dead. They cannot be killed by force of arms. They must not become a spreading cancer in the breast of humanity. They must be cut out and exposed . . . ."

Chapter 14, Statue of Security

1. Portions of this chapter are adapted from Annas, G.J., Blinded by Bioterrorism: Public Health and Liberty in the 21st Century, *Health Matrix* 2003; 13: 33–70; and Annas, G.J., Puppy Love: Bioterrorism, Civil Rights and Public Health, *Florida Law Review* 2003; 55: 1171–90.

2. *See generally* Jonathan M. Mann, Sofia Gruskin, Michael Grodin, and George J. Annas, eds., *Health and Human Rights: A Reader*, New York: Routledge, 1999, 7–20.

3. Gostin, L.O., When Terrorism Threatens Health: How Far Are Limitations on Personal and Economic Liberties Justified?, *Florida Law Review* 2003; 55: 1105–69.

4. *Smallpox Vaccination Plan*: Hearing Before the Senate Appropriations Committee, Subcommittee on Labor, Health & Human Services, and Education, 108th Congress, 2nd Session (January 29, 2003) (statement of Julie L. Gerberding,

Director, Centers for Disease Control and Prevention); *see also* Enserink, M., and Kaiser, J., Has Biodefense Gone Overboard?, *Science* 2005; 307: 1396.

5. Smith, S., Anthrax vs. the Flu: As State Governments Slash Their Public Health Budgets, Federal Money Is Pouring in for Bioterror Preparedness, *Boston Globe*, July 29, 2003, C1.

6. McClain, W., Pulitzer-winning Cartoonist Draws from "Anti-Stupid" Angle, *The Daily Cardinal* (University of Wisconsin-Madison), October 28, 2004, 1.

7. Cohen, H.W., et al., The Pitfalls of Bioterrorism Preparedness: The Anthrax and Smallpox Experiences, *American Journal of Public Health* 2004; 94: 1667.

8. Florida Health Emergency Act, Fla. Stat. Ann. § 381.00315 (West 2004).

9. Id.§ 381.00315(1)(b). " 'Public health emergency' means any occurrence, or threat thereof, whether natural or man made, which results or may result in substantial injury or harm to the public health from infectious disease, chemical agents, nuclear agents, biological toxins, or situations involving mass casualties or natural disasters."

10. *See* Emergency Powers, Minn. Stat. Ann. § 12.39 (West 2005).

11. The original medical examination and treatment sections of the model act contained the following provisions:

> *Section 502*: Any person refusing to submit to the medical examination and/or testing is liable for a misdemeanor. If the public health authority is uncertain whether a person who refuses to undergo medical examination and/or testing may have been exposed to an infections disease or otherwise poses a danger to public health, the public health authority may subject the individual to isolation or quarantine. . . . Any [healthcare provider] refusing to perform a medical examination or test authorized herein shall be liable for a misdemeanor. . . . An order of the public health authority given to effectuate the purposes of this subsection shall be immediately enforceable by any peace officer.

> *Section 504*: Individuals refusing to be vaccinated or treated shall be liable for a misdemeanor. If by reason of refusal of vaccination or treatment, the person poses a danger to the public health, he or she may be subject to isolation or quarantine . . . . An order of the public health authority given to effectuate the purposes of this section shall be immediately enforceable by any peace officer.

Quoted in Annas, G.J., Bioterrorism, Public Health, and Civil Liberties, *New England Journal of Medicine* 2002; 346: 1337–41. On the genesis of the "model act" *see* David Rosner and Gerald Markowitz, *Are We Ready?: Public Health Since 9/11*, University of California Press: Berkeley, 2006, 138–39.

12. Memorandum from John Auerbach, Commissioner of Public Health on *False Rumors Regarding Mandatory Vaccination for H1N1 Influenza*, September 2, 2009. The memo also included the following sentence in bold letters and italics: "Mandatory vaccination is not and has never been part of the plan or discussion in Massachusetts' pandemic response." The memo concluded, "For up-to-date, accurate information about H1N1 and the Commonwealth's response, go to our webpage at http://www.mass.gov/dph/swineflu or contact us at (617) 624–5200. New York state was the only jurisdiction to attempt to mandate flu vaccination for

anyone in the fall of 2009–and the Governor instructed the state health commissioner to withdraw the requirement in late October, 2009. It had drawn extensive criticism from healthcare professionals. McNeil, D.G. and Zraick, K., New York Health Care Workers Resist Flu Vaccine Rule, *New York Times*, September 21, 2009, A17. As is almost always the case, the public health problem was not gaining more power to coerce people into getting treatment, but how to supply treatment to those who wanted it. Stolberg, S.G., Vaccine Shortage is Political Test for White House, *New York Times*, October 29, 2009, Al.

13. *See* Fink, S., The Deadly Choices at Memorial, *New York Times Magazine*, August 30, 2009, 28–46. *See also* Cyril Wecht, *A Question of Murder*, Amherst, NY: Prometheus Books, 2008, 243–310.

Chapter 15, Pandemic Fear

1. Portions of this chapter are adapted from Annas, G.J., The Statue of Security: Human Rights and Post-9/11 Epidemics, *Journal of Health Law* 2005; 38: 319–51. The McConnell quotations are taken from McConnell, J., Influenza Begs Many Questions, *Lancet* 2009; 373: 1590.

2. John M. Barry, *The Great Influenza: The Epic Story of the Deadliest Plague in History*, New York: Viking, 2004. His very reasonable updated thinking is summarized in Barry, J.M., Pandemics: Avoiding the Mistakes of 1918, *Nature*, 2009; 459: 324–25.

3. Annas, G.J., Bush's Risky Flu Pandemic Plan, *Boston Globe*, Oct. 8, 2005. *See generally*, Marc Siegel, *False Alarm: The Truth About the Epidemic of Fear*, New York: John Wiley, 2005, and Philip Alcabes, *Dread: How Fear and Fantasy Have Fueled Epidemics from the Black Death to Avian Flu*, New York: Public Affairs, 2009. *See also* on H1N1, President's Council of Advisors on Science and Technology, *Report to the President on U.S. Preparations for 2009-H1N1 Influenza*, August 7, 2009 (discussing a "plausible scenario" for H1N1 in the United States that could infect 30 to 50% of the population, lead to 1.8 million hospitalizations, and cause 30,000 to 90,000 deaths).

4. Andrew J. Bacevich, *The Limits of Power: The End of American Exceptionalism*, New York: Metropolitan Books, 2008.

5. *See, e.g.*, Shane, S. and Stetler, B., Coast Guard Drill, Misunderstook, Sets Off 9/11 Scare, *New York Times*, September 12, 2009, A8; Milbank, D., For Coast Guard and CNN, an Exercise in Embarrassment, *Washington Post*, September 12, 2009 ("Here's some advice: Don't pretend to shoot terrorists near the Pentagon on Sept. 11 with the president nearby.")

6. Chang, L. and Wonacott, P., SARS Measures in China Add to Air of Panic, *Wall Street Journal*, April 25, 2003, B7; Hutzler, C., China Reverts to Top-Down Rule with Heavy Hand to Fight SARS, *Wall Street Journal*, May 8, 2003, A8; *See* Rothstein, M., et al., *Quarantine and Isolation: Lessons Learned from SARS* (A Report to the Centers for Disease Control and Prevention, 2003) available at http://archive.naccho.org/documents/Quarantine-Isolation-Lessons-Learned-from-SARS.pdf.

7. Id.

8. Pottinger, M., et al., Quarantine Quandary, *Wall Street Journal*, April 1, 2003, B1; Eckholm, E., Thousands Riot in Rural Chinese Town over SARS, *New York Times*, April 28, 2003, A1.

9. Altman, L.K., Fearing SARS, Ontario Urges Wider Quarantines, *New York Times*, April 18, 2003, Al.

10. "Bed Chains" for Canada SARS Violators, *BBC News*, June 1, 2003.

11. Cohn, M.R., Nations Must Stay on SARS Alert: WHO, *Hamilton Spectator* (Ontario, Canada), June 18, 2003, D1.

12. Personal communication, July 16, 2003. *See also* Gully, P., National Response to (SARS): Canada, Presentation to WHO Global Meeting, July 17, 2003.

13. Guidelines previously posted on the CDC website.

14. Boston Public Health Commission, Factsheet, SARS – Colleges and Universities, 2003. *See also*, Smith, S., US allows for SARS Quarantines, *Boston Globe*, April 5, 2003, A2.

15. Id.

16. Altman, L.K., Public Health Fears Cause New York Officials to Detain Foreign Tourist, *New York Times*, April 28, 2003, A5; and personal communication with M. Layton and W. Lopez, July 24, 2003.

17. Press release, CDC Says Possible SARS Patient Test Results Are Negative for SARS, Dallas County Department of Health and Human Services, July 14, 2003.

18. Department of Health and Mental Hygiene, New York City Board of Health, Notice of Adoption of Amendments to Sections 11.0l and 11.55 of the New York City Health Code.

19. *See In re Smith*, 146 N.Y. 68, 77 (1895) ("While he was vested with great and extensive powers, in order, in the presence of danger, to act summarily for the preservation of the public health, he was bound to show a state of facts which justified such an exercise of those powers"). On San Francisco, *see* A Science Odyssey, *Bubonic Plague Hits San Francisco: 1900–1909*, Public Broadcasting System (PBS), available at www.pbs.org/wgbh/aso/databank/entries/dm00bu.html. "In the summer of 1899, a ship sailing from Hong Kong to San Francisco had had two cases of plague on board. Because of this, although no passengers were ill when the ship reached San Francisco, it was to be quarantined on Angel Island. When the boat was searched, 11 stowaways were found—the next day two were missing. Their bodies were later found in the Bay, and autopsy showed they contained plague bacilli . . . . But rats from the ship probably had something to do with the epidemic that hit San Francisco nine months later. On March 6, 1900, a city health officer autopsied a deceased Chinese man and found organisms in the body that looked like plague . . . . Disinfection campaigns were the order of the day. In some places they ran carbolic acid through sewers, actually spreading the disease faster because it flushed out rats that had lived there . . . . [In] San Francisco, however, political issues vied with scientific efforts. Anti-Chinese feeling ran strong in the city then, and the first step taken was to quarantine Chinatown."

20. Gerberding, J., *CDC Telebriefing on SARS: Genetic Sequencing of Coronavirus*, April 14, 2003.

21. Mariner, W.K., Public Health and Law: Past and Future Visions, *Journal of Health Politics, Policy and Law*, 2003; 28: 525; 550.

22. New York Academy of Medicine, *Redefining Readiness: Terrorism Planning through the Eyes of the Public*, September 14, 2004 (prepared by Roz D. Lasker), available at www.nyam.org.

23. Zakaria, F., Beyond Bush: What the World Needs Is an Open, Confident America, *Newsweek*, June 11, 2007, 22–29.

24. Ron Suskind, *The One Percent Doctrine: Deep Inside America's Pursuit of Its Enemies Since 9/11*, New York: Simon & Schuster, 2006.

25. Jack Goldsmith, *The Terror Presidency: Law and Judgment Inside the Bush Administration*, New York: W.W. Norton, 2007.

26. Stein, R., Swine Flu is Suspected in Region: WHO Warns of Likely Pandemic, *Washington Post*, April 30, 2009, Al.

27. Brown, D., The Two Faces of Tuberculosis: Lawyer's Illness Brings the World's Public Health Woes Home, *Washington Post*, June 19, 2007, HE01.

28. New York Academy of Medicine, *With the Public's Knowledge, We Can Make Sheltering in Place Possible*, 2007.

29. Gostin, L.O., Bayer, R., and Fairchild, A.L., Ethical and Legal Challenges Posed by Severe Acute Respiratory Syndrome, *JAMA* 2003; 290: 3229–37. *See also* Gostin, L.O., When Terrorism Threatens Health: How Far Are Limitations on Personal and Economic Liberties Justified?, *Florida Law Review* 2003; 55: 1105–69.

30. Mariner, W.K., Annas, G.J., and Parmet, W.K., Pandemic Preparedness: A Return to the Role of Law, *Drexel Law Review* 2009; 1:341–82. *See also* Annas, G.J., Mariner, W.K., and Parmet, W.E., *Pandemic Preparedness: The Need for a Public Health—Not a Law Enforcement/National Security—Approach*, published as American Civil Liberties Union (ACLU) policy on their website, January 2008 (http: www.aclu.org/privacy/pdfs/pemic_report.pdf).

Chapter 16, Bioidentifiers

1. This chapter is adapted from Annas, G.J., Protecting Privacy and the Public: Limits on Police Use of Bioidentifiers in Europe, *New England Journal of Medicine* 2009; 361: 196–201, and Annas, G.J., Family Privacy and Death: Antigone, War and Medical Research, *New England Journal of Medicine* 2005; 352: 501–506.

2. *S. and Marper v. The United Kingdom*, [2008] ECHR 30562/04.

3. Joseph Wambaugh, *The Blooding*, New York: William Morrow, 1989. It is worth noting that in some popular literature DNA profiles are metaphorically referred to—inaccurately—as "DNA fingerprints." This term should never be used because of the confusion it causes, and in this chapter the term "fingerprints" refers exclusively to the impression left on a surface by a person's fingertips after they have been coated with ink or another coloring agent. This is also the way the European court uses the term.

4. McCartney, C., The DNA Expansion Program and Criminal Investigation, *British Journal of Criminology* 2006; 46: 175–92.

5. Williams, R. and Johnson, P., Circuits of Surveillance, *Surveillance & Society* 2004; 2: 1–14.

6. Simoncelli, T. and Steinhardt, B., California's Proposition 69: A Dangerous Precedent for Criminal DNA Databases, *Journal of Law, Medicine & Ethics* 2006; 34: 153–64.

7. National Research Council, *Bits of Power: Issues in Global Access to Scientific Data*, Washington, D.C.: National Academies Press, 1997.

8. *R (on the application of S) v. Chief Constable of South Yorkshire; R (on the application of Marper) v. Chief Constable of South Yorkshire*, [2002] EWCA Civ. 1275.

9. Editorial DNA and Human Rights: Throw It Out, *Economist*, Dec. 6, 2008, 73–74.

The United States has the largest collection, with 6.7 million DNA profiles in its National DNA Index System, usually referred to as CODIS. Moore, S., In a Lab, an Ever-Growing Database of DNA Profiles, *New York Times*, May 12, 2009, D3. *See also*, Moore, S., FBI and States Vastly Expanding Databases of DNA, *New York Times*, April 19, 2009, A1 (minors are required to provide DNA samples in 35 states upon conviction, and in some states upon arrest; 16 states now take DNA from some who have been found guilty of a misdemeanor).

10. Sturcke, J., DNA Pioneer Alec Jeffreys: Drop Innocent from Database, *Guardian*, April 15, 2009, 1.

11. Cole, S.A., Fingerprint Identification and the Criminal Justice System: Historical Lessons for the DNA Debate (in) David Lazer, ed., *DNA and the Criminal Justice System: The Technology of Justice*, Cambridge: MIT Press, 2004, 63–89. *See also* Duster, T., Selective Arrests, an Ever-expanding DNA Forensic Database, and the Specter of an Early-twenty-first-century Equivalent of Phrenology (in) David Lazer, ed., *DNA and the Criminal Justice System: The Technology of Justice*, Cambridge: MIT Press, 2004, 315–34.

12. Rothstein, M.A. and Talbott, M.K., The Expanding Use of DNA in Law Enforcement: What Role for Privacy? *Journal of Law, Medicine & Ethics* 2006; 34: 153–64.

13. Hsu, S.S., New Rule Expands DNA Collection to All People Arrested, *Washington Post*, December 12, 2008, A1. Some want to "perfect" the DNA technology so it can provide a sketch of the suspect—much like an artist's sketch—but based on DNA that, for example, codes for eye color, skin color, and other physical characteristics. *See* Naik, G., To Sketch a Thief: Genes Draw Likeness of Suspects, *Wall Street Journal*, March 27, 2009, A9. *And see* M'Charkek, A., Silent Witness, Articulate Collective: DNA Evidence and the Inference of Visible Traits, *Bioethics* 2008; 22: 519–528.

14. Rosen, J., Genetic Surveillance for All: What If the FBI Put the Family of Everyone Who Has Ever Been Convicted or Arrested into a Giant DNA Database?, *Slate*, posted March 17, 2009 (at 5).

15. I have been guilty of oversimplifying the relationship between DNA profiles and fingerprints myself. *See* Annas, G.J., Privacy Rules for DNA Databanks: Protecting Coded 'Future Diaries,' *JAMA* 1993; 270: 2346–50.

16. Green, R.C. and Annas, G.J., The Genetic Privacy of Presidential Candidates, *New England Journal of Medicine* 2008; 359: 2192–93.

17. http://thinkprogress.org/2008/04/16/chertoff-fingerprints/

18. The Privacy Office, US Department of Homeland Security, *Privacy Impact Assessment: Official Guidance*, Washington, D.C.: US Department of Homeland Security, 2007.

19. Letter to Stockwell Day, April 11, 2008. *See* supra note 16 and http://www.privcom.gc.ca/media/nr-c/2008/let_080411_e.asp.

20. Kaye, D.H. and Smith, M.E., DNA Databases for Law Enforcement: The Coverage Question and the Case for a Population-wide Database (in) David Lazer, ed., *DNA and the Criminal Justice System: The Technology of Justice*, Cambridge: MIT Press, 2004, 247–83.

21. Glantz, L.H., A Nation of Suspects: Drug Testing and the Fourth Amendment, *American Journal of Public Health* 1989; 79: 1427–31. *See also* James Bradford, *The Shadow Factory: The Ultra-Secret NSA from 9/11 to the Eavesdropping on America*, New York: Doubleday, 2008.

22. Editorial, Watching Big Brother: The World Is Sleepwalking into a Surveillance Society, *Nature* 2008; 456: 675–76.

23. Annas, G.J., Rules for Research on Human Genetic Variation—Lessons from Iceland, *New England Journal of Medicine* 2000; 342: 1830–33; Kaiser, J., Cash-Starved deCODE is Looking for a Rescuer for its Biobank, *Science* 2009; 325: 1054 ("Icelanders' genetic data could be moved to another European Union country, but all personal identifiers would have to be removed or made anonymous, says Sigrun Johannesdottir, director of the Icelandic Data Protection Authority.").

24. *Guomundsdottir v. Iceland, Icelandic Supreme Court*, No. 151/2003.

25. Abbott, A., Icelandic Database Shelved as Court Judges Privacy in Peril, *Nature* 2004; 429: 118. *See also*, Merz, J.F., McGee, G.E., and Sankar, P., "Iceland Inc."? On the Ethics of Commercial Population Genomics, *Social Science & Medicine* 2004; 58: 1201–09; and Kaiser, supra note 23.

26. Another infamous case explores family privacy in the context of death more directly. As President Clinton wrote in his autobiography, in July 1993, his lifelong friend and White House counsel, Vincent W. Foster, Jr., committed suicide using "an old revolver that was a family heirloom." Foster left a note, which read, in part, "I was not meant for the job in the spotlight of public life in Washington. Here ruining people is considered sport." He was found dead in Fort Marcy Park. The park police conducted the initial investigation and took photographs of the scene, including ten color photographs of Foster's body. Despite five separate investigations that determined that Foster's death was a suicide, conspiracy theorists were skeptical. One of them, Allan Favish, sought the public release of the photographs of the death scene under the Freedom of Information Act, arguing that the government's investigations of Foster's death were "grossly incomplete and untrustworthy." Foster's widow and sister joined the case, arguing against disclosure. A lower court ultimately granted Favish access to five of the photographs, ruling that exception 7(c) to the Freedom of Information Act—that records can be withheld from the public if they "could reasonably be expected to constitute an unwarranted invasion of personal privacy"—did not apply to the Foster photographs.

The case was appealed to the US Supreme Court, which unanimously reversed the ruling. The Court made it clear that the members of the Foster family were not attempting to enforce Vincent Foster's own privacy interests. Instead, Foster's family had the right to "invoke their own right and interest to personal privacy" and to "seek to be shielded by the exemption [7(c)] to secure their own refuge from a sensation-seeking culture for their own peace of mind and tranquility, not for the sake of the deceased." In a sworn declaration, for example, Foster's sister noted that she was "horrified and devastated" by a photograph that had already been leaked to the press: "I have nightmares and heart-pounding insomnia as I visualize how he must have spent his last few minutes and seconds of his life." She added, "Releasing any photographs would constitute a painful unwarranted invasion of my privacy."

As the Court construed it, the question was whether Congress had intended that the phrase "personal privacy" be read "to permit family members to assert their own privacy rights against public intrusions long deemed impermissible under the common law and in our cultural traditions." The Court found in US "case law and traditions the right of family members to direct and control disposition of the body of the deceased and to limit attempts to exploit pictures of the deceased family member's remains for public purposes," and concluded that Congress intended to continue family privacy in this regard. The Court also found that the invasion of their privacy was "unwarranted" because no evidence of governmental impropriety was presented in regard to the investigation of Foster's death. The Court therefore ruled that the Foster photographs could be kept from the public on the basis of family privacy. *National Archives and Records Administration v. Favish*, 541 U.S. 157 (2004).

27. Parker, M. and Lucassen, A.M., Genetic Information: A Joint Account? *British Medical Journal* 2004; 329: 165–67. *See also* Offit, K., Groeger, E., Turner, S., Wadsworth, E.A., and Weiser, M.A., The "Duty to Warn" A Patient's Family Members About Hereditary Disease Risks, *JAMA* 2004; 292: 1469–73, and Annas, G.J., Reforming Informed Consent to Genetic Research, *JAMA* 2001; 286: 2326–28.

28. Editorial, An Afternoon at UK Biobank, *Lancet* 2009; 373: 1146.

29. Quoted by Rosen, supra note 14.

Chapter 17, Genetic Genocide

1. This chapter is adapted from Annas, G.J., Bioethics and Genomics (in) Andrew Clapham and Mary Robinson, eds., *Realizing the Right to Health*, Zurich: Ruffer & Rub, 2009, 321–9.

2. *E.g.*, Maxwell J. Mehlman, *Wondergenes: Genetic Enhancement and the Future of Society*, Bloomington, Indiana: 2003.

3. Advisory Committee on Health Research, *Genomics and World Health: Report of the Advisory Committee on Health Research*, Geneva: World Health Organization, 2002.

4. University of Toronto Joint Center for Bioethics, *Top 10 Biotechnologies for Improving Health in Developing Countries*, Toronto: University of Toronto Press, 2005.

5. Editorial, Watson's Folly, *Nature* 2007; 449: 948; Milmo, C., Fury at DNA Pioneer's Theory: Africans Are Less Intelligent than Westerners, *The Independent*, October 17, 2007, 24. Watson has apologized many times for these remarks, but his apologies only serve to demonstrate his ability to talk without thinking. For example, on October 31, 2009, on the Charlie Rose Show, Rose asked him how "someone as smart as you [could] say what you did?" Watson replied, "Oh, I was saying something to a girl—I never thought of her as a reporter . . .".

6. *See, e.g.*, Baruch, S. and Hudson, K., Civilian and Military Genetics: Nondiscrimination Policy in a Post-GINA World, *American Journal of Human Genetics* 2008; 83: 435–44; and, Hudson, K., Holohan, M., and Collins, F., Keeping Pace with the Times: The Genetic Information Nondiscrimination Act of 2008, *New England Journal of Medicine* 2008; 358: 2661–63.

7. This is a proposal my colleagues Leonard Glantz and Winnie Roche and I made with the Genetic Privacy Act of 1995 discussed in George J. Annas, *Some Choice: Law, Medicine and the Market*, New York: Oxford University Press, 1998, 109–11.

8. Schwartz, J., DNA Pioneer's Genome Blurs Race Lines, *New York Times*, December 12, 2007, A24. In her disturbing and evocative novel of post apartheid South Africa, *The House Gun*, Nadine Gordimer writes of Harold and Claudia Lindgard (the parents of a young man who has killed his friend):

> The Lindgards were not racist, if racist means having revulsion against skin of a different color, believing or wanting to believe that anyone who is not your own color or religion or nationality is intellectually and morally inferior. Claudia [a physician] surely had her proof that flesh, blood, and suffering are the same, under the skin. Harold surely had his proof in his faith that all humans are God's creatures in Christ's image, none above the other. Yet neither had joined movements, protested, marched in open display, spoken out in defense of these convictions. They thought of themselves as simply not that kind of person; as if it were a matter of immutable determination, such as one's blood group, and not failed courage.

Gordimer was the headliner on the 2001 UNESCO panel at UN Racism Conference in Durban at which the original version of this chapter was first presented. It took direct action to overcome apartheid. Although the Lindgards seemed to believe in behavioral genetic determinism, there is no gene (or blood characteristic) that codes for or excuses inaction in the face of actual or threatening human rights abuses.

9. *See, e.g.*, Kraft, P. and Hunter, D., Genetic Risk Prediction: Are We There Yet?, *New England Journal of Medicine* 2009; 360: 1701–03. Public health can also be a handmaiden of the new genetic discrimination, rather than a force for social justice and human rights in this new regime. As epidemiologist Philip Alcabes has put:

> We all agree that race doesn't exist biologically. There is no DNA signal that reproducibly encodes blackness or whiteness. But talk of risk makes it seem that it does. To identify African American "ethnicity" as a correlate of susceptibility to prostate cancer, as a recent report in *Nature Genetics* does, or to license a heart-failure medication for African Americans only, as the Food and Drug Administration has done, is to create a biological race where none exists. To claims, as a recent article in the *American Journal of Epidemiology* does, that race is associated with higher levels of "risk behaviors" (in this case, smoking cigarettes and marijuana, and drinking alcohol) is not only to misappropriate the idea of risk in order to condemn disapproved activities;

it also reifies race by associating it with presumptively noxious, morally reproved behaviors. Alcabes, P.; What Ails Public Health?, *Chronicle of Higher Education*, Nov. 9, 2007, B6-8.

10. National Research Council, *Evaluating Human Genetic Diversity*, Washington, D.C.: National Academies Press, 1997.

11. For more on this project see https://www3.nationalgeographic.com/genographic/ (accessed April 23, 2009).

12. Juengst, E., Groups as Gatekeepers to Genomic Research: Conceptually Confusing, Morally Hazardous, and Practically Useless, *Kennedy Institute of Ethics Journal* 1998; 8: 183–200.

13. *See* Commentary: Should Scientists Study Race and IQ?, *Nature* 2009; 457: 786–89. (Steven Rose argues "no" and Stephen Ceci and Wendy Williams argue "yes.")

14. Quoted in Gregory Stock and John Campbell, eds., *Engineering the Human Germline: An Exploration of the Science and Ethics of Altering the Genes We Pass to Our Children*, New York: Oxford University Press, 2000, 79. Watson has also consistently argued against any sort of international agreement on genetic engineering: *E.g.*, "I think it would be complete disaster to try and get an international agreement. I just can't imagine anything more stifling. You end up with the lowest possible denominator. Agreement among all the different religious groups would be impossible. About all they'd agree upon is that they should allow us to breath air . . . . I think our hope is to stay away from regulations and laws whenever possible" (Id. at 87).

15. Quoted in Richard Reeves, *John Stuart Mill: Victorian Firebrand*, London: Atlantic Books, 2007, 284.

16. John Harris, *Enhancing Evolution: The Ethical Case for Making Better People*, Princeton: Princeton University Press, 2007, 23–25. Although one of the major problems with germline genetic engineering is the ethics of risky research on children (and would-be children), Harris dismisses this issue out of hand by arguing that parents should be able to make research decisions for their children, and that humans in general have a "duty" to be research subjects. The former argument is, I think, simply untenable, and the latter has been refuted by Brassington, I., John Harris' Argument for a Duty to Research, *Bioethics* 2007; 21: 160–68. *See also* Ronald Bailey, Transhumanism and the Limits of Democracy, April 28, 2009 (available at www.reason.com), who argues that our suggestion (previously published in note 17, infra) is an "over-the-top scenario" that should be taken "down a notch or two." On the prospect for genetic genocide, Bailey argues that "It is an unfortunate historical fact that plenty of unenhanced humans have been quite capable of believing that millions of their fellow unenhanced humans were inferiors who need to be eradicated." He agrees that future genocides are possible, but that the risk is greatly outweighed by the benefits, such that banning enhancement technologies would involve "huge social costs."

17. Annas, G.J., Andrews, L., and Isasi, R., Protecting the Endangered Human: Toward an International Treaty Prohibiting Cloning and Inheritable Alterations, *American Journal of Law & Medicine*, 2002; 28: 151–78. Updated in

George J. Annas, *American Bioethics: Crossing Human Rights and Health Law Boundaries*, New York: Oxford University Press, 2005, 43–58.

18. Wills, C., Evolution Theory and the Future of Humanity (in) Nick Bostrom and Milan Cirkovic, eds., *Global Catastrophic Risks*, New York: Oxford University Press, 2008, 64. The quotation from Evans is from his Health Care in the Age of Genetic Medicine, *JAMA* 2007; 298: 2670–72.

19. Supra note 1, *See also* Annas, G.J., The ABCs of Global Governance of Embryonic Stem Cell Research: Arbitrage, Bioethics and Cloning, *New England Law Review* 2005; 39: 489–500; Isasi, R. and Annas, G.J., Arbitrage, Bioethics, and Cloning: The ABCs of Gestating a United Nations Cloning Convention, *Case Western Reserve Journal of International Law* 2003; 35:397-414; *and* International Bioethics Committee of UNESCO, *Report of the IBC on Human Cloning and International Governance,* June 9, 2009 ("IBC is of the position that, although it may be premature for the international community to engage now in the elaboration of a new binding normative instrument aimed at harmonizing both practices and principles in this area, the issues surrounding the international governance of human cloning cannot be ignored and a focused international dialogue is crucially needed."). The proposed Convention would also prohibit the use of so-called synthetic biology techniques to create a genetically-modified child. *See, e.g.,* Specter, M., A Life of its Own: Where will Synthetic Biology Lead Us?, *New Yorker*, September 28, 2009, 56–65.

20. Editorial, Time to Connect, *Nature* 2009; 459: 483, and Cyranoski, D., Marmoset Model Takes Center Stage, *Nature* 2009; 459: 492.

21. Sasaki, E. et al., Generation of Transgenic Non-human Primates with Germline Transmission, *Nature* 2009; 459: 523–27.

22. Schatten, G. and Mitalipov, S., Transgenic Primate Offspring, *Nature* 2009; 459: 515–16.

23. *E.g.,* the Raelians. *See* Rael, *The True Face of God* (published by the Raelian Religion, 1998), and *see also generally,* Joel Garreau, *Radical Evolution: The Promise and Peril of Enhancing our Minds, Our Bodies—and What it Means to be Human*, New York: Doubleday, 2004, and Maxwell Mehlman, *The Price of Perfection: Individualism and Society in the Era of Biomedical Enhancement*, Baltimore: Johns Hopkins University Press, 2009.

24. Tachibana, M., Sparman, M., Sritanaudomchai, H. et al., Mitochondrial Gene Replacment in Primate Offspring and Embryonic Stem Cells, *Nature* 2009; 461: 367–76.

25. Editorial, The Ethics of Egg Manipulation, *Nature* 2009; 460: 1057, *and see* Shoubridge, E.A., Asexual Healing, *Nature* 2009; 461: 354–55.

26. Kurt Vonnegut, *Breakfast of Champions*, New York: Dell, 1973, 187. Margaret Atwood's character, Adam One, describes our predicament poetically: "Then they [we] fell from a joyous life in the moment into the anxious contemplation of the vanished past and the distant future." *The Year of the Flood*, New York: Doubleday, 2009, 188.

Index